RT 86.73 .N86 1984

Nurses, patients, and pocketbooks

DATE DUE

DISCARD

THE HISTORY OF AMERICAN NURSING

Edited by

Susan Reverby, Wellesley College

A Garland Series

NURSES, PATIENTS, AND POCKETBOOKS

A Study of the Economics of Nursing by the Committee on the Grading of Nursing Schools

Edited by
May Ayres Burgess

GARLAND PUBLISHING, INC.
NEW YORK • LONDON
1984

CARROLL COLLEGE LIBRARY
HELENA, MONTANA 59625

For a complete list of the titles in this series see the final pages of this volume.

This facsimile was made from a copy in the Yale University School of Nursing Library.

Library of Congress Cataloging in Publication Data

Main entry under title:

Nurses, patients, and pocketbooks.

(The History of American nursing)
Reprint. Originally published: New York : Committee on the Grading of Nursing Schools.
1. Nursing—Economic aspects—United States. 2. Nursing—Economic aspects—United States—Statistics. 3. Nurses—Supply and demand—United States—Statistics. I. Burgess, May Ayres. II. Committee on the Grading of Nursing Schools. III. Series.
[DNLM: 1. Economics, Nursing. WY 16 C7343n 1928a]
RT86.73.N86 1984 338.4′7362173 83-49181
ISBN 0-8240-6507-7 (alk. paper)

The volumes in this series are printed on acid-free, 250-year-life paper.

Printed in the United States of America

RT
86.73
.N86
1928

NURSES, PATIENTS, AND POCKETBOOKS

Report of

A STUDY OF THE ECONOMICS OF NURSING CONDUCTED BY THE COMMITTEE ON THE GRADING OF NURSING SCHOOLS

MAY AYRES BURGESS, *Director*

10176

NEW YORK CITY
1928

Copyrighted, 1928
Committee on the Grading of Nursing Schools

COMMITTEE ON THE GRADING OF NURSING SCHOOLS

WILLIAM DARRACH, M.D., *Chairman*, 632 West 168th Street, New York City

MAY AYRES BURGESS, PH.D., *Director*, 370 Seventh Avenue, New York City

MARY M. ROBERTS, R.N., *Consultant, Editor, American Journal of Nursing*, 370 Seventh Avenue, New York City

MEMBERS

THE NATIONAL LEAGUE OF NURSING EDUCATION:

ELIZABETH C. BURGESS, R.N., *Assistant Professor of Nursing Education*, Teachers College, Columbia University, 525 West 120th St., New York City.

LAURA R. LOGAN, R.N., *Dean, Illinois Training School for Nurses*, 509 South Honore Street, Chicago, Illinois.

THE AMERICAN NURSES' ASSOCIATION:

HELEN WOOD, R.N., *Director, Rochester University School of Nursing*, Crittenden Boulevard, Rochester, N. Y.

SUSAN FRANCIS, R.N., *Superintendent, The Children's Hospital of Philadelphia*, 18th and Bainbridge Streets, Philadelphia, Pa.

THE NATIONAL ORGANIZATION FOR PUBLIC HEALTH NURSING:

KATHARINE TUCKER, R.N., *General Director, Visiting Nurse Society*, 1340 Lombard Street, Philadelphia, Pa.

GERTRUDE E. HODGMAN, R.N., *Assistant Professor, School of Nursing, Yale University*, 62 Park Street, New Haven, Conn.

THE AMERICAN MEDICAL ASSOCIATION:

WILLIAM DARRACH, M.D., *Dean, College of Physicians and Surgeons, Columbia University*, 632 West 168th St., New York City.

WINFORD H. SMITH, M.D. (*Alternate*), *Director, The Johns Hopkins Hospital*, Baltimore, Md.

THE AMERICAN COLLEGE OF SURGEONS:

MALCOLM T. MACEACHERN, M.D., *Associate Director, American College of Surgeons*, 40 East Erie Street, Chicago, Ill.

BOWMAN C. CROWELL, M.D.* (*Alternate*), *Associate Director, American College of Surgeons*, 40 East Erie Street, Chicago, Ill.

THE AMERICAN HOSPITAL ASSOCIATION:

JOSEPH B. HOWLAND, M.D., *Superintendent, Peter Bent Brigham Hospital*, 721 Huntington Avenue, Boston, 17, Mass.

BERT W. CALDWELL, M.D.* (*Alternate*), *Executive Secretary, American Hospital Association*, 18 East Division Street, Chicago, Ill.

THE AMERICAN PUBLIC HEALTH ASSOCIATION:

CHARLES-EDWARD A. WINSLOW, D.P.H., *Professor, Public Health, Yale University*, New Haven, Conn.

LEE K. FRANKEL, PH.D. (*Alternate*), *Vice-President, Metropolitan Life Insurance Co.*, 1 Madison Ave., New York City.

MEMBERS AT LARGE:

MRS. CHESTER C. BOLTON, *Representing the Patient and the Hospital Trustee*, Franchester Place, Richmond Rd., South Euclid, Ohio.

SISTER DOMITILLA, *Director of Nursing Education, St. Mary's Training School for Nurses*, Rochester, Minnesota.

HENRY SUZZALLO, PH.D., *Trustee, Carnegie Foundation for the Advancement of Teaching*, 522 Fifth Avenue, New York City.

SAMUEL P. CAPEN, PH.D., *Chancellor, University of Buffalo*, Buffalo, New York.

EDWARD A. FITZPATRICK, PH.D., *Dean, Graduate School, Marquette University*, 115 Grand Avenue, Milwaukee, Wis.

W. W. CHARTERS, PH.D., *Professor of Education, University of Chicago*, Chicago, Ill.

NATHAN B. VAN ETTEN, M.D., *General Practitioner*, 300 East Tremont Avenue, New York.

---

* Dr. Crowell was appointed to succeed Allan Craig, M.D., and Dr. Caldwell to succeed William H. Walsh, M.D., in the fall of 1927.

TABLE OF CONTENTS

TABLE OF CONTENTS

TABLE OF CONTENTS

TABLE OF CONTENTS

TABLE OF CONTENTS

TABLE OF CONTENTS

PART II

TABLE OF CONTENTS

LIST OF TABLES

LIST OF TABLES

LIST OF TABLES

LIST OF TABLES

LIST OF TABLES

LIST OF DIAGRAMS

LIST OF DIAGRAMS

LIST OF DIAGRAMS

LIST OF DIAGRAMS

LIST OF DIAGRAMS

IN ACKNOWLEDGMENT

Many people have helped in the making of this book. It would be difficult to name them all, for they include not only those who have worked over the manuscript, but the numbers who through stimulating questions, criticisms, and suggestions, were responsible for the form in which the study grew. Visitors who have taken the time to come to the central office, and correspondents who have written concerning local reactions to the work, have helped us to think in terms of a nation-wide problem. Nurses, physicians, and hospital administrators who have talked with the Director in the field, and spent generous hours in teaching her to see something of the problems involved in their work have contributed more than they could know. Of especial help have been the long conferences with busy members of the medical profession, who have taken so seriously the work in hand, and have been so generous in their offers of cooperation.

The Committee on the Grading of Nursing Schools consists of twenty-one men and women, each one of whom is leading an active life, saturated with strong professional interests. Almost every problem which comes before the Committee for consideration has a direct, and often a vital, bearing upon projects for which some or most of the members are being held professionally responsible. Theirs is no academic interest! It is direct and personal. To one who has been privileged to watch the Grading Committee in action, knowing a little of what each member must have at stake when radical discussion is in progress, it has been an inspiring thing to see the way in which the members have come to work together. Representing, as they do, such varying responsibilities, and holding, as they did at the outset, such widely divergent theories as to the problems the Committee was facing, they have nevertheless laid personal emotions and prejudices aside and approached the work of the Committee in the spirit of true research, to quite an extraordinary degree.

The result of this studying together for a common purpose has been that they have brought to every problem on which the Director has asked their help a minute, sympathetic, and expert consideration which has immeasurably increased the effectiveness of the work under way. In matters having to do with the details of statistical and office administration they have delegated authority to the Chairman and the Director, working together; but on matters involving questions of fundamental policy they have accepted full responsibility. They have made decisions and adopted plans. It is this particularly helpful type of supervision (which has left the hands of the Director free, and yet has given her the constant assurance of support, understanding, and thoughtful guidance from the whole Committee) that has made it possible to gather and present so many facts in so short a time.

It was a fortunate decision on the part of the Grading Committee that the central office should be located at 370 Seventh Avenue. Four parent organizations—The American Nurses' Association, The National League of Nursing Education, The National Organization for Public Health Nursing, and The American Public Health Association—have their headquarters in the same building. The opportunity thus afforded for frequent and informal contact with the directors and staff members of these organizations and with the editors of the nursing magazines housed on the same floors, has been a daily source of help. Almost every diagram in this book, for example, has been tried out first, in rough draft, on Miss Geister, Miss Pfefferkorn, Miss Allen, Miss Carr, or Miss Roberts (and sometimes, where they disagreed, on all of them, in series), before it was allowed to assume formal shape. Their frank and penetrating comments have been of greatest value.

For advice and assistance with the many statistical problems encountered in the course of the work the author is indebted to Miss Jessamine Whitney, Colonel Leonard P. Ayres, Dr. Robert W. Burgess, and Dr. W. Randolph Burgess. While the author must accept sole responsibility for the statistical processes actually followed, she is most grateful to these four counsellors for helping her through difficulties and saving her from pitfalls.

As the time for writing this report drew near, Miss Mary M. Roberts, R.N., Editor of the American Journal of Nursing, was asked by the Committee to act as editorial consultant. Miss Roberts has been generous with her help since the first days of the Committee's work, and during the past six months she has devoted uncounted hours to incisive criticism and skilful suggestions which have greatly increased the effectiveness with which the material is presented.

It is an unfortunate characteristic of the questionnaire type of inquiry that text cannot be written until computations are made; computations cannot be made until data are tabulated; and tabulation cannot begin until all the questionnaires which are to be included in any one

CARROLL COLLEGE LIBRARY
HELENA, MONTANA 59625

part of the study have been received and coded. Because of this essential sequence and the fact that many returns were delayed, the staff of the central office suddenly were faced with the necessity of doing in a few weeks' time a volume of work which would normally require many months. It should be a source of real professional satisfaction to each member of the staff to realize with what cheerful determination, and with what untiring and swift precision, they carried the work through, and made it possible to publish the report by the date set.

Finally, as agent for the members of the Grading Committee, and the organizations they represent, the author wishes to express sincere appreciation to the many thousands of nurses, physicians, patients, registrars, and public health and hospital administrators who received the questionnaires of the Committee, read the questions, answered them, and, sending them promptly back, provided the raw material of which this book is made.

Because the questionnaire method makes possible the gathering of statistical data and personal testimony in a variety, quantity, and representative quality almost unavailable through any other device, it has become extremely popular, and is being used for many purposes by many different investigators. The result is that busy people are bombarded with questionnaires; and sometimes are strongly tempted to toss each new appeal of this sort into the waste basket, unanswered. Had all the people who received questionnaires from the Grading Committee yielded to that natural human impulse, Nurses, Patients, and Pocketbooks could never have been written. Consequently, every individual who took the time and trouble to send back a completed questionnaire to the Committee may with full justice regard himself as field agent of the Committee and contributor to the book. To each of them the Committee, and the author, owe a special vote of heartfelt thanks.

MAY AYRES BURGESS

April 27, 1928 370 Seventh Avenue, New York City

HOW TO READ THIS BOOK

Many people will ultimately read all of this book—and reread it. If, when it first comes, it seems too long to read straight through, the following suggestions may be helpful.

The Introduction and Chapter 1 tell why the Committee on the Grading of Nursing Schools made this study. They are short chapters. Every one should read them.

Chapters 2, 3, 4, 6, 8, 10, 12, 14, and 16 are full of facts and figures. Readers will find it worth while to look at the diagrams, and to read at least the summary statements at the close of each chapter.

Chapters 5, 7, 9, 11, 13, 15, and 17 consist of quotations taken verbatim from reports sent to the Committee. Readers should read parts of these, especially to get the viewpoints of people in situations other than their own.

Chapters 18, 19, 20, 21, 22, 23, 24, 25, 26, 27, and 28 discuss the implications of this study. Every one should read these chapters carefully. They are not long.

This book is a reference book. It should be kept quickly available. Readers should become sufficiently familiar with its contents so that whenever discussions arise which involve facts as to the economics of nursing they will know where to look for the data they need.

The chief purpose of the book is to stimulate constructive thought and discussion. The facts are believed to be valid as presented. But the conclusions to be drawn from these facts must be determined by each reader for himself.

INTRODUCTION—A STATEMENT FROM THE COMMITTEE

On April 18, 1928, the Committee on the Grading of Nursing Schools authorized the publication of the report contained in this volume. The Committee took this action after many hours of careful discussion. The final decision was unanimous and earnest. The Committee believes that in authorizing the printing of Mrs. Burgess' book it has taken a decisive step towards the completion of its ultimate purpose, which, as readers of its program* will remember, was defined as being

"the study of ways and means for insuring an ample supply of nursing service, of whatever type and quality is needed for adequate care of the patient, at a price within his reach."

The actual grading of schools, it was decided, could safely rest only upon a foundation of broad and careful study. The program reads:

"Grading implies the ultimate adoption of certain minimum standards which must be met if the school is to harvest crops of graduates properly prepared for nursing. It is impossible to decide what these minimum standards are until we know what qualities the graduates should have; and we cannot know that until we know what they will be called upon to do. So we come back again to the decision . . . that grading must be founded upon and accompanied by a careful inquiry into the underlying facts of nursing employment."

* A Five Year Program for the Committee on the Grading of Nursing Schools. Plan and Budget submitted by May Ayres Burgess, Director, Nov. 18, 1926, 370 Seventh Avenue, New York City. Price, 25 cents.

It is the results of this inquiry which are presented in this book. While the members of the Committee are in substantial agreement with the ideas suggested in the text, they do not wish to imply, through the fact that they have authorized its publication, that each member has bound himself to unqualified approval of every word and phrase. The presentation is Mrs. Burgess' own; but the Committee has gone on record as stating that "It presents in our judgment a substantially accurate picture of the problems with which the Committee deals."

Nurses, Patients, and Pocketbooks is the report on a nation-wide study of supply and demand in nursing service. It has been under way for eighteen months. By the time the book is in print it will have cost (exclusive of other projects upon which the Committee has been working) in the neighborhood of $35,000. The Committee hopes and expects that it may prove worth many times that sum.

The book is the first of three such volumes contemplated by the Committee in connection with its three projects:

1. The supply and demand of nursing service
2. What nurses need to know, and how they may be taught
3. The grading of schools of nursing

As will be seen by an examination of the list of members, the Committee on the Grading of Nursing Schools consists of 21 members, of whom 14 are officially appointed by national organizations to represent them, and 7 are elected as members at large. It is working on a $200,000 budget and a five-year program. The work was started through the generosity of a member of the

Committee, Mrs. Chester C. Bolton, and funds for its continuation are being contributed by the parent organizations, the Rockefeller Foundation, the Commonwealth Fund, and—in generous amounts—by nurses all over the country.

The plan of the Committee is to gather certain essential facts and make them available in a form which every one can use. It believes that the seven parent organizations may be counted upon to help nursing put itself on a sound professional basis if they can have the necessary facts so that they can agree upon what ought to be done and who ought to do it. Most of the work of the Committee will be a combination of scientific research and simple, readable presentation.

The first book illustrates what the Committee is trying to do. It is in two parts: Part 1 gives the facts which the Committee has gathered. Part 2 discusses what they probably mean. Part 1 is full of diagrams and tables, and a wealth of individual quotations from nurses, physicians, patients, registrars, hospital superintendents, and public health administrators. Part 2 attempts a friendly but penetrating analysis of their implications; and asks of some of them, "What should be done? What can be done?"

Some people have wondered why the Committee (a committee definitely appointed for the purpose of grading schools of nursing) should have felt it necessary to spend the first 18 months of its active study not in grading but in studying the economics of nursing. They will not wonder after they have read this book. It deals with supply and demand in nursing service, but it leads directly to considerations of deep educational import to the profession and of deep economic import to the hospitals and to patients. It raises the challenge, "Have hospitals any social justification for running any but very high type schools in the face of an apparent overproduction of nurses, not all of whom are reasonably acceptable to society?" Grading takes on new significance in the light of the findings in this first report.

The original program adopted by the Committee called for the first grading of schools to precede the publication of the supply and demand monograph. As returns on the economic situation began to come in, however, it was apparent that all possible haste must be made to gather the essential facts and make them public. With serious unemployment reported from all parts of the country, with testimony from physicians and patients that there is no numerical nursing shortage, and with over 18,000 new graduates coming into the field this year, it was clear that attention of the seven parent organizations, and of others interested in nursing, must be focussed upon the question of supply and demand in the immediate future. The publication of this report has therefore been pushed forward, and given precedence over all other activities of the Committee.

It is a bulky volume. The members of the Grading Committee decided that nothing of importance should be cut from the original manuscript. There are 61 diagrams and 70 statistical tables. Not all of them are essential to a general understanding of the principal economic problems discussed in this book; but they have been included for two reasons.

First, the text suggests changes. It criticizes existing practices, and points the need for radical adjustments. If accepted, many people will be faced with new and exceedingly difficult professional problems; and they have the right, therefore, to know in detail the statistical material upon which these suggestions have been based. The second reason for including all of the significant material gathered in the course of this study is that there will be uses for it other than those for which it was originally gathered. The nursing profession has voluntarily submitted itself to almost microscopic analysis. It should be put in possession, for whatever use it sees fit, of the findings resulting from such a study.

Seven chapters consist entirely of quotations from the more lengthy comments written on the backs of questionnaires. Statistics, by themselves, are, to most people, dry and lifeless. It is only when they can be interpreted in the light of human emotions that their significance can be fully comprehended. On the Grading Committee, the thousands of confidential communications, from every source and type, have had an extraordinarily illuminating effect. They have furnished color and life. They have changed the impersonal concepts of "totals" and "per cents," "averages" and "medians," into so many hundreds of living, breathing people, each trying to do his job, and struggling against heavy odds.

The 819 quotations included in this book are selected, not because they are unusual, but because they are characteristic of the great mass of individual testimony which has poured into the Committee's hands. Some of it will strike home to every reader as being the sort of thing he, himself, would have said—perhaps did say. Some of it will seem incredibly at variance with what he believes possible. Nursing, while essentially sound at the core, is so many sided; its heights are so lofty and its depths so low; its colors so bright and its shadows so dark, that no one person can begin to know them all.

Yet unless a real attempt is made by thoughtful people to understand, not only the economic facts brought out in this book, but the living reactions of individuals to them, it will be difficult to know how to bring needed changes about. If the various professions adopt plans for the improvement of conditions in nursing, those plans must be carried through, not by some vague cohesive unemotional membership, but by the nurses, physicians, patients, registrars, public health administrators, and superintendents of hospital and nursing services, who are quoted in these chapters. It is these very people, and thousands like them, who will in the last analysis decide the fate of nursing. They must be taken seriously.

It has been difficult for the Director, and for the members of the Grading Committee, to avoid the temptation of offering tentative answers to the questions raised in this report. At the beginning of its work, however, the Committee agreed that it was not a legislative or administrative body. If it has desires, it has no power to enforce them. Its function is to gather facts, make recommendations, ask questions. The answers to the questions must be found by those who have the power to act. Some recommendations the Committee hopes to make. The problems are so complex and so difficult that it cannot make them at this time. It must take further time to think.

This volume is, essentially, a report from the Grading Committee to the members of the seven national organizations by whom it is officially sponsored. It is not a confidential report, but is printed and placed on sale, so that the full findings may be available to every interested reader. In the foreword of its original program, adopted November 18, 1926, the statement appears:

INTRODUCTION

"*The Committee plans to keep its cards on the table, face up.*"

That policy has been adhered to in this book.

The Committee believes that in planning and carrying through the supply and demand study, and in presenting the findings in the pages which follow, Dr. Burgess has drawn an accurate, illuminating, and helpful picture. It authorizes the printing of the entire report, and recommends its broad and deep consideration to all who are concerned with nursing problems.

WILLIAM DARRACH, M.D.
Chairman

CHAPTER 1

WHY THIS BOOK WAS WRITTEN

Physicians talk about "nurses!" and "My nurses!" Nurses talk about "doctors" and "My doctors!" There is apparently a world of difference for the members of both professions between those who belong to each other and those outside.

Nurses and physicians—some of them—probably know the finest sort of comradeship there is, the close, intensely loyal understanding which comes through perfect team-play for high stakes—the highest of all stakes—the saving of human life. Nurses and physicians in the operating room of the hospital are not separate people, they are members of a highly organized, intensely alert, team, working together with intelligent precision for a single purpose. Nurses and physicians fighting together for the life of a desperately ill patient are, again, not individuals. They are partners, bound together by their invincible determination to pull that patient through.

√ If all nurses and all physicians could have worked together, often, in this finest of all professional comradeships, the chances are that this book would never have needed to be written. But not all physicians and all nurses understand each other; nor do they all understand the hospitals, or the hospitals all understand them. Physicians say, "Hospital charges are outrageous. My patient is paying $19 a day, $9.50 each, for special nurses alone. Nurses shouldn't be allowed to get such prices!

And the hospital ought to provide enough nursing service so that specials wouldn't be needed!"

Special nurses answer, "Do you want to run us out of nursing? With cases as scarce as they are, do you begrudge us our $8 a day for 12 hours of work? We don't get that extra $1.50. The hospital gets it. It's supposed to pay for food we often never eat. This hospital could feed its entire dining room from the fees it collects and blames on us!"

Hospitals answer, "Specials? Do you think we *like* to have that incessant shift and change in workers? Your patients insist on having specials. We couldn't possibly extend our nursing service to cover their demands. And do you expect us to *lose money* on our pay patients' specials?"

The argument continues around the circle, each stating the truth as he sees it; but there is no common ground of accepted fact upon which the three can meet.

The Committee believes that nursing education cannot be placed upon a sound professional basis without the close cooperation of the medical and nursing professions and of the hospital which is the laboratory for nursing practice. Nursing and medicine are, and apparently always have been, separate professions. But since they are working, even though their techniques are radically different, for exactly the same object—the health of the patient—it is essential that they work in harmony. Neither can succeed without the support of the other, and—although the proposition would hardly receive general acceptance—this applies to the educational systems of both professions almost as truly as it applies to the procedures of the operating room and the bedside.

Physicians who, after leaving medical college, have had experience in hospitals which are proud of their high grade nursing service, carry out with them into the field something of an understanding of what good nursing can contribute to the recovery of the patient. Medical students, sometimes even before their hospital experience, learn something about nursing from the more thoughtful of their teachers, or even occasionally, in the very modern school, from regularly planned nurse instruction. Sometimes physicians out in the field learn through practical experience the difference between a woman who is merely kind and willing, and a woman who is a skilful nurse; but apparently there are large numbers of physicians who, never having had extended hospital experience, or other special contacts with really skilful nurses, have only the vaguest notion of what the nursing profession regards as its important contribution to the care of the sick. There is nothing in the ordinary medical course, or in the ordinary medical practice afterward (nor even in the fact that a man gives ten lectures a year to student nurses) which miraculously makes a physician an authority on nursing. He must have known real nurses before he can intelligently talk about them. Probably there are some physicians who have never seen an example of good nursing in their lives.

Many nurses are about equally uninformed as to what medical education implies. Some of them would have greater sympathy for physicians, and a better understanding of the problems they are facing, if they did know a great deal more about the processes of medical education. The outstanding difference between the two professions, however, is that, while nurses never worry very much about how the medical student is trained, physicians are continually concerned over the education of the nurse. And many physicians are not and never have been sufficiently close to nursing to make them safe advisers on so difficult and technical a subject.

It has, then, seemed of first importance to the Grading Committee that a careful study be made of the fundamental facts which must lie at the basis of nursing education, and of the economic facts surrounding the employment of nurses, so that physicians and nurses could have immediately available a common basis for discussion. The Committee is convinced at the close of its first 18 months of study, even more definitely than it was at the beginning, that physicians and nurses are fundamentally in agreement. They are working for the same purpose—the welfare of the patient—and where there seems to be conflict between the two groups the difficulty does not arise from warring principles, but is rather based upon lack of understanding of the facts involved. The Committee hopes that in presenting the data which follow, it may be rendering a real service to both the nursing and medical professions, and therefore, of course, to the patient.

In the original program of the Grading Committee this monograph was planned for a publication date some six months later than has since been chosen, and it was to have been preceded by the first of the gradings of nursing schools. The plan was changed, to give precedence to the publication of the supply and demand figures. It is believed that when the first grading studies are completed, their results will be of considerably greater interest and help to educators in the nursing field because they can be interpreted in the light of the economic findings of this preliminary study.

When the Grading Committee first started its work, many of the members believed that there was a real nursing shortage; and some of the earliest statistical studies were, in fact, directed towards discovering new sources from which student material might be drawn. Since the Committee had adopted at the outset, however, the policy of gathering facts before attempting to draw conclusions, it was decided to study the actual production of nurses, the length of their professional life, and the conditions under which they worked, before attempting to study the kinds and quantities of educational experience they needed in order to fit them for professional success.

The results have been—for most of the Committee—unexpected and disturbing. The implications of the figures seem so clear as to be unavoidable. Yet if they are carried forward to their logical conclusions they raise questions which are almost overwhelming in their seriousness. They seem to call upon the nursing profession for wide-spread revisions in organization; and for the development of a much more comprehensive educational philosophy. They bring home to the medical profession responsibilities which have not yet been wholly faced. They seem to demand from the public, cooperation and financial support hitherto unknown. They call upon the entire hospital world for drastic changes in policy and increased financial responsibilities.

This book does not cover the field. It is being written rapidly, in the belief that it is more important to make the facts immediately available than to present a scholarly treatise upon them. The Committee believes that if the various professions are put in possession of the facts, they may be relied upon to carry the discussion to whatever lengths are necessary to reach a satisfactory conclusion; and it has accordingly devoted the greater part of this volume to the direct presentation of evidence; including at the end only a few brief chapters of discussion which may perhaps serve to stimulate the broader and deeper consideration which the findings seem to demand.

SUMMARY

To summarize what has been said:

a. This book presents the results of a study, made by the Committee on the Grading of Nursing Schools, of the economic factors which most directly affect nursing education.

b. The study was primarily undertaken in order to furnish nurses, physicians, and hospitals with the facts they must have for their thinking.

c. The Committee believes that the nursing and medical professions are in accord on essential principles; and that if they can agree upon the facts which are involved they will proceed to work harmoniously for needed developments in nursing education.

d. The results presented in this monograph are startling and profoundly significant. Carried to their logical conclusions they seem to call for radical adjustments in practically all groups concerned with the education and employment of graduate nurses.

e. The book has been prepared and published with all possible speed in order that its findings may be immediately available to the members of the professions which the Grading Committee represents. The Committee urges upon all readers deep and thoughtful consideration of the problems raised by the facts in the pages which follow.

PART I

WHAT THE COMMITTEE HAS LEARNED

The chapters in this section present the statistical data gathered by the Grading Committee in its study of the supply and demand of nursing service; together with typical comments upon the nursing situation from those who have cooperated in the work.

CHAPTER 2

HOW FAST HAS NURSING GROWN?

The whole nursing problem is so intimately bound up with the economic problems of the hospital that the Grading Committee was afraid to take any decisive action towards the grading of nursing schools until it knew definitely first, whether the country was suffering from a nursing shortage or a nursing surplus, and second, whether the kind of nurse the hospitals want is really the kind of nurse the public needs. This second question cannot be answered until information is at hand to answer the questions:

Are more nursing schools needed, or are there too many now?

Should entrance requirements be lowered in order to divert girls from industry into nursing?

Or should they be raised in order to attract fewer but higher grade workers?

Would raising entrance requirements actually mean fewer students?

Are there now enough graduate nurses to take care of the sick in hospitals?

Or would hospitals have to go out of business if they decided to stop being educators?

Why do hospitals run nursing schools? Is it to provide graduates for local needs? Or to maintain a stable hospital nursing service? Or to save money?

The answers to these questions are not yet complete;

but the facts reported in the chapters which follow will serve at least to illuminate the discussion.

It is generally accepted, in educational circles, that attempts to raise educational standards may succeed if they are made at a time when the profession is well supplied with workers, but are almost doomed to failure if they are vigorously pressed at a time when there is a real shortage. Since the grading of nursing schools will inevitably result in active discussions of educational standards, it seemed essential for the Grading Committee to discover, at the outset, the answer to the question, "Is there a nursing shortage?" Part of the answer to the question will be found in this chapter.

1. Nursing and Medical Schools

The earliest nursing school of which the Committee has record is that of the Woman's Hospital at Philadelphia, which apparently started its nursing education about 1861. The New England Hospital for Women and Children established its school in 1872, and in 1873 the schools of Bellevue, New Haven, Massachusetts General, and the Prospect Heights of Brooklyn were organized. The numbers of nursing and medical schools and the numbers of graduates from them have been compiled from 1880 to date. There is evidence to indicate that these records, especially between 1890 and 1910, do not include all of the nursing schools, so that the figures which are given in the following table may be taken as conservative statements for nursing schools and graduates.*

* Practically all figures for nursing schools were taken from the various reports of the United States Bureau of Education; those for graduates of medical schools and colleges from the files of the Journal of the American Medical Association.

TABLE 1. MEDICAL AND NURSING SCHOOLS AND GRADUATES, 1880–1926

	Medical schools	Nursing schools	Medical graduates	Nursing graduates
1880	100	15	3,241	157
1890	133	35	4,454	471
1900	160	432	5,214	3,456
1910	131	1,129	4,440	8,140
1920	85	1,775	3,047	14,980
1926	79	2,155	3,962	17,522

The accompanying diagram shows the numbers of medical and nursing schools at each ten year period as shown in the preceding table. It will be noted that the numbers of medical schools grow steadily until 1900. Shortly after that date, however, there was an awakening wave of interest in the problems of medical education which resulted in a definite undertaking on the part of thoughtful members of the medical profession to raise the standards for admission and graduation.

The result was a sharp decrease in the numbers of medical schools and medical graduates which continued for the next twenty years. Recently the numbers of graduates have been again increasing, but in 1926 had not yet reached the totals for thirty years earlier. In nursing education, however, there has apparently never been any nationally accepted policy for the control of the numbers of nursing schools or the standards for admission and graduation.

2. Nurses and Physicians per Population

A striking change in the relative supplies of nursing and medical service has come about through the policy of controlling and limiting entrance to the medical profession while there has been almost complete freedom of

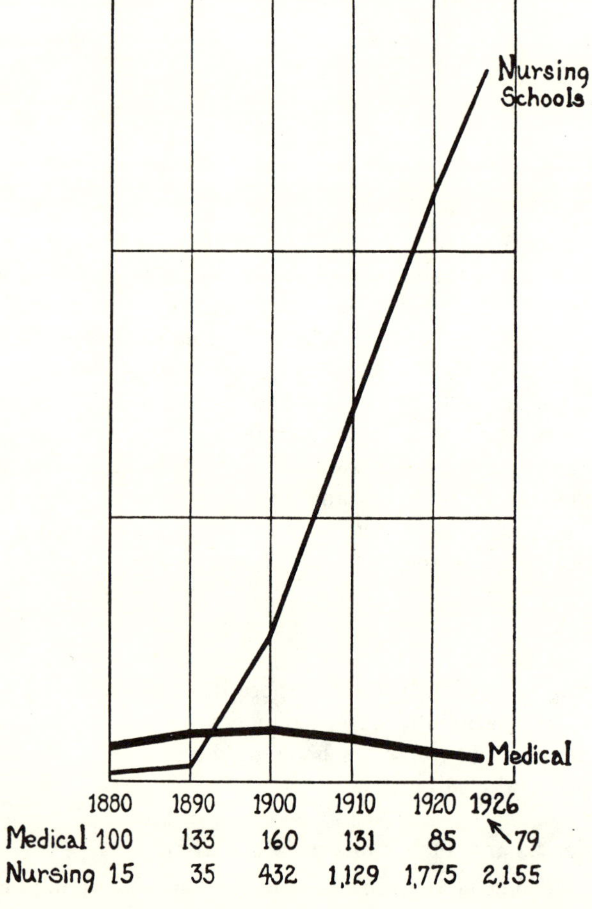

Diagram 1.—Medical and nursing schools in the United States at 10-year periods

access to the nursing profession. The United States Census began, in 1900, to separate its reports of nurses into "untrained" and "trained." The following table shows the numbers of trained nurses and physicians for each 100,000 people in the United States, as given in the United States Census for 1900, 1910, and 1920:

TABLE 2. NURSES, PHYSICIANS, AND POPULATION IN THE UNITED STATES IN 1900, 1910, AND 1920; AND NURSES AND PHYSICIANS FOR EVERY 100,000 PEOPLE IN THOSE YEARS

	1900	1910	1920
Population of the United States	75,602,515	91,972,266	105,710,620
Graduate nurses	11,804	82,327	149,128
Physicians	131,030	151,132	144,977
Nurses per 100,000 population	16	90	141
Physicians per 100,000 population	173	164	137

The figures in the preceding table are presented graphically in Diagram 2, in which it will be seen that *in proportion to the population of the United States* the numbers of physicians have steadily decreased and the numbers of nurses steadily increased, until, in 1920, there were more nurses than physicians. While figures are not available for 1928, there is every reason to believe that the relative excess of nurses over physicians is by this time considerably greater.

3. Practicals vs. Trained

An attempt was made to secure figures on the numbers of practical nurses in the United States. The Census returns are for trained and untrained nurses, and the latter figure includes both practical and domestic, so that the number of untrained nurses making their livings by taking care of sick people cannot be definitely calculated from these figures. Diagram 3, however, shows the best calculation the Committee has been able to make.

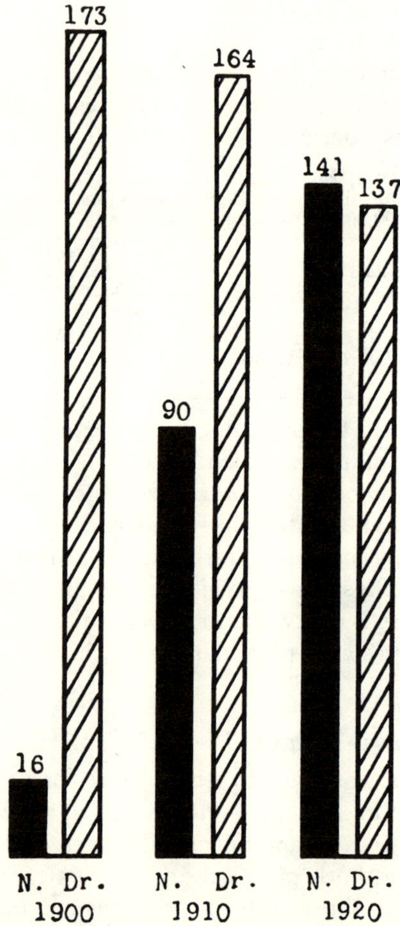

Diagram 2.—Nurses and doctors for every 100,000 people in the United States, as given in the Census for 1900, 1910, and 1920

It will be noted that the rate of growth of practical nurses apparently decreased markedly after 1900, at which period the sudden spurt in the numbers of trained nurses began. Apparently in 1920 there were just about the same numbers of practical and trained nurses in the United States, and the diagram would seem to suggest that by 1930 practicals will be very much less numerous. The figures in the diagram are exceedingly interesting as a basis for speculation, but they serve rather to raise questions than to furnish any decisive answers. People who have looked at the diagram have suggested:

(a) That as graduate nurses became more numerous, the demand for practicals decreased.

(b) That the drop in the rate for practical nurses was due to the movement of women of the servant class away from domestic or practical nursing and into industry.

(c) That women of the servant class have found it to their social advantage to enter training schools and make themselves trained nurses rather than practicals.

This report will not attempt to discuss any of these three hypotheses, but it is to be hoped, as time goes on, that the implications of the figures may become more definitely clear.

4. Nurses per Physician

The nursing and medical professions are mutually dependent. Since this is true, it becomes important to measure how closely the numbers of nurses are corresponding to the numbers of physicians. These figures as shown in the United States Census are as follows:

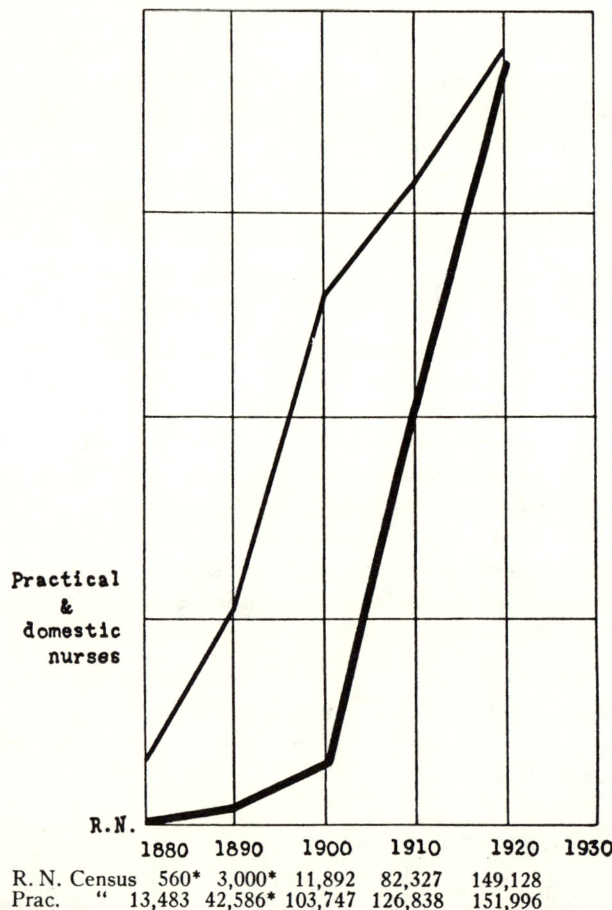

		1880	1890	1900	1910	1920
R. N.	Census	560*	3,000*	11,892	82,327	149,128
Prac.	"	13,483	42,586*	103,747	126,838	151,996

Diagram 3.—Trained and untrained nurses as counted in each census period

* *Estimated.*

TABLE 3. NURSES AND PHYSICIANS IN THE UNITED STATES IN 1900, 1910, AND 1920; AND THE NUMBER OF NURSES FOR EVERY 1,000 PHYSICIANS IN THOSE YEARS

	Physicians	Nurses	Graduate nurses for every 1,000 physicians
1900	131,030	11,804	90
1910	151,132	82,327	545
1920	144,977	149,128	1,029

These figures are shown in Diagram 4 and indicate, as was shown in another form by Diagram 2, that by 1920 there were more nurses than physicians in the United States. Just how many more there will be when the 1930 census is taken is an interesting matter for speculation.

5. Growth in Individual States

Table 4 is a detailed statement, by states, of the proportion of nurses and physicians to the population, and to each other, in 1900, 1910, and 1920. An examination of the table indicates that in 1900 not only were there very few nurses in comparison with the total population, but there were large portions of the country in which the scarcity was much more marked than in others. In general, in 1900 the New England, Middle Atlantic, and Pacific States had more nurses per population than other parts of the country. By 1910 these discrepancies were beginning to be ironed out, and by 1920, while there were still certain parts of the country—notably the East South Central and the West South Central—in which there were comparatively few nurses per 100,000 population, the differences between the various parts of the country had become far less marked than in the two earlier decades. Changes in the supply of nurses in relation to

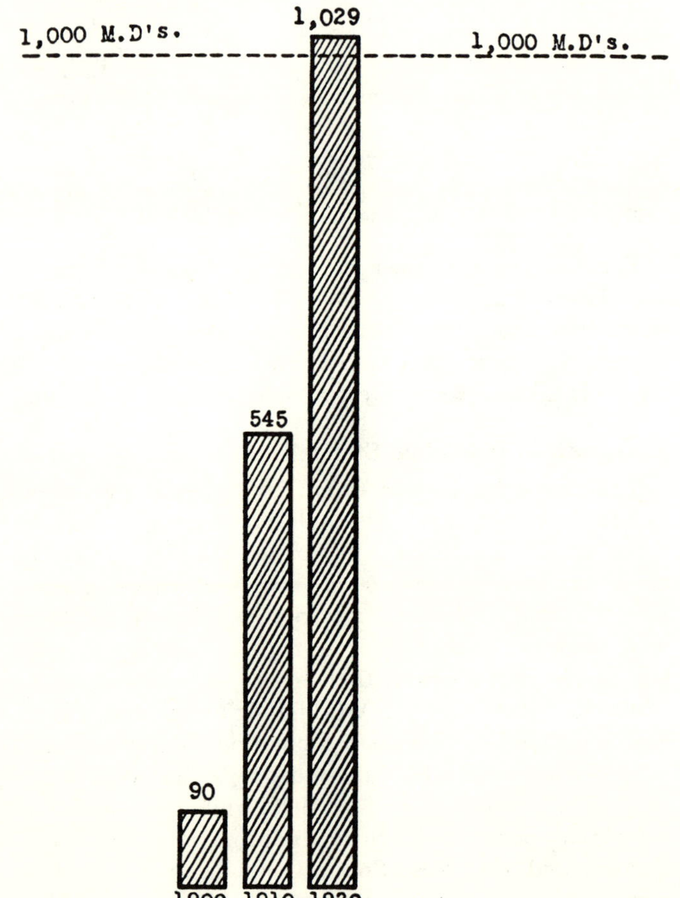

Diagram 4.—Graduate nurses for every thousand physicians, as shown in the U. S. Census for 1900, 1910, and 1920

physicians (rather than population) become even more impressive, as, for example, in Delaware, where within the short period of twenty years the condition has changed from one in which there were almost twelve times as many physicians as nurses, to one in which there are only about half as many.

TABLE 4. PHYSICIANS AND NURSES PER 100,000 PEOPLE AND NURSES PER 1,000 PHYSICIANS, IN EACH STATE, IN 1900, 1910, AND 1920

State	Physicians per 100,000 population			Nurses per 100,000 population			Nurses per 1,000 physicians		
	1900	1910	1920	1900	1910	1920	1900	1910	1920
Maine	174	175	144	20	110	172	114	629	1200
New Hampshire	191	173	143	21	139	202	112	803	1411
Vermont	215	204	161	18	132	198	86	648	1230
Massachusetts	196	185	156	28	172	257	145	927	1646
Rhode Island	158	147	122	30	137	168	193	927	1370
Connecticut	167	147	125	27	139	218	161	946	1747
Total New Eng.	186	175	146	26	152	227	140	870	1562
New York	190	176	163	38	152	221	198	867	1358
New Jersey	137	127	111	26	106	138	193	840	1241
Pennsylvania	164	156	131	24	101	152	144	643	1160
Total Middle Atlantic	173	162	143	31	126	182	177	778	1274
Delaware	152	133	123	14	85	100	89	642	1807
Maryland	177	171	162	26	140	197	145	819	1211
District of Columbia	336	347	280	67	267	416	200	770	1482
Virginia	114	115	104	13	70	109	110	611	1046
West Virginia	145	144	118	2	56	81	14	391	687
North Carolina	92	90	84	4	44	79	47	489	943
South Carolina	86	85	81	8	37	74	86	434	915
Georgia	132	124	114	7	55	84	53	444	734
Florida	130	142	148	5	52	105	41	365	711
Total S. Atlantic	128	126	116	11	69	109	85	545	943
Ohio	203	178	137	11	81	119	55	457	869
Indiana	212	195	146	9	60	94	43	306	647
Illinois	205	188	166	15	93	157	73	493	947
Michigan	180	160	122	11	83	129	63	519	1063
Wisconsin	120	121	106	9	71	129	74	582	1217
Total E. N. Cen.	191	174	141	12	81	130	61	464	926

TABLE 4. PHYSICIANS AND NURSES PER 100,000 PEOPLE AND NURSES PER 1,000 PHYSICIANS, IN EACH STATE IN 1900, 1910, AND 1920—*Continued*

State	Physicians per 100,000 population			Nurses per 100,000 population			Nurses per 1,000 physicians		
	1900	1910	1920	1900	1910	1920	1900	1910	1920
Kentucky	170	168	127	10	38	62	59	224	483
Tennessee	183	169	138	7	42	71	35	248	511
Alabama	116	121	97	3	33	56	30	274	583
Mississippi	107	116	93	2	19	39	19	165	421
Total E. S. Cen.	147	145	115	6	34	58	40	232	504
Minnesota	121	130	119	9	105	198	78	807	1660
Iowa	180	188	148	8	82	150	43	436	1011
Missouri	231	209	178	11	71	124	48	338	700
North Dakota	99	113	84	5	72	122	51	635	1451
South Dakota	121	133	102	13	56	124	105	420	1215
Nebraska	163	171	150	9	79	132	57	461	881
Kansas	204	182	144	6	62	103	28	340	714
Total W. N. Cen.	182	174	145	9	78	141	49	446	974
Arkansas	203	183	135	2	23	39	12	124	286
Louisiana	112	125	108	6	47	73	52	377	678
Oklahoma	187	188	130	2	29	59	11	152	451
Texas	195	164	131	3	40	73	18	243	556
Total W. S. Cen.	177	165	127	4	36	64	21	219	504
Montana	146	152	115	14	114	151	93	748	1313
Idaho	134	153	111	4	78	114	28	509	1021
Wyoming	162	162	134	2	80	115	13	494	858
Colorado	275	257	189	26	156	225	95	606	1194
New Mexico	98	166	117	8	62	83	78	376	706
Arizona	181	142	114	11	95	122	63	670	1066
Utah	110	132	112	7	64	124	66	486	1105
Nevada	198	252	198	5	101	133	24	403	673
Total Mount.	180	186	138	14	105	150	77	565	1091
Washington	185	191	146	12	137	194	67	718	1323
Oregon	201	211	159	9	124	178	47	586	1124
California	297	254	199	46	204	297	155	806	1492
Total Pacific	256	230	180	33	173	255	127	754	1413
Total U. S.	173	164	137	16	90	141	90	545	1029

6. How Many Nurses are Needed?

It would be desirable at this point to devote a few paragraphs to the discussion of how many nurses are actually needed for each 1,000 physicians or for each 100,000 of the population. Unfortunately, at the present time no adequate figures are at hand upon which such a discussion can be safely based. On the one hand, it is clear that many patients are not receiving skilled nursing care who could be greatly benefited by it. This is also true, of course, of patients who need and are not receiving medical care. On the other side is the fact that even under present conditions there are apparently many thousands of nurses unemployed for months at a time, and there is every prospect that the numbers will grow larger.

The problem which the Committee faces at the moment would seem to be not only whether, under some theoretically ideal condition, more nurses could be utilized to the advantage of the public, but also, and more important, whether, if present tendencies continue, there will be work enough, and money enough, so that future graduates can have a reasonable hope of being self-supporting.

The medical profession is giving considerable thought to these problems as they apply to physicians. It is particularly stressing the need for better methods for the distribution of medical service, and, as will be seen from the following quotation, taken from the report of the Commission on Medical Education published in January, 1927, it is evidently more interested in a proper distribution of service than in increasing the numbers of physicians in the profession. The quotation follows:

"It is important that the medical schools will be able to produce sufficient numbers of well trained physicians for the future needs of the country. There is general agreement that we now probably have a sufficient number of physicians for our population."

The report then proceeds to discuss with great care, but with no apparent evidences of anxiety, an educational program for the future which would cut the supply of physicians per 100,000 population one-third or more below the 1920 figure.

7. SUMMARY

The outstanding findings of this chapter may be listed about as follows:

a. In the opinion of the Committee, the grading of schools of nursing could not safely be undertaken until information was available to show how closely the supply of nursing service corresponds to the demand. Accordingly, the supply and demand study was undertaken as the first project for the Committee.

b. The medical profession, for the past quarter century, has followed a definitely recognized policy of enforcing high standards for graduation, and as a result, limiting the numbers of medical schools and students.

c. The nursing profession has not as yet adopted any similar generally accepted policy for the limitation of schools or students, or the enforcement of adequate standards.

d. In 1900 there were 160 medical schools and 432 nursing schools. In 1926 there were 79 medical schools and 2,155 nursing schools.

e. In 1900, for every 100,000 people in the United States, there were 173 physicians and 16 nurses. In 1920, there were 137 physicians and 141 nurses.

f. In 1900, for every 1,000 physicians there were 90 nurses. In 1920, for every 1,000 physicians there were 1,029 nurses.

g. The Committee would be glad to know how much nursing care 100,000 people really need. But the chief concern of the Committee, at this time, is not *primarily*, "How much do people need?" but rather, "How much can they be persuaded to buy?" If nursing is to be a self-supporting, self-respecting profession, the number of nurses must, it would seem, bear some direct relation to the amount of work available and paid for at reasonably adequate rates.

h. The medical profession is considering similar problems as they relate to its own members. Nurses may find it profitable to note that while the medical profession is quick to acknowledge its responsibility for providing adequate medical service to the community, it is stressing as means towards this end not an increase in the number of physicians, but rather the importance of new and better methods of distribution. According to recent studies, the present numerical ratio of physicians to population is considered adequate, and plans for the future involving drastic reductions in the ratio of physicians to population are being seriously discussed.

CHAPTER 3

HOW FAR IS IT GOING?

This chapter estimates that 37 years from now there will be nine or ten nurses for every two physicians. At the present time there are probably about three nurses for every two physicians. In the Report of the Commission on Medical Education, reference to which was made in the preceding chapter, there are included careful estimates of the numbers of physicians who will probably be in active service at ten-year intervals from 1925 through 1965, and these estimates are compared with Dr. Raymond Pearl's estimates of population in the United States for the same years.

These figures are given in several different sets according to different hypotheses concerning the probable growth of medical school graduates. The following table shows the estimated population, and the lowest and highest estimates for physicians in active practice.

TABLE 5. LOWEST AND HIGHEST ESTIMATES OF NUMBERS OF PHYSICIANS IN THE UNITED STATES FROM 1925 THROUGH 1965, TOGETHER WITH ESTIMATED POPULATION

Years	Population	Estimated physicians		Estimated physicians per 100,000 population	
		Lowest	Highest	Lowest	Highest
1925	115,000,000	129,000	129,000	112	112
1935	129,000,000	122,000	136,000	95	105
1945	142,000,000	114,000	136,000	80	96
1955	154,000,000	118,000	147,000	77	95
1965	164,000,000	130,000	164,000	79	100

Although it involved a serious amount of work, as will

be seen from the account in the pages which follow, it seemed worth while to attempt to get corresponding figures for the future numbers of nurses in the profession.*

1. Making a Professional Life Table for Nurses

The first step towards making a table of average expectancy of professional life was to secure individual records for as many graduate nurses as possible. Accordingly requests were sent to 1630 superintendents of nurses asking, "Have you kept a record of past graduates of your school so that you could easily tell for each graduate (a) The year she was graduated? (b) Whether she is married or single? (c) Whether she is still alive? (d) Whether she is actively nursing or retired?"

Eight hundred ninety-three, or 55 per cent, of these postals were returned by the superintendents, and of these some 607 reported that the lists of graduates for their schools could be used for the purposes described. Accordingly a letter was sent to these superintendents, giving a detailed description of the types of notation needed against the name of each graduate on the list. The Committee offered to pay the expenses incurred in

* In order to secure these figures the Committee had to find the answers for the following questions:

(a) What is the "average expectancy of professional life" for nurses who have been graduated from training school each number of years?
(b) How many of the nurses who were counted as in active practice by the 1920 Census will still remain in active practice at each year thereafter?
(c) If present tendencies in the nursing profession continue, how many nurses will probably be graduated from the profession each year from now until 1965?
(d) Taking the number of nurses active in the profession in 1920, adding the number of new graduates each year, and striking out the number who will probably leave the profession each year, how many nurses will thus be found remaining in active practice each year from 1925 through 1965?

having the graduate lists annotated and copied, and the hope was expressed that it might be possible to secure lists of graduates from as many as 50 schools. The surprise and gratification of the Committee may be understood when it is stated that of the 607 schools to whom requests for these detailed lists were sent 423, or 70 per cent, replied by sending the desired material!*

These lists included separate statements for 73,271 graduates, and in many cases it was evident that either the superintendent herself or some one of her assistants had spent many hours in careful checking and annotation of the lists. In spite of the Committee's sincere offer to defray clerical expenses involved, only one hospital in the entire group presented a bill, and that bill was for only $5.00. The Committee believes that the tables presented on the following pages offer a contribution which will have profound significance to the nursing profession, and it therefore is confident that these superintendents of nurses and their assistants will never regret the many hours of careful overtime work which made the study possible.

When the lists of graduates were received, each entry on each list was tabulated by hand. The results are shown in Table 6, which gives the total number of graduates for whom individual records have been secured for each year from 1875 through 1927; and of these, the number who are still active in the nursing profession.

The table also gives the total years elapsed since graduation for those groups. The fifth column in the table should be read: "Of each 1,000 nurses who were graduated less than a year ago, 942 are still in the profession at the beginning of the next year." "Of each 1,000 nurses who were graduated over one year but less than two years

* Three arrived too late for tabulation.

TABLE 6. SURVIVORS AMONG 73,271 GRADUATES FROM 420 SCHOOLS OF NURSING, 1875–1927

Year of graduation	Years since graduation	Total graduates	Still nursing	Still nursing of each 1,000 graduated	
				Crude	Smoothed
1927	0–1	5,032	4,740	942	941
1926	1–2	4,686	4,062	867	870
1925	2–3	4,735	3,686	778	779
1924	3–4	4,462	3,173	711	708
1923	4–5	3,463	2,266	654	647
1922	5–6	3,381	2,039	603	597
1921	6–7	3,873	2,155	556	555
1920	7–8	3,701	1,962	530	521
1919	8–9	3,385	1,668	493	494
1918	9–10	3,196	1,480	463	472
1917	10–11	2,812	1,226	436	456
1916	11–12	2,630	1,099	418	443
1915	12–13	2,433	1,094	450	432
1914	13–14	2,196	957	436	423
1913	14–15	1,994	859	431	415
1912	15–16	2,013	851	423	407
1911	16–17	1,850	765	414	400
1910	17–18	1,685	701	416	394
1909	18–19	1,513	606	401	389
1908	19–20	1,322	530	401	384
1907	20–21	1,290	512	397	379
1906	21–22	1,110	436	393	373
1905	22–23	1,078	438	406	366
1904	23–24	959	381	397	357
1903	24–25	941	335	356	348
1902	25–26	862	291	338	338
1901	26–27	727	241	331	328
1900	27–28	654	222	339	318
1899	28–29	641	195	304	308
1898	29–30	658	210	319	298
1897	30–31	562	158	281	287
1896	31–32	540	168	311	276
1895	32–33	461	123	267	265
1894	33–34	397	96	242	252
1893	34–35	307	90	293	237

TABLE 6. SURVIVORS AMONG 73,271 GRADUATES FROM 420 SCHOOLS OF NURSING, 1875–1927—*Continued*

Year of graduation	Years since graduation	Total graduates	Still nursing	Still nursing of each 1,000 graduated	
				Crude	Smoothed
1892	35–36	296	69	233	220
1891	36–37	254	56	220	201
1890	37–38	198	38	192	180
1889	38–39	163	29	178	157
1888	39–40	152	21	138	132
1887	40–41	116	11	95	108
1886	41–42	81	6	74	85
1885	42–43	85	11	129	65
1884	43–44	66	3	45	47
1883	44–45	63	1	16	32
1882	45–46	47	1	21	21
1881	46–47	57	5	88	13
1880	47–48	41	3	73	6
1879	48–49	42	2	48	2
1878	49–50	30	1	33	1
1877	50–51	12			
1876	51–52	13			
1875	52–53	6			

ago, 867 are still in the profession at the beginning of the second year," and so on.

The last column gives the same figures, but has been "smoothed." If the numbers of nurses still in the profession are plotted on diagram paper, the line will show many ups and downs caused, first, by the fact that in the earlier years the graduating classes were very small, and accidental differences are, therefore, given undue weight, and second, by the fact that this is a line based on history. Space does not permit a careful analysis of the historical implication of these figures, but it has been an interesting study to compare the hills and hollows of the line with the economic conditions of the country three years earlier when the graduates of that year were entering school. While there are exceptions, in general the line shows that the numbers of graduates have tended to increase from two to four years after marked periods of panic or depression in this country, and have tended to decrease sharply following marked periods of prosperity. The influence of the Spanish and World Wars is clearly indicated in the returns; and shortly following the close of the World War there came a decided break in the numbers of graduates which was not made up until three years later.

In order to secure a series of figures which would represent the rate at which nurses would normally drop out of their profession regardless of wars, panics, or periods of prosperity, the crude figures of graduates were "smoothed" by various mathematical processes, and the resulting figures are given in the last column of the table which is under discussion.

Diagram 5 is based upon the smoothed figures in the last column of Table 6; but instead of showing the number remaining in the profession, it shows, for every 1,000 who start, the number who will drop out each year. The heavy professional mortality in the early years, the long plateau of low mortality, and the quick rise again as nurses who are 35–45 years out of school (55–65 years old) drop out in larger numbers are clearly shown.

By a series of mathematical procedures, the Committee then found how many years of professional life each of these theoretical 1,000 nurses had had before dropping out of the profession. The figures so derived are shown in Table 7.

In this table the first column shows the total professional life for the average nurse who was graduated each number of years ago and who still remains in the profession. The second column shows the number of years which she has already spent in the profession, and the third the years which remain ahead for her. In other words, for the nurse who has been graduated less than one year there is an average professional life of 17.34

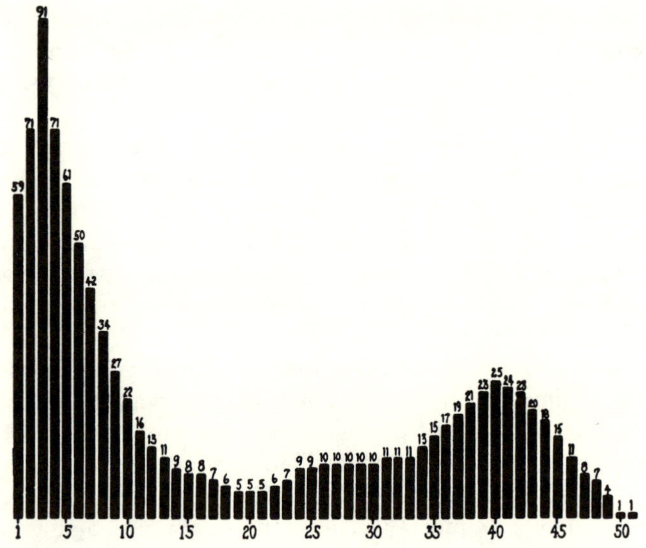

Diagram 5.—Nurses who drop out each year, from 1,000 who start

years. She may stay in the profession longer than that or she may drop out earlier, but she has more chance of remaining in the profession 17.34 years than for remaining in it any other particular number of years. If she has just been graduated, and therefore has no years behind her, the whole of her 17.34 years lie ahead. The nurse, however, who was graduated five years ago has a total

TABLE 7. AVERAGE PROFESSIONAL LIFE STILL AHEAD FOR NURSES WHO HAVE REMAINED IN THE PROFESSION EACH NUMBER OF YEARS. (BASED ON INDIVIDUAL RECORDS OF 73,271 GRADUATES FROM 420 SCHOOLS, 1875–1927)

Average yrs. of professional life	Years past	Years ahead	Average yrs. of professional life	Years past	Years ahead
17.34	0	17.34	35.50	25	10.50
18.40	1	17.40	37.86	26	11.86
19.78	2	17.78	38.20	27	11.20
21.80	3	18.80	38.54	28	10.54
23.63	4	19.63	38.87	29	9.87
25.43	5	20.43	39.18	30	9.18
27.10	6	21.10	39.52	31	8.52
28.66	7	21.66	39.83	32	7.83
30.04	8	22.04	40.14	33	7.14
31.22	9	22.22	40.48	34	6.48
32.23	10	22.23	40.86	35	5.86
33.00	11	22.00	41.27	36	5.27
33.37	12	21.37	41.73	37	4.73
33.90	13	20.90	42.22	38	4.22
34.33	14	20.33	42.76	39	3.76
34.72	15	19.72	43.38	40	3.38
35.09	16	19.09	44.02	41	3.02
35.42	17	18.42	44.71	42	2.71
35.69	18	17.69	45.38	43	2.38
35.91	19	16.91	46.11	44	2.11
36.13	20	16.13	46.84	45	1.84
36.33	21	15.33	47.52	46	1.52
36.57	22	14.57	48.23	47	1.23
36.84	23	13.84	49.00	48	1.00
37.18	24	13.18	50.00	49	1.00
			50.50	50	.50

professional life of 25.43 years. If she has already spent five of those years, she may look forward, reasonably, to 20.43 ahead. The other entries in the table may be read in the same way.

If a nurse has actually remained in the profession for ten years, she is very apt to stay in for twenty-two years longer. The reason for this is that in the first years after graduation so many young nurses drop out of the profession that the average rate of dropping out is very high. The average expectancy of life increases from graduation until the tenth year out. From then on it decreases.

In speaking of these life tables, it should be borne in mind that the figures are for duration of *professional* life and not for human life. A nurse who has been ten years in the profession may expect to remain in the profession 22.2 years longer, but even if she drops out at that point, she may continue to lead a happy and useful life in some other field of endeavor for many years thereafter.

These two tables will probably be the basis for considerable discussion in the nursing ranks. The mortality in nursing in the early years after graduation is very high. More than one-fourth of the nurses drop out by the end of the third year, and half of them have dropped out by the end of the eighth year. From that point on, however, the mortality is low, so that the median years of service and the average years of service for the entire group are very far apart.

2. Estimating for the Future

Because the estimates of the Committee are startling in their implications, it has seemed necessary to go into some detail in showing the processes by which they were derived. Readers whose interest in statistical methodology is mild may perhaps profitably skip the next few paragraphs, and turn to page 62, where Section 3 summarizes the results of the calculations.

After having constructed the life table showing the average expectancy of life for nurses who have been out of training each number of years, the next step in the long process towards discovering how many nurses there will be in 1965 was to analyze the total number of nurses shown as active on January 1, 1920, by the United States Census. This number—taken as 150,000—was first distributed into the approximate number which had probably been graduated each preceding year. This distribution was made on the assumption that the *ratio of nurses still in the profession to the total number being graduated in the same year* was the same in the 1920 census group as for the 73,271 graduates of whom we had individual record.

The second assumption was that the *ratio of each succeeding group of graduates to the one before it* was approximately the same for the 1920 group as had been found to hold true for the 73,271. On these two assumptions the 150,000 survivors counted by the Census in 1920 were distributed back according to the years in which they probably were graduated. The total probable number of graduates each year was estimated from these figures of the survivors.

Finally the theoretical total graduates were distributed according to the number which would theoretically survive for each year from 1920 on. It was found, according to these calculations, that in the year 1965 there would be 367 of the original 1920 census group still in the profession, and in each previous year the numbers would be considerably larger.

The next problem was to make a reasonably conservative estimate of how many new graduates there would be each year. The first question in this main problem was, "At what rate are the annual crops of nurse graduates being produced?" We knew the numbers of graduates for certain years and had, or could make, reasonable estimates for others. The ordinary arithmetical process of plotting the successive crops of graduates on arithmetic paper and drawing a straight line through to show where the group would be in succeeding years gave a total so far beyond any reasonable hypothesis that it was clear much more careful methods would have to be instituted.

Accurate records of the annual graduates from 1875 to date could not be secured. There are in existence some lists purporting to give these figures, but there is rather convincing evidence that at certain periods these estimates had been considerably too low. It was decided, therefore, to take the total graduates for each year as gathered by the Committee and to multiply by a constant which would bring the number of graduates in the Grading Committee's list into agreement with the numbers actually known in certain years for which accurate figures were available.

This process was probably unduly conservative, because the list gathered by the Grading Committee is for schools now in existence, many of which date from very far back, but it cannot include the graduates from the unknown numbers of schools which have been started, graduated nurses for a few years, and have then closed their doors. Since no better figures apparently exist, however, it was decided that this process was reasonably safe.

The resulting estimates of graduating classes from 1875 on were then plotted upon semi-logarithmic paper. The property of semi-logarithmic paper is that in the vertical scale equal distances imply equal units, not of addition, but of multiplication. The distance between 10 and 100, for example (being equal to 10 × 10), is the same as the distance from 100 to 1,000 (10 × 100) or 1,000 to 10,000

(10 × 1,000), or 10,000 to 100,000 (10 × 10,000). Data plotted on such a scale will lie in a straight line if they are progressing at a steady rate. Figuratively speaking, if the driver is putting on the gas, the curve swings up and away from the straight line, and if he is putting on the brakes, it swings towards or under the straight line.

Diagram 6 shows in the irregular line the plottings of successive crops of graduates from 1875 through 1926. It will be seen that in the early years, nursing schools were rapidly accelerating their speed, but that as the years went on, although the actual numbers of nurses increased with astonishing rapidity, the rate of increase shows a definite tendency to slacken. Instead of leaping straight upward toward the sky, the curve of progress is apparently approaching the top of the hill, and in the not too distant future, unless conditions change, will reach its height and remain there on a steady level of annual production.

The dashed line in the diagram shows where the present tendencies in the rate of production are apparently carrying the profession. Each point in this line is carefully computed on the basis of a logarithmic formula which gives a prediction for the future based on the actual performances of the data in the past.*

The logarithmic curve just described made it possible to predict, in what seems to be a reasonably conservative manner, the probable number of nurse graduates in each succeeding year from now until 1965. This prediction, of course, is based on the assumption that conditions in the profession continue approximately as they are now and

* For advice and assistance in computing this trend line the Committee is indebted to Dr. Robert W. Burgess, author of "The Mathematics of Statistics." The formula he used is:

$$\log y = 4.4723 - 1.1756 \times 10^{-.011486x}$$

where y = number of graduates in year x, and x = 0 in 1912.

that no attempt will be made to control nursing education or to limit the numbers of graduates.

Having ascertained the probable size of each successive graduating class from 1920 through 1965, computations were then carried through for each graduating group in

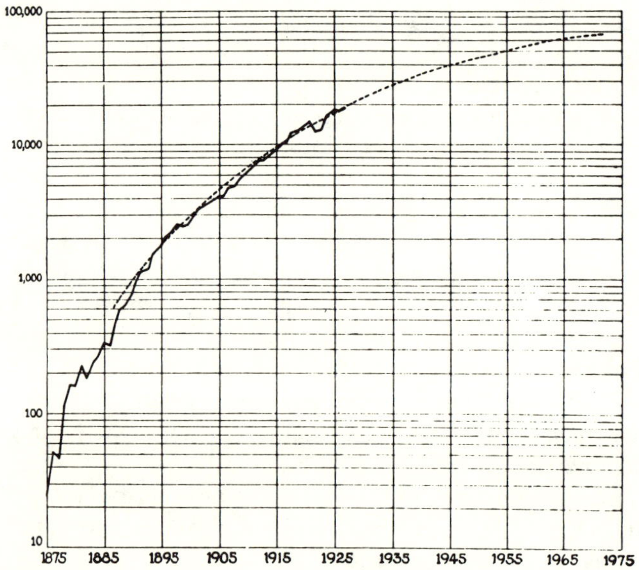

Diagram 6.—Nurses graduated each year in the past ——— and in the future - - - - - -. The logarithmic trend line is derived from the estimated graduates each year from 1886 through 1926

order to estimate the probable number of those graduates who would remain in the profession for each year after graduation. The results were then combined, so that the survivors from the nurses counted by the Census in 1920 were added to the survivors from each succeeding graduating class. The results are shown in Table 8, which gives, first, the year, second, the estimated total graduates in that year, and third, the estimated total nurses in service in the United States.

It should be noted that the "estimated total nurses in service" does not include any allowance for nurses immigrating from other countries after graduation; nor for married nurses continuing actively in the profession without the knowledge of their superintendents of nurses. (See Chapter 12, Sec. 3, 4.) The total estimates as given may, therefore, be taken as exceedingly conservative.

TABLE 8. ESTIMATED GRADUATES FROM NURSING SCHOOLS, AND ESTIMATED TOTAL NURSES ACTIVELY ENGAGED IN NURSING EACH YEAR FROM 1920 THROUGH 1965

Year	Nurse graduates	Nurses in profession January 1	Year	Nurse graduates	Nurses in profession January 1
1920	13,980	150,000	1943	35,451	362,135
1921	14,649	154,732	1944	36,574	375,742
1922	12,624	159,972	1945	37,696	389,457
1923	13,050	163,238	1946	38,839	403,547
1924	16,686	166,900	1947	39,981	417,920
1925	17,753	174,027	1948	41,123	432,551
1926	17,521	181,876	1949	42,265	447,442
1927	18,907	189,071	1950	43,408	462,559
1928	19,853	197,198	1951	44,550	477,895
1929	20,798	205,796	1952	45,653	493,468
1930	21,763	214,751	1953	46,776	509,225
1931	22,728	224,106	1954	47,898	525,167
1932	23,709	233,805	1955	49,041	541,351
1933	24,698	243,830	1956	50,163	557,818
1934	25,702	254,195	1957	51,286	574,534
1935	26,746	264,857	1958	52,389	591,494
1936	27,809	275,902	1959	53,492	608,748
1937	28,881	287,286	1960	54,595	626,202
1938	29,956	298,997	1961	55,697	643,907
1939	31,039	311,015	1962	56,800	661,854
1940	32,142	323,354	1963	57,903	680,001
1941	33,245	335,990	1964	58,987	698,344
1942	34,356	348,920	1965	60,000	716,794

3. The Result—In 1965

This long series of calculations finally resulted in two simple statements:

1. If present conditions continue, the graduating class of 1965 will contain 60,000 members.
2. If present conditions continue, a census taken in 1965 would find approximately 717,000 nurses actively at work in the profession.

These estimates were then compared with Dr. Raymond Pearl's predicted population of the United States at ten-year periods from 1925 through 1965, and the predictions of Dr. Rappleye and the Commission on Medical Education of the maximum numbers of physicians in the profession for those years. Table 9 shows the comparative results secured.

TABLE 9. ESTIMATED POPULATION, AND ESTIMATED ACTIVE PHYSICIANS AND ACTIVE NURSES, 1925–1965

Years	Population	Physicians	Nurses	Physicians per 100,000 population	Nurses per 100,000 population	Nurses per 1,000 physicians
1925	115,000,000	129,000	174,000	112	151	1,349
1935	129,000,000	136,000	264,900	105	205	1,948
1945	142,000,000	136,000	389,500	96	274	2,864
1955	154,000,000	147,000	541,400	95	351	3,683
1965	164,000,000	164,000	716,800	100	437	4,371

If, instead of taking the maximum figure for physicians, the minimum were taken, we should then have 79 physicians and 437 nurses for each 100,000 population, and 5,541 nurses for each 1,000 physicians.

These various figures must be taken not as definite assurances, but rather as the best estimates which the

Committee has been able to make. They seem to offer a reasonably safe basis, however, for saying that unless some radical control is exercised in the near future by which the numbers of nurses allowed to enter training schools are greatly diminished, or unless the numbers of medical schools and the size of medical graduating classes are markedly increased, we shall have in this country in 1965 between four and five times as many nurses as there are physicians. These figures are illustrated in Diagram 7, which shows the number of nurses and the number of physicians who at the present rate will be in active practice in the United States at each ten-year period from 1925 through 1965.

In the light of the facts given in this chapter, the reader will find of particular interest such portions of the succeeding chapters as deal with present conditions of employment—and unemployment—among nurses; and the wide-spread testimony from physicians that the present supply of nurses (which is probably about three nurses to every two physicians—January 1, 1928) is so ample that, while there is often an unsatisfactory distribution, there is from the medical viewpoint no "nursing shortage."

4. SUMMARY

The outstanding points in this chapter are:

a. Because estimates were already available for the probable number of physicians, and for the general population at ten-year intervals until 1965, it was decided to make similar estimates for nurses.
b. The first step towards this end was to construct a Professional Life Table.
c. Through rather remarkable cooperation on the part

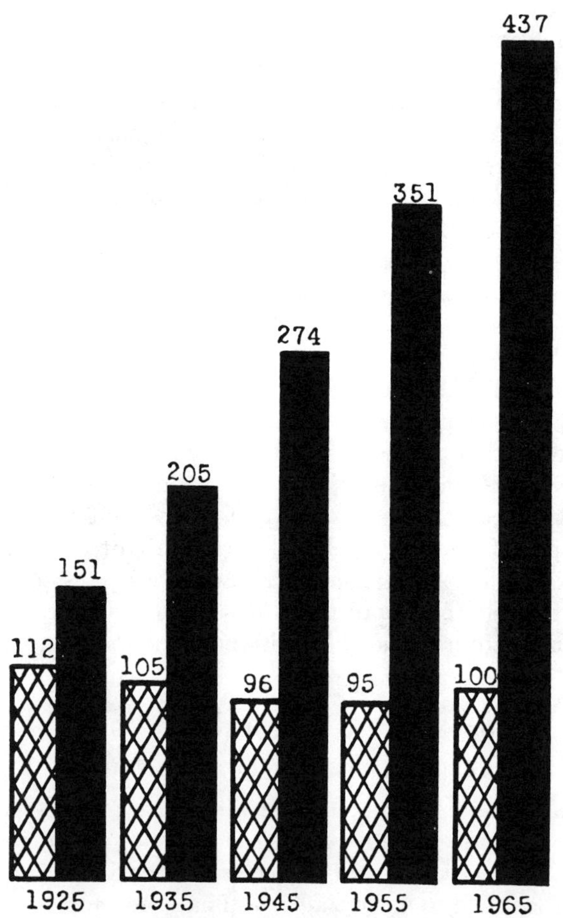

Diagram 7.—Nurses ▬ and physicians ▨ for each 100,000 people in the United States estimated for 1925–1965

of superintendents of nursing schools and their assistants, individual, annotated records were secured of 73,271 graduates of 420 training schools.

d. From these records a table was constructed by means of which it is possible to predict how much longer nurses each number of years out of training school may expect to remain in the profession.
e. By a lengthy and somewhat complicated series of mathematical computations estimates were made oı the probable number of nurses actively in the profession each year from 1920 through 1965.
f. These computations indicate that if present tendencies continue
    (1) The graduating class of 1965 will number 60,000 members.
    (2) A census in 1965 would find about 717,000 active nurses in the profession.
    (3) The nurses will outnumber the physicians by four or five to one.
g. In the light of the facts given in this chapter, the reader will find it worth while to read with particular care such parts of succeeding chapters as deal with the alleged "nursing shortage."

CARROLL COLLEGE LIBRARY
HELENA, MONTANA 59625

CHAPTER 4

IS THERE UNEMPLOYMENT NOW?

The registries are the best possible source of information on the employment of private duty nurses. In the middle of January, 1928, sixteen hundred thirty-eight return postals were mailed to superintendents of nurses asking for the addresses of hospitals having registries. Of the 873 (or 54 per cent) who replied, 373 reported that they had registries, and were therefore put on the list. In addition, the names and addresses of 69 central professional registries were secured from the pages of the American Journal of Nursing. Finally, through the courtesy of the American Telephone and Telegraph Company, access was secured to the Red Books or telephone business directories of all cities where such directories are published in the United States, and the names and addresses of 437 nurse registries advertised in these books were copied.

This procedure provided the Committee with the names and addresses of 879 registries. Some of these undoubtedly were duplicates, since it is a common custom for a registry to use more than one name in the telephone book, and since central professional registries and hospital registries frequently cannot be distinguished from commercial registries in these lists. The fact that 414 questionnaires came back, which gives a 47 per cent return on the original number sent out, probably means that the actual per cent of return is considerably higher.

It is a matter of real misfortune, for the purposes of this study, that there was no way in which a difference could be made in tabulating the returns between commercial registries and central professional registries. In many cities there is no method by which addresses can be separated to indicate which of the registries are actually sponsored by the local nursing organizations, and there is reason to suspect that some registries which are really commercial have been reported in this study as being sponsored by the district nurses' association. In one instance known to be a commercial registry, where the registrar signed his name and address, the registry is checked as being under the control of the district nurses' association and the name of the registry, which is one of the largest in the country, reads "The Nurses' Official Registry of . . . State," which would certainly mislead many nurses unfamiliar with local conditions.

The first question on the report blank read: "Is the registry under the control of a Hospital, an Alumnæ Association, a District Nurses' Association, a Nurses' Club, a Medical Society, a Health Center, a Women's Club, a private individual, a business firm, or some other authority?" If the check mark indicated that control was under the district nurses' association, the return had to be tabulated in that way. It was also found that the distinction between control by the "district nurses' association" and by a "nurses' club" was not clear in the minds of some people who made returns, and the two groups, therefore, had to be thrown together. We have, then, 81 returns checked to indicate that they are officially controlled by the district nurses' association and 12 controlled by local nurses' clubs, making a total of 93 registries which would seem to be classed as central professional registries, although the official list includes only 69 registries, and presumably not all of these answered.

In all the figures which follow it should be remembered that "Hospital Registries" include 220 registries conducted by hospitals and 25 by alumnæ associations; "District" includes central professional registries, registries conducted by nurses' clubs, and at least a few successful commercial registries. Registries listed as "Individuals" include 36 registries conducted by individuals and 4 by small business firms, and the classification "Other" includes a few registries conducted by medical societies, health centers, women's clubs, etc.

1. Where are the Registries and on What Basis Do They Operate?

Of the 414 returns from registries, 389 are filled out in detail, and the figures which follow will be based upon that number. Thirty-four per cent of these registries are in the North Atlantic States, 38 per cent in the North Central, 10 per cent in the South Atlantic, 8 per cent in the South Central, 10 per cent in the Western States. The location of registries in cities of each population group is as follows:

TABLE 10.—PER CENT OF REGISTRIES IN CITIES OF EACH SIZE

500,000 and over	18%
100,000 to 500,000	15
25,000 to 100,000	31
10,000 to 25,000	19
Under 10,000	17
	100%

Registries are controlled as follows:

Controlled by	Registries	Per cent
Hospital or alumnæ association	245	63
District assn., nurses' club, commercial	93	24
Individuals or small firms	40	10
Other	11	3

Of the total group of registries 66 per cent have their homes in the hospital or nurses' home, 21 per cent in the registrar's home, 6 per cent in a business building, 4 per cent in a "club," and 3 per cent elsewhere. It is of special interest to note the per cent of registries which are conducted in the registrar's own home, since this usually means a small, personal affair, lacking most of the attributes of the serious business office. Among the hospital and alumnæ associations 2 per cent of the registries are located in the registrar's home, among district, club, and some of the commercial registries 43 per cent, and among the registries controlled by individuals 83 per cent.

As has been the rule with practically all of the Grading Committee studies, the people giving the report were not asked to sign their names. The result was a fairly frank discussion of the financial status of the registries. The following table shows the per cent of all registries reporting as shown for 1927:

TABLE 11. PER CENT OF REGISTRIES OF EACH TYPE, SHOWING DIFFERENT FINANCIAL CONDITIONS FOR 1927

	Hospital alumnæ	District, club, com.	Individual	Other	All
Deficit	2%	11%	29%	33+%	7%
Break even	7	39	37	33+	17
Profit	5	35	34	33+	15
Don't know	40	9	..	..	28
Charge nominal fee	5	1	..	..	4
Make no charge	41	5	..	..	29
	100%	100%	100%	100%	100%

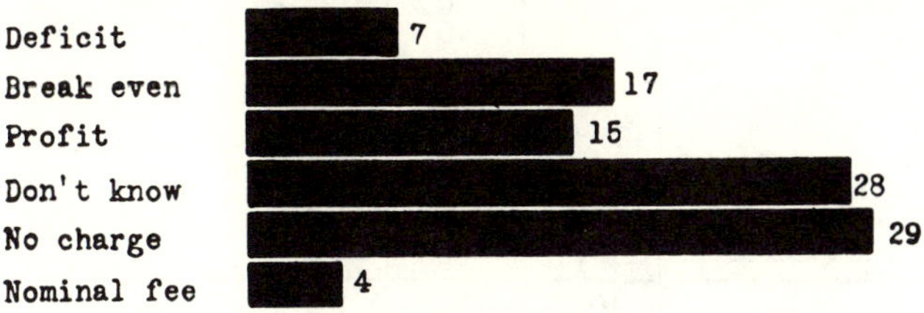

Diagram 8.—Per cent of registries in each financial group

2. Who Handle the Registries?

Registrars run all the way from drug store clerks, elevator operators, and telephone girls, through nurses who happen to be off duty at the time, to regularly appointed and paid administrators. Almost three-fifths of all the registries report that they have no regular full time employee who is responsible for the work of the registry.

The per cent of registries employing helpers is as follows:

58% report no full time person
26% report 1 full time person
10% report 2 full time people
4% report 3 full time people
2% report 4 or more full time people

In this last group are included two registries, one of which employs 15 and the other 16 full time people. As might be expected, most of the registries which report that they do not employ a single full time person responsible for registry work are in the hospital group. Eighty-six per cent of all the hospital registries report no full

TABLE 12. PER CENT OF REGISTRIES CONDUCTED BY EACH TYPE OF REGISTRAR

	Hospital or alumnæ	District, club, commercial	Individual	Other	All
Physicians	0%	0%	3%	0%	.2%
Registered nurses	87	90	43	10	82.5
Graduates but not registered	1	2	3	0	1.7
Practical nurses	0	2	19	0	2.6
Business men or women	8	2	24	80	8.6
Social workers	0	1	5	0	.9
Other	4	3	3	10	3.5
	100%	100%	100%	100%	100%

time person employed. Fourteen per cent of the district registries report no full time person employed, and 3 per cent of the individual registries.

Ninety-eight per cent of all the registrars are women, and 2 per cent are men. The preceding table shows the types of both paid and unpaid registrars.

The registries were asked whether the registrar received a regular salary, or a share in the profits, or whether she worked without pay. The no-pay cases were separated to include those in which the statement was definitely made that the registrar received no pay and the others in which the conduct of the registry was such an incidental activity that no special person was in charge and therefore no payment was asked for. The returns to the question are as follows:

TABLE 13. PER CENT OF REGISTRIES PAYING REGISTRARS AS INDICATED

Registry	Regular salary	Share profits	No pay	Incidental activity	Total
Hospital, Alumnæ.	6%	2%	36%	56%	100%
District Assn., Club, Commercial.....	81	5	9	5	100
Individual........	20	65	15	..	100
Other............	80	10	10	..	100
All............	27%	8%	27%	38%	100%

3. Who are Enrolled on the Registry?

While hospital registries frankly exist for the most part in order to secure special nurses of the types wanted for cases in their own hospitals, it is interesting to note that only 20 per cent of the hospital and alumnæ registries limit registration to their own graduates. Eighty per cent admit graduates from other hospitals, although in many cases the note is added: "Of course, preference is given to our own graduates."

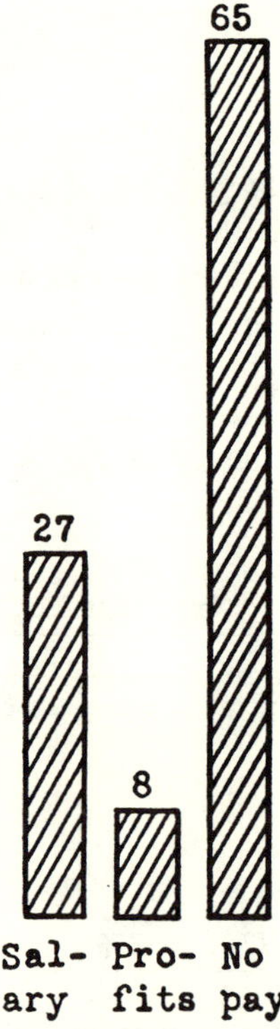

Diagram 9.—Per cent of registries where the registrar receives a regular salary, or a share in the profits, or no pay at all

Among the registries grouped under district, club, and commercial, 40 per cent limit enrollment to their own members while 60 per cent admit members from outside. It seems probable, although there is no direct evidence to this effect, that if the records could be clarified so that commercial registries were dropped from the district and club group, the per cent limiting enrollment to their own members would be considerably larger.

TABLE 14. PER CENT OF REGISTRIES ENROLLING EACH NUMBER OF TYPES OF WORKERS

Workers	Hospital	Dist., etc.	Indi-vidual	Other	All
1 type only	65%	32%	7%	..	49%
2 types	26	17	10	10%	22
3 types	7	25	28	10	13
4 types	1	18	25	40	9
5 types or more	1	8	30	40	7
Total	100%	100%	100%	100%	100%

TABLE 15. NUMBER AND PER CENT OF REGISTRIES IN EACH GROUP ENROLLING WORKERS FOR EACH SPECIFIED TYPE

	Hospital alumnæ		District, club, com.		Indi-vidual		Other		All	
	No.	%	No.	%	No.	%	No.	%	No.	%
R.N.	233	100	91	100	40	100	10	100	375	100
Graduates, not R.N.'s	51	22	33	36	30	75	8	80	122	33
Male nurses	24	10	43	47	24	60	9	90	100	27
Practical nurses	27	12	50	55	34	85	10	100	121	32
Hospital maids	1	..	2	2	3	8	..	..	6	2
Orderlies	3	1	5	6	5	13	1	10	15	4
Domestic servants	1	..	..	..	1	3	..	..	2	1
Physicians	2	1	4	4	7	18	2	20	15	4
Others (teachers, etc.)	1	..	7	8	10	25	5	50	23	6

The smallest hospital or alumnæ registry reported two members enrolled on the registry. The middle reported 24; and the highest reported 650. The smallest of the "district, club, and commercial" registries had an enrollment of 11 nurses, the middle 140, and the largest 3,720. Among the registries run by individuals, the smallest had an enrollment of 15 nurses, the middle 75, and the largest 300.

The registries were given a list of different sorts of workers and were asked to check which groups were admitted to their own registry. It was found that hospital registries were much more restricted in the sorts of service they furnish than are the others.

It is of particular interest to note what sorts of workers are being enrolled by these different groups.

4. Calls Received and Filled

The registries were asked to report the total calls received and filled during the week just finished, which, for most of the registries, was the last week in January, 1928.

It is a surprising fact that many registries keep no monthly record of calls filled, and most registries keep no monthly record of calls received. Of the 389 registries, only 200 were able to answer both questions even for the preceding 7 days! From these 200, however, we have a total of 9,696 calls received and 9,574 filled. Of the calls received, 7,659 (or 79 per cent) were for hospital and 2,037 (or 21 per cent) were for home service. The records show that 99.4 per cent of the hospital calls were filled and 96.3 per cent of the home calls. Letters from registrars support these figures, and indicate that although home calls are harder to fill than hospital calls, nevertheless almost all of the calls actually received were filled by the registries. Nurses may hesitate to take home calls, but they do take them. Calls actually unfilled amount to a very small per cent of the total.

It is interesting to note that of every five calls four are for hospital duty, and only one for home duty. This is partly because about three-fifths of the registries studied are controlled by hospital or alumnæ associations, which make very little pretense of catering to the demand of patients in the home. It is not at all strange that "hospital specialing" and "private duty" are synonymous in the minds of most nurses enrolled on these registries. In registries controlled by private individuals the per cent of home calls is much larger.

Registries were asked which calls were *easier to fill*—hospital calls or home calls. Table 16 and Diagram 10 show the results.

TABLE 16. PER CENT OF REGISTRIES REPORTING EACH TYPE OF CALL AS "EASIER TO FILL"

Which easier to fill?	Hospital	District	Individual	Other	All
Hospital calls	91%	86%	37%	67%	84%
Home calls	1	1	52	16	6
No difference	8	13	11	17	10
Total	100%	100%	100%	100%	100%

Diagram 10.—"Which are easier to fill, calls from hospitals or from homes?"

The registries run by private individuals show quite a different story. There seems to be a fair number of small registries run by private individuals expressly for the purpose of supplying nursing service to the home.

It was thought that the size of the city in which the registry was located might make some difference as to whether hospital or home calls were easier to fill. The tabulation was, therefore, made on the basis of population and it was found that in cities of 500,000 and over there are evidently many registries which make a specialty of filling home calls. A possible explanation may be that nurses flock to the largest cities in such numbers, and many of them with such inadequate preparation, that they cannot hope to find regular employment in the hospitals and therefore must either accept home calls or remain idle. Whatever the true cause, it is astonishing to note that 20% of the registries in cities of over 500,000 report that "home calls are easier to fill" as compared with 4, 3, and 2% in cities of smaller size.

Registries were asked to tell what sorts of calls were the hardest for them to fill. The following table shows their answers:

TABLE 17. PER CENT OF REGISTRIES OF EACH TYPE, SPECIFYING EACH KIND OF CALL AS "HARDEST TO FILL"

	Hospital alumnæ	District, club, com.	Individual	Other	Total
Home calls	48%	31%	19%	25%	40%
Country calls	42	51	15	50	42
Contagion	17	31	15	75	22
Night	8	9	15	25	9
24-hour	4	4	8	13	4
Hospital floor	2	10	12	13	5
Obstetric	5	4	8	25	5
Mental, nervous	5	9	..	13	6
Alcoholic	2	8	..	..	3
Other	5	9	27	..	8

5. Reports from Private Duty Nurses

In addition to the reports secured directly from the registries, certain data were compiled from the reports given by private duty nurses earlier in the study. It is interesting to compare the statements of the registries as to calls which are hardest to fill with the statements of private duty nurses of "What they register against." Thirty-nine per cent of the private duty nurses report that they do not "register against" any sort of service; 35 per cent registered against one type; and 20 against two. Only 6 per cent registered against more than two types. The commonest "registrations against" are shown in the accompanying diagram:

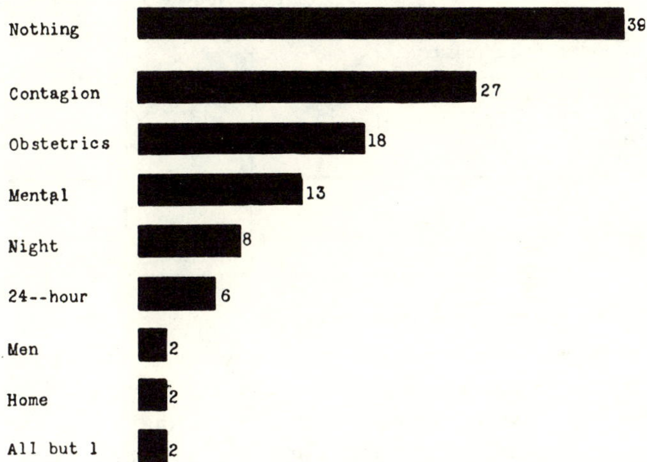

Diagram 11.—Per cent of nurses "registering against" each type of call. Four out of ten private duty nurses do not register against anything. The most unpopular cases are contagion, obstetrical, and mental and nervous. Many nurses have had little or no training along these three lines

The following table shows the sources through which private duty nurses secured their cases, and divides the nurses into two groups—those who received their training in the same state in which they are now practising and those who were trained in some other state. It will be seen that nurses who were trained in some other state tend to receive their cases through central or commercial registries more frequently than do nurses trained in the same state.

TABLE 18. PER CENT OF PRIVATE DUTY NURSES TRAINED IN THE SAME STATE OR IN SOME STATE OTHER THAN THAT IN WHICH THEY ARE NURSING, WHO RECEIVED THEIR CASES THROUGH EACH SPECIFIED SOURCE

	Trained in same state	Trained in outside state	All
Through hospital registry...	38%	24%	35%
Central professional.......	23	39	26
Commercial...............	3	6	3
Physician.................	15	13	14
Friend....................	20	16	20
Other.....................	1	2	2
	100%	100%	100%
Total nurses..............	2,406	581	2,987
Per cent..................	80.5%	19.5%	100%

6. The Demand for Practicals

The registrars were asked "For which is there more demand, for graduates or for practical nurses?" The vote was overwhelmingly to the effect that there was more demand for graduate nurses. This might be expected for hospital registries, but it holds true for most of the others as well. For all registries combined 93 per cent said that there was more demand for graduates than for practical nurses. When the groups are separated it is found that 99.1 per cent of the hospital registries and 98.7 per cent of the district, club, and commercial registries give the same answer. The registries run by single individuals, however, report in half the cases that there is more demand for graduate nurses and in the other half that there is more demand for practical nurses.

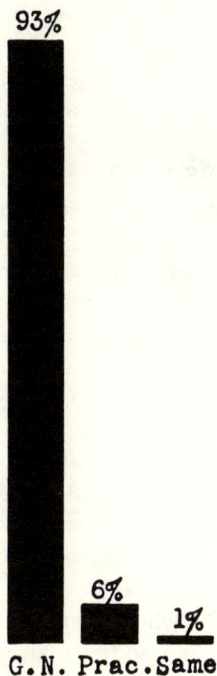

Diagram 12.—"For which do you have more demand, for graduate nurses or for practical nurses?"

When the registries are separated into geographical groups, it is found that:

91% of registries in the North Atlantic States 94% of registries in the North Central States 94% of those in the South Atlantic States 96% in the South Central States 94% in the Western States	Report more demand for Graduates than for Practicals

Twenty-one per cent of the registries reported that the demand for practicals seems to be growing, 46% that it is falling off, and 33% that it remains about the same. Forty-five per cent of the registries in cities of over 500,-000, down to only 12% in cities of 10,000, say that the demand is growing; while 28% in cities of over 500,000, up to 63% in cities of 10,000, say that it is falling off.

7. "Do You Want More Nurses?"

Probably the most significant question which was asked in the entire study was, "Would you like to have more nurses encouraged to move to your city?" The response was immediate and overwhelming. Registrars not only answered in the space allowed, but in many instances wrote long paragraphs of comment and emphasis upon the backs of the questionnaires. The question was directly answered by 353 of the 389 registries. Of these 353, 325 said "No" while only 28 said "Yes." Some 21 of those 28 registries are hospital registries connected, apparently, with institutions where the supply of alumnæ graduates is not yet sufficient to meet the needs for specials within the hospital walls.

Of the 325 registries who answered "No," many underlined the "No." Some added marginal notes telling of the large numbers of nurses still on the waiting list. Several registrars wrote in substance, "Until recently we have been anxious to secure more nurses, but now the hospitals in our own city have such large graduating classes that we have more local nurses than we know what to do with." The answers divided according to the type of registry are shown in Table 19.

The registrars were asked how many nurses were waiting for calls on the day when the questionnaire was filled

IS THERE UNEMPLOYMENT NOW?

Diagram 13.—Answers of 353 nurse registries to the question, "Would you like to have more nurses encouraged to move to your city?"

out. Of the 331 who answered that particular question, a few reported no nurses on call, but the average registry reported between 18 and 19 nurses. The hospital registries have fewer nurses on call than do the others. Half the hospital registries had four or less waiting for cases and the highest waiting list for a hospital registry was 78. For the "district, club, and commercial" group half the registries had at least 26 nurses on call, and the highest reported 231 on call that day. For registries conducted by individuals and small business firms, half had at least 13 nurses waiting on call, and the highest reported 200.

TABLE 19. PER CENT OF REGISTRIES OF EACH TYPE ANSWERING THE QUESTION "WOULD YOU LIKE MORE NURSES ENCOURAGED TO MOVE TO YOUR CITY?"

Registry	Yes	No	Total
Hospital, alumnæ	10%	90%	100%
District, club, com.	4	96	100
Individual	6	94	100
Other	12	88	100
All	8%	92%	100%

There is some reason to believe that hospital registries, perhaps unconsciously, but rather automatically, limit the number of nurses enrolled to approximately the number which the hospital can keep successfully employed. This probably occurs through the fact that as soon as the hospital registry reaches what is, for its own purposes, a satisfactory enrollment, it seems rather inclined to give ample employment only to the more satisfactory of its people, with the result that less satisfactory alumnæ find few cases coming through the hospital registry and gradually seek other channels for employment. The statistical evidence here is not conclusive, but the fact that the number of nurses waiting for employment in hospital registries is so markedly below the numbers for other sorts of registries, gives color to the theory. The suggestion is also supported by the reports from registrars and from private duty nurses. Many of the latter complain that they are no longer able to secure employment through their own hospitals. In some cases special pleas for help have reached the Grading Committee from nurses who thus find themselves "discriminated against."

8. Present Employment Conditions

There seems no question that, at the time this text is being written (March, 1928) employment conditions for private duty nurses are extremely bad. The data given in the previous section show that registries do not want to have more nurses encouraged to move to their localities. The American Journal of Nursing reports that for some time past notices have been received for insertion in its pages from official district registries saying in effect, "We do not wish to seem inhospitable, but employment conditions in this region are so poor that we urge upon nurses in other cities to investigate before coming here." These conditions are not confined to one or two sections of the country, but seem to be rather general.

Two questions were asked concerning present employment conditions which at first seemed to have resulted in mutually contradictory answers. The first was: "Is your registry receiving more or less calls now than it did a year ago?"; and the second: "Are present employment conditions better or worse than they were a year ago?"

Of all the registries combined, 56% said that they were receiving fewer calls; while at the same time 63% said that conditions were either the same, or better.

An analysis of the returns, however, showed that the returns from hospital registries were markedly different, in each case, from those of the other sorts of registries. Some 54% of hospital registries are getting as many or more calls, but only 28% of the other registries. Similarly 20% of the hospital registries say that present conditions are definitely better, as compared with 13% of the other registries.

The picture apparently is something like this. Hospital registries are getting more calls, either because they have more patients, or because the patients are willing to pay for special nurses as they were not a few years ago. To the head of a hospital registry, employment conditions are "good" if the hospital can get enough nurses (preferably from among its own alumnæ) to meet its own demands for specials and if its own alumnæ are reasonably well employed. As the number of its own alumnæ grows, the hospital naturally does not have to call upon the outside registries, and accordingly the business of these registries drops.

For many of the outside registries, the fact that the hospitals are now meeting their own nursing needs from their own alumnæ, has meant a serious drop in business. For these registries last year there was a real unemployment problem. For the coming year there will, apparently, be a worse one.

The figures indicate that conditions are becoming especially serious in the large cities. In cities of 500,000 or over only 9% of the hospital registries, and 3% of the outside registries report that conditions are "better," whereas 43% of the hospital registries and 68% of the outside registries report that they are definitely worse. The ideal state from the hospital viewpoint would probably be one in which the hospital had so many alumnæ that it never had to go outside for its supply of specials; and yet did not have so many alumnæ that it could not provide employment for all of them within its own walls. So long as the hospital remains in this ideal middle ground, employment conditions will be "good," but, if either it has too few, or too many alumnæ, conditions become unsatisfactory. The returns seem to indicate that many hospitals in the largest cities have reached or are close to reaching the third stage where they are unable to offer adequate employment to large numbers of their own graduates.

The following comment from the superintendent of a large metropolitan hospital illustrates what is happening.

> "In 1925 and 1926 we had a yearly average of practically 7,000 calls. About 4,300 of these calls were covered by our own graduates, but about 2,000 calls went to nurses in outside registries, and another 700 went unfilled. We usually had a daily average of 250 nurses enrolled.
>
> "In 1927, however, although we had practically the same number of calls (nearly 7,000) we were able to fill well over 6,000 of them from our own alumnæ. We employed only 734 outside nurses, and had only 34 calls unfilled. One of the reasons for this change was that by 1927 the daily average of nurses enrolled on our registry had increased from 250 to 329."

Knowing that this hospital graduates in the neighborhood of 80 new nurses a year, one wonders how long it will be before its supply of alumnæ becomes an embarrassment of riches! Yet the figures gathered by the Grading Committee strongly suggest that something like this situation is already developing in many different schools.

9. Vocational Guidance

The registrars were asked, "During the month of December, 1927, about how many trained nurses consulted you as to the advisability of their changing from one branch of nursing to another?"

In each group one or more registries reported that no one had asked for advice. In the hospital and alumnæ registries there is apparently practically no tradition calling for vocational guidance among the alumnæ enrolled on the registry. Half of these registries reported only one consultant or less during the month of December, and three-fourths had had no more than two. The highest number of vocational discussions for a single hospital registry during the month of December was ten.

In the "district, club, and commercial" registries, however, and in the registries conducted by individuals or small business firms, half of the registries had had at least four nurses consult them about changing during the month, and in one registry there were over 219 such consultations.

10. SUMMARY

a. Generally speaking, about 69 nurse registries in the United States are probably conducted by central nursing organizations; about half the rest by hospitals; and the other half by commercial firms or individuals. This study, however, contains a somewhat higher proportion of hospitals than is probably normal.

b. It was impracticable for the Committee to discover which registries are officially sponsored by nursing organizations, and which by commercial firms, because no distinguishing names or emblems have been adopted to point the difference.

c. Hospital and alumnæ registries are rather frankly run by the hospitals for their own convenience. They are usually located in the hospital or the nurses' home. They rarely charge a fee for enrollment. They do not ordinarily employ a special registrar and therefore do not pay her any salary. The typical enrollment on the registry is 24 nurses.

d. Outside registries seem to belong to two general types—the more or less businesslike organization (which includes district, club, and the larger commercial registries) and registries which are the private ventures of individuals.

e. The "district-club-commercial" group are ordinarily housed either in the nurses' club, the home of the registrar, or in a business building. Three-fourths of them either "break even" or make a profit. They usually employ at least one full time registrar, who is a registered nurse, to whom they pay a regular salary. The typical registry of this type enrolls 140 nurses.

f. Registries run by individuals as private enterprises are usually conducted in the registrar's own home. About 3 out of 10 ran on a deficit in 1927. The others either broke even or made a profit. Besides the proprietor there is usually one extra full time worker. Of each 10 registries, four are run by registered nurses; two by practical nurses; three by business men or women; and one by a social worker, a doctor, or a graduate unregistered nurse. Seven of the 10 share in the profits, two are on salary, and one carries on the work without pay. The typical private registry enrolls 75 nurses.

g. Sixty-five per cent of the hospital registries enroll R.N.'s only, as compared with 32% of the "district-club-commercial" registries and 7% of the privately run registries.

h. About one-eighth of the hospital registries, over half of the "district-club-commercial," and nearly nine-tenths of the privately run registries enroll practical nurses.

i. For all registries, eight out of ten calls are for hospital cases and only two for home cases. The privately owned registries, however, receive a much larger proportion of home calls.

j. It is not at all strange, therefore, that "hospital specialing" and "private duty" are synonymous in the minds of most nurses enrolled on registries.

k. All except the privately or individually run registries report overwhelmingly that hospital calls are easier to fill than home calls. For privately run registries the vote is about 50–50.

l. There seems to be less difficulty in persuading nurses to accept home calls in the largest cities than elsewhere.

m. Practically all calls received, by all kinds of registries, are filled.

n. The hardest calls to fill are home calls, country calls, and calls for contagious cases.

o. Except in the privately conducted registries where the vote is 50–50, there is a 99% vote to the effect that graduate nurses are more in demand than practicals.

p. There seems to be more demand for practicals in large cities than in small ones.

q. Of 353 registries, 325 do not want any more nurses encouraged to move to their cities. Most of them are emphatic in their protest against the suggestion.

r. There is evidence to suggest that

(1) Hospitals are increasingly able to fill their own needs for specials from their own alumnæ.

(2) Outside registries which have existed largely by catering to hospitals are finding it difficult to place the nurses on their lists.

(3) Enrollments are rapidly growing.

(4) Some hospitals are no longer able to keep their own alumnæ busy.

(5) These conditions seem to be most acute in the largest cities.

CHAPTER 5

WHAT REGISTRARS SAY

A huge volume of frank and illuminating testimony was secured by suggesting that no names need be signed to the returned questionnaires, and by leaving plenty of empty space, in which those who were cooperating in the Supply and Demand study could write freely anything which they felt might promote understanding.

While only the briefest excerpts can be made from what has proved a gold mine of material, it has seemed worth while, following each main division of this report, to insert a chapter made up of these comments. The quotations have been selected not because they are unusual, but because they express quite vividly opinions or experiences which are apparently rather common to the whole group. In every instance they are chosen from a considerable number of similar import.

1. Control of Registry

Many of the registries which replied indicated a really astonishing lack of sound business organization.

> OHIO.—We keep a registry for our own convenience and that of the nurse and doctor. There is no one person in charge. We have no special rules or regulations and for the service there is no charge to either our graduates or outside nurses.

> KANSAS.—In reality we do not run a registry. We simply reserve a corner of the "Patient's Register" for the names of our own graduates and the two or three other graduates who live in this town and will work part of the time.

SOUTH CAROLINA.—When the registry was first organized, it was kept in her home by a graduate nurse who had married. The nurses had many complaints, chiefly that they were not registered promptly, and the nurse would go out in the afternoon leaving the registry with a cook who could not read nor write. When the doctor would call for nurses he could not be given the information correctly nor promptly. So they asked that it be put back in the hospital.

MASSACHUSETTS.—There is no commercial registry but a drug store has a list of names. Practical nurses, attendants, etc., are also registered there, but there is no one to answer night calls from 10 p. m. until 8 a. m.

MASSACHUSETTS.—When I took over the hospital, graduate and practical nurses were registered at the local drug store. You can imagine it—young drug clerks sending out nurses! So I asked our board if I could take it over (at the request of the local nurses' club). We charge a nominal fee of $1.00 and have the work done by the office help. The doctors and graduate nurses, also the patients, get very satisfactory service, but, of course, the hospital has to stand the loss except that it is an indirect gain for us to know just where all the graduate nurses are.

2. Registrar's Problems

There is evident need for a better understanding of what the job of the Registrar involves, and what the relations should be between the Registrar and her Board, on the one hand, and the nurses enrolled on the registry, on the other.

TEXAS.—We feel that if the nurse registries had more and better cooperation from the hospitals, it would mean better service not only to the hospital, but to the doctor, the nurse, and the layman. If every nurse who is graduated would be required to register at the Nurse Registry, and every hospital would call its nurses through the registry (with the understanding that the registry would endeavor to reach the nurse specified by the hospital), we feel that one of the greatest problems confronting the nurse registry today would be solved.

CONNECTICUT.—My problem is to know how to get the local nurses into line so that they will understand that a registry is a background to them and of real help to them at all times.

MICHIGAN.—The present registry conditions are far from satisfactory, mostly, I would say, because we *seem* to be in control of the private duty nurses we register, but actually *are not.* The candidates are, first of all, not carefully enough selected but, especially, are not checked up after acceptance. The official registries claim a superiority over the commercial registries in that our members are carefully scrutinized and in that they are always well selected nurses whom we can recommend and whom we will sponsor.

I am afraid we do not, or cannot, maintain this claim without some form of "advisory service" or "supervisory service" (if I may use that term). I believe with the 1,200 registrants here, that if we had some form of advisory service, whereby we could have at the registry office a closer contact with every one of them, close enough to be of guidance, and an organization with a controlling board, frequent regular meetings when an advisory service could be rendered, that we would probably reach some method of control.

When a situation continues such as is the case here, where nurses who are in no sense able to meet nursing demands remain on the registry year after year (and this means about 30% of the registrants), our high standards are not maintained. It seems so difficult, almost impossible, to keep the unfit weeded out, where we do not have an organized way of taking care of them. "No chain is stronger than its weakest link," and as long as the private duty nurses, the largest number in our association, remain unorganized—mostly disorganized—we can hardly expect much progress, and our most difficult problems remain unsolved.

OHIO.—Outside nurses coming here are not taken readily into the hospitals for the reason that the supervisors do not recognize the name and therefore pass over her or take a nurse off a case and put her on the new case rather than chance the new nurse. This nurse waits indefinitely on the registry.

Again, the power of selection of nurses in the hospitals is very much overdrawn. Personal feelings play a large part, and it is almost impossible to call nurses fairly. Also, when a hospital or a doctor blacklists a nurse, it is next to impossible to get a written statement to the effect, thus making it impossible for us to approach the girl. We have several foreign nurses here who repeatedly, for various reasons, dodge the State Board, and yet, because they are such good nurses, are called directly by doctors and supervisors and given work in the hospital, while other "registered" nurses are waiting a call on the registry.

OREGON.—The greatest problem of the nurses' registries, we consider, is lack of cooperation between the nurses and doctors.

ARIZONA.—This being a general vocational and technical bureau handling only the highest type of help—we exclude labor and domestic help—we find the lack of responsibility on the part of nurses toward accepting positions offered very distressing, to say the least. Our main findings might be expressed as follows:

(1) The eastern, Canadian, and foreign trained nurses are most reliable. As you also know, they are

among the most highly educated previous to and during training.

(2) The western nurse usually is accepted into training with only some high school education. While there is a scattering of nurses who have all or some college education, they are so few that they are examples.

Our conclusion:

(1) The same general educational qualifications in all training schools, raising the standard as near as possible to that of a college education, thereby nullifying this irregularity.

(2) Any placements lost in the nurses' department we charge off to the fact that we are unable to make the connections with the proper type and that we must not try to sell to the employer a person we ourselves are not sold upon.

We furnish to the mining companies, for example, their managers, engineers, office help, teachers, doctors, and nurses. Therefore the latter must be able to meet the same demand that other trained people do.

We do not give our opinion in any but a helpful attitude although critical. We shall be glad to hear from your office at any time relative to nurses who are interested in locating here.

Massachusetts.—Conditions governing the problems of a registry should be adjusted with the appreciation of the fact that the registrar is an executive and not a subordinate.

It would be well for the registrar to meet with her governing board at least once a year. In this way adjustments which mean much to her in the daily successful conducting of affairs would not be so likely to be forgotten, neglected or indefinitely postponed —perhaps for years in some instances. To ask for improved conditions now and then is a sign of progress.

A registrar is expected to keep up with the times

in the profession but when she has only 11 days off out of 365 (not counting her vacation) how can she be expected to be very enthusiastic about attending conventions? There are at least four important meetings in a year which she would like to attend. The question arises whether it would not be a paying proposition for her to be sent at least once a year with expenses paid from the treasury.

A word of approval or commendation for work well done would promote a feeling of happiness and content. It is much easier to accomplish anything if one knows her efforts are appreciated and her endeavors looked upon with the spirit of sympathetic good will.

Registries have a way of growing and progressing out of the old-time routine. Membership increases, fees are changed, service in hospitals forms the bulk of the work of the nurse. The cases increase greatly in number but are shorter in duration. This means great increase of labor in our registries. Have our committees been alert in recognizing that fact, and do they take care to see that their registrars are not overworked?

I might suggest that it is the women who have given years of faithful service who should be given special consideration, rather than the new comers who have not been doing this kind of work long enough to become tired out.

MASSACHUSETTS.—The great difficulty, of course, is the long hours. Shorter hours, even with smaller compensation, would go a great way towards making a happier and healthier nurse.

TEXAS.—The need is for well qualified nurses prepared to hold administrative and supervisory positions. Quite a few requests are received annually from other hospitals for women to fill these positions.

CALIFORNIA.—In regard to consultation as to the advisability of changing from one branch of nursing to another, the common desire expressed in all interviews is for a regular schedule of hours and salary—not less than $125 without maintenance. There is not a thorough grasp of the fact that such employment would mean restrictions to a stated vacation each year of from 2 to 4 weeks. There is a desire expressed also for at least one day off in each week included in salary. *There is remarkable reluctance to give up bedside nursing.*

3. Floor Duty

Registrars agree in testifying that general floor duty is not eagerly sought by graduate nurses.

WASHINGTON.—Many of the nurses coming are floaters, though a great many do become permanent, but the largest number by far are here for a time and then go on to greener fields.

We find that we are filling our general duty positions almost entirely from this floating group of nurses. The local nurses do not seem to care to take that work as a rule, and it gives the outside nurse a chance to become acquainted, should she desire a little later to do private duty.

ILLINOIS.—A great many nurses have expressed dissatisfaction with private duty nursing but dislike general floor duty as much, and, since special fields require further preparation, they continue private duty nursing in a discontented spirit.

NORTH DAKOTA.—Our state tuberculosis sanitorium calls for general duty nurses frequently and we seldom succeed in getting any one for them. Nurses who have not been working refuse to go even for a short time. Reasons given are, "Isolated place," "Low salary," "Do not care to leave town."

4. Nurses' Choice of Work

The large amount of evidence showing that private duty nurses tend to prefer hospital special duty raises a ques-

tion as to whether the training, which is almost entirely hospital training, is at fault.

Ohio.—Every call from the community is filled. We manage some way to get a nurse.

Vermont.—All the nurses prefer hospital cases and it is very difficult at times to get a nurse to go out of town.

Pennsylvania.—I dread to ask any graduate to take a case outside of the hospital. Only a small percentage are willing to do so.

Illinois.—Our graduates do not care to go on call away from their own hospital which in time will bring difficulties as we are graduating fair sized classes every year.

North Dakota.—We find it almost impossible to get nurses to go out of town, either to home calls or small hospitals.

Alabama.—We have difficulty in getting nurses to take cases in private homes; they all prefer hospital nursing. A very few will take obstetrical nursing.

Vermont.—We find among the younger graduates a tendency to refuse out of town calls and also calls for contagious work.

Pennsylvania.—We have little or no trouble with registering our own nurses. The only difficulty is in inducing nurses to take patients in homes for two reasons:

1. It is easier in the hospital where equipment is handy, assistance easily secured, and the hours are definite. The nurses often have apartments near hospital and it is easy for them to go back and forth. Salary is assured because it is paid by hospital check whether patient pays or not.

2. The hospital patients are usually acutely ill or else operation patients and work is more interesting and varied. The work in the home is more of

the personal maid work, so spoken of by the nurses. Most acutely ill patients are sent to the hospital, probably because of the convenience to the doctor who can there see six or seven patients in the same time that it usually takes to drive to a house, see the patient, and drive to the next house. Operations are practically never done now in private homes.

PENNSYLVANIA.—Our nurses are most independent and want to choose their cases. They all want to nurse in the hospital.

OHIO.—We find nurses willing to assume charge of any kind of case offered, namely, communicable disease, in the country, or anywhere the registrar has a call for service. This is quite an improvement over some of the objections they made several years ago.

STATE NOT KNOWN.—There are two hospitals in our city. Each employs its own nurses first. Girls graduating from hospitals in other cities have to take the home cases or the overflow from the hospitals, consequently they get discouraged with their work and are constantly changing or returning to town in which they trained, where they will have a better chance to take hospital work which all graduate nurses prefer.

IOWA.—We find many of the recent registered nurses choosing only certain kinds of cases and choosing only hospital work. During the winter months it is difficult to obtain nurses for country cases and these sometimes are obtained only after much persuasion, coaxing, and begging.

CONNECTICUT.—We find rural calls very hard to fill. We do not seem to have as much trouble placing nurses in homes as in former years although the younger graduates need some coaxing to take their first home case as they do not feel fitted to cope with situations outside of hospitals.

5. Holiday Calls

Nurses have an extraordinary sense of group loyalty in many things, but there is an almost total lack of esprit de corps in relation to the registries, no sense of a group obligation to maintain its prestige and its service. This may be due to a lack of leadership on the part of the registries.

VIRGINIA.—Calls coming in Saturday night and Sunday are hardest to fill. Also suspected contagious diseases and night duty.

PENNSYLVANIA.—With exception of holiday season, have been able to meet demands.

CALIFORNIA.—The inability to fill all of the requests in December was due to all of the nurses going "off call" for the Christmas holidays.

NEW YORK.—We were unable to fill 12 calls owing to Christmas holidays.

ILLINOIS.—There are enough nurses in the city to take care of practically all calls if some arrangement could be made to take care of the calls at holiday times and during vacations. The unfilled calls were during the summer vacations and many were from small nearby towns.

PENNSYLVANIA.—The nurses all go away over the holidays. It is almost impossible to get nurses over Thanksgiving or Christmas or Easter, often during summer, and always over the foot-ball season.

NEW YORK.—In this particular community the summer months are our busiest time of the year, owing to the heavy tourist traffic going through our city and to the fact that bootleggers travel nightly over the highway and driving recklessly, occasion many an accident. The majority of these accidents come here. We also have many visitors at our summer hotels and camps who may fall ill, and many of these are also brought to our hospital. The majority of these people have wealth and request special nurses. The hospital employs usually from three to six extra graduates for relief during summer vacations, and this too must be taken into consideration when trying to regulate the supply and demand for special nurses. The nurses on our registry are more or less familiar with these conditions, and yet a good many take their vacations during this time and then during the latter part of September, October, November, and December they are idle because we are not busy, and they have to wait days and sometimes weeks for a call. Whereas if they would take their vacation at this time and be on call during the busy months, they would not be so much out of pocket. January and March are our busiest months.

6. Floaters

There is abundant evidence that the floating nurse is a nation-wide problem.

TEXAS.—Floaters are our problem. They stream by, stopping over to work for short time and have their cars repaired. They see doctors and get a call or two if they cannot get on the registry. Registered nurses who do qualify wander from city to city. I have them come and show cards from three or four registries in other places. I am swamped with inquiries and have a form letter telling them not to come, as we have more nurses than we can find work for and usually have a hundred on our waiting list. The social service agencies and the Red Cross call me frequently about application for assistance or transportation. We have a special relief fund and prefer to assist nurses who are in distress, by means of our association committee.

NEW YORK.—I prefer to get my nurses by interview —what I mean by that is—have a nurse come to me from a good reliable registered school. I find the tramp nurse is more a roving spirit and cannot be relied upon. The tramp nurse is one who comes in a town or city and stays long enough to get money to go on to the next town, regardless of the position in which she leaves the Registry she has connected herself with. My experience has been such they would come to me asking to come on my registry, without means to pay the fee. I would as a sister nurse give them cases and they in return would go away without ever paying me or thanking me for my courtesy. I feel myself justified in calling nurses of that type "Tramp Nurses."

MISSOURI.—Hospitals occasionally graduate the kind of nurses they do not care to call back on cases themselves.

CALIFORNIA.—We are finding many nurses who, undesirable presumably in their own schools, drift on or travel and we are constantly being made aware that greater care is required by the Registrar in selection before enrolling. There is much to be said in criticism of such a group in the matter of appearance, quality of work, reliability and personality, who find they cannot make good in the localities from which they come to us.

7. Want More Nurses?

The registries not only had a more than adequate supply of nurses in January, 1928, but indicated that the oversupply was not a recent thing; from which it may be assumed that the general economic conditions throughout the country were not the basic cause of the surplus.

WISCONSIN.—We are in a community where people cannot always afford a graduate R.N. at the price she is charging today, hence the girls do not get all the work they need and have migrated to more remunerative fields.

COLORADO.—Economic conditions in mine section of Colorado are such that people can hardly get necessary hospital, general care, and so quite naturally special nurses are *not* employed. There just isn't any money.

Rhode Island.—We have sent out more nurses in the last few months than in the corresponding months last year, but we have a longer list, and fewer calls in proportion.

Indiana.—Almost all our graduates stay right here, and the result is that now we have more nurses than the field needs.

D. C.—I do not think there is need of any nurses being sent here. Nurses are leaving here seeking work elsewhere.

Pennsylvania.—Infinitely worse this year.

Iowa.—Our city has an oversupply of registered nurses, consequently there is much "waiting time" between cases for the majority.

Kentucky.—Would state emphatically that we do not need more nurses in Louisville. Heretofore with only four training schools, there was a shortage and we begged for more to come. In the last three years, with four more large training schools added and pouring out students, we are having a problem, and woe betide the stranger in our midst. This year many more students are coming out, crowding off the older and strange nurses.

New York.—I have conducted the central registry for nurses for the past fourteen years, and this is the worst business year I have experienced, last year being very little better. I have from seven to ten nurses daily, mostly graduates or undergraduates, from all over the country either writing me or calling on me for nursing either in private homes or in institutions or hospitals, even at a reduced price in order to make a living. Every case I received during 1927 I could have filled four or five times over, as we had so many nurses of all kinds waiting for cases. Have hundreds more than I can use.

MINNESOTA.—Some of our graduates have left to do private duty elsewhere, as there is not enough here to keep them busy.

MICHIGAN.—Nursing conditions have never before in my three years duty as registrar been so "slack." Nurses have become quite discouraged, in the past few months some going to their homes, others leaving city seeking institutional positions elsewhere. Modern facilities attract the sick to hospitals, where students care for them, unless in a more serious case where a graduate is called in. Her stay is of short duration—returns again and registers. Where once we only boasted of hospitals in a fair sized city, we have them every few miles now—like Standard Oil Gas Stations.

UTAH.—The last five months with exception of two weeks in January, work has been poorer than at any other time in history of registry.

NEW JERSEY.—We are always glad to register new nurses, but during 1927 we did not have work for our own nurses, with the exception of part of August. Last year we refunded the fee to a number of recent graduates, so they could return to their own hospitals, rather than have them remain here without money or employment.

GEORGIA.—I hate not to seem hospitable in wanting more nurses, but we are already overcrowded, and it keeps me miserable as they cannot all keep busy here. We graduate at least 100 here every year.

NORTH CAROLINA.—This city has four general hospitals with training schools, and these hospitals turn out a number of graduates each year, and most of these nurses stay in the city, so with the nurses who were already here we are having an oversupply. Many nurses who want to come here write to find out something of the nursing conditions here, and those I can warn, but others come before investigating and are sorry that they did not write.

OHIO.—Do not have any objection to out-of-town nurses when business conditions are good, but in the past year, due to the percentage of unemployment, feel it an injustice to local nurses to encourage the out-of-town nurse.

ILLINOIS.—Employment conditions among nurses last year bad, this year worse. Personally I think this is owing to the large number of nurses coming here from other states. Work for nurses has been so poor the past year, that many nurses have taken up other lines of employment.

WISCONSIN.—There are times in the fall of the year that one half of the total number of nurses on my list are waiting for work. Our dull period was not quite as long this year as some years, but I had more nurses in at one time than ever before.

CONNECTICUT.—We are most fortunate in having our supply of nurses just about meet the demand, and sending any more to this city, I feel, would not be a good policy just now.

MASSACHUSETTS.—Usually this is the best time of the year and more calls are received than can be filled. However, this year is the reverse in the case, and there are more nurses on the list than there are positions.

NEW YORK.—Last year we were often troubled about getting enough nurses. This year so many of our 1927 graduates went on the registry here that we have often this winter had from 12 to 18 on call over days at a time.

WEST VIRGINIA.—We have far too many here now. Some have not had a call for four weeks. Work here is so scarce for R.N.'s that I'm surprised we have any girls taking up the profession.

Oklahoma.—With four training schools in the city there are enough nurses graduating every year with what few come unannounced to fill the demand.

California.—This part of California, having delightful climate, attracts more nurses than we are able to give employment.

South Dakota.—We would not appreciate having nurses move to this locality as we have more than we can keep busy now, and we graduate from three to six each year, providing too many for the demand here.

Florida.—Since November, 1927, we have had a third of the nurses on call most of the time. I have had several tourist nurses here wanting to register, but I explained to them the situation, so they moved on.

Missouri.—We have many idle nurses in the city. We have had too many nurses for over a year now. The hospitals are not calling as many specials as formerly. Schools are filled to capacity. For two years we have had a great many nurses here. Our schools have turned out large classes, larger than for many years, we find ourselves with too many. Some have eliminated themselves, taken up other work, or left the City.

Nebraska.—There have been so many short cases —from one to two days only.

Pennsylvania.—With three hospitals graduating a class each year, what would your answer be? Never receive calls from hospitals as each one has their own registry.

CHAPTER 6

IS THERE A PUBLIC HEALTH NURSE SHORTAGE?

At the same time that the ten state study of private duty nursing was being made, in March, 1927, report blanks were sent to every public health nursing organization in those ten states which had more than one staff member. Of the 246 organizations thus addressed, replies were received from 108, or 44 per cent. The following pages give a summary of the answers given by these 108 public health administrators. The purpose of this study was not to cover the general field of public health nursing, but, rather, was limited to an inquiry concerning employment conditions at the time when the study was being made, in March, 1927.

The organizations studied ranged in size from many in which there were only two or three workers, up to one which included a staff of 232 workers. The sizes of staff were as follows:

42% of the organizations had from 2 to 5 members
19% of the organizations had from 6 to 10 members
12% of the organizations had from 11 to 15 members
11% of the organizations had from 16 to 20 members
16% of the organizations had 21 members and over

100% Total

1. Extras Employed?

March, 1927, was, so far as that particular year was concerned, a period of reasonably heavy sickness, although like the corresponding month in 1928, there were no serious epidemics. The Committee desired to find how many of the public health organizations were obliged to secure extra workers in order to help carry the heavy load of spring illness. Of the 108 organizations, only 27 reported that they had hired any extras during the month just closed, 66 reported that they had not, and 15 left the question unanswered. There is a marked tendency for people filling in questionnaires to assume, when the answer to a question is "No," that the fact may be so indicated by leaving a blank space, and it therefore seems probable that the fifteen organizations which left this question unanswered probably all belong to the "no" group, which did not employ any extra workers. In all tabulations for the Supply and Demand study, however, unanswered questions are tabulated as "not stated," and are omitted in computations of per cents.

The twenty-seven organizations employed among them forty-nine extra workers, and the number of extra workers did not seem to be affected by the size of staff. The population, however, made a genuine difference, since no extras were employed in cities of over 500,000, and only two of the forty-nine were in cities of less than 25,000. The chief need for extra workers seemed to be in cities of 25,000 to 100,000. Of the extra workers employed to help out during the rush period, the directors reported that if they had had places for them, they would have been glad to keep about three-fifths. The other two-fifths proved not wholly fitted for the work. Slightly over half of the extras employed had had no previous public health experience.

2. Applicants for Regular Staff Vacancies

The directors of public health organizations were also asked:

"During the past month how many *staff* vacancies for nurses have you had? How many have you filled?"

Of the total 108 organizations reporting, 37 reported one or more staff vacancies, 69 reported no vacancies, and 2 did not answer the question specifically, but in all probability should be included in the group which had no vacancies. The 37 organizations had 70 vacancies during the month, of which 53 were filled, and 17 were not. The number of applicants for the 17 unfilled positions is not known, but for the 53 vacancies which were filled, there were 289 applicants, an average of 5.5 applicants for each position filled.

The number of applicants was apparently considerably greater in the larger organizations than in the smaller. The average applicants per organization were as follows:

Organizations with	workers had an average of	applicants for appointment
2 to 5	1.4	
6 to 10	2.5	
11 to 15	5.4	
16 to 20	4.2	
21+	11.4	

The directors were asked:

"Do you usually have more applicants for staff positions than you need, or is this true only at certain seasons of the year, or is it almost never true?"

TABLE 20. PER CENT OF DIRECTORS OF PUBLIC HEALTH ORGANIZATIONS REPORTING THAT THEY USUALLY, SOMETIMES, OR ALMOST NEVER, HAVE MORE APPLICANTS FOR STAFF POSITIONS THAN THEY NEED

Nurses on staff	Usually	Some times	Almost never	All
2– 5	69%	9%	22%	100%
6–10	55	25	20	100
11–15	100	0	0	100
16–20	50	25	25	100
21+	75	12+	12+	100
All	69%	14%	17%	100%

IS THERE A PUBLIC HEALTH NURSE SHORTAGE?

Diagram 14.—"Do you usually have more applicants for staff positions than you need?" Per cent of Directors of Public Health Nursing in 10 states who gave each type of answer

Of the 108 organizations, 65 reported that they usually had more applicants than they needed, 13 reported that this was true at certain seasons of the year, and 16 that it was almost never true. Fourteen organizations did not answer the question. Size of staff apparently makes comparatively little difference in this condition.

3. Reasons for Refusing Applicants

The directors were asked as to the reasons why applicants were considered ineligible for the positions. Twenty-seven organizations reported the reasons why 134 applicants had been refused. Since some applicants were refused for more than one reason, no grand total can be given here.

Reasons for refusing applicants	Applicants	Per cent
Had not had enough theoretical courses in public health work	45	34
Had not had enough practical public health experience	32	24
Did not have academic background needed	27	20
Had not had broad enough general nursing experience	25	19
Had personality difficulty	17	13
Seemed to lack understanding of what public health work stands for	16	12
Did not seem physically strong enough to do the work	15	11
Came from too small nursing schools	14	10
Seemed to be poor bedside nurses	10	7
Seemed to lack professional viewpoint	7	5
Came from the wrong section of the country	6	4
Other	13	10

4. Bedside Nursing Technique

The Committee was especially interested in following up the question of whether or not bedside technique is important in applicants for public health work, and how adequately they prepared along that line. The question was asked:

"When you secure new workers for regular staff duty, are you usually able to rely upon their having satisfactory bedside nursing technique or must you teach them that, as well as the educational and preventive aspects peculiar to the public health field?"

Of the 108 directors, 24 did not answer this question, and 2 others definitely stated that in their work no particular bedside technique was necessary. Of the 82 directors who were definitely interested in the bedside technique of applicants for staff positions, 59 said that most applicants had satisfactory bedside nursing technique, and 23 that it was ordinarily necessary to provide special instruction along that line. The organizations with staffs of more than 11 people were less satisfied with the bedside technique of applicants than were directors of organizations with a fewer number of workers.

5. Supervision

The directors were also asked, "Do inexperienced nurses resent supervision? Do the more experienced nurses?" For all the directors combined, 23 per cent said that the non-experienced nurses resented supervision, and 15 per cent that the experienced did so. The difficulty in introducing the concept of supervision to non-experienced workers is apparently considerably greater in small staffs than in larger ones. In staffs with five members or less, over half reported that non-experienced workers often or sometimes resented supervision.

6. Means for Holding Workers

The directors were finally asked:

"Which of the following do you consider particularly important as means of keeping good workers contentedly on the staff?"

The checked list, together with the per cents of affirmative votes from directors of organizations of each size, is given in the following table:

Table 21. Per Cent of All Directors in Organizations of Each Size Who Checked Each Specified Item as Particularly Important for Holding Good Workers Contentedly on the Staff

	Staff 2–5	Staff 6–10	Staff 11–15	Staff 16–20	Staff 21+	All
Vacations on pay	90%	100%	100%	100%	100%	99%
Regular hours	90	95	100	92	100	97
Sympathetic supervision	65	84	100	92	100	83
Staff courses and conferences	53	95	100	83	93	78
A sliding salary scale	68	84	85	67	87	78
Hope for promotion to supervisory jobs	35	37	46	67	67	46
Opportunity for bedside nursing without idle time on duty	28	32	46	25	47	35
Frequent shifts in assignments of work	15	16	8	17	93	17

7. SUMMARY

This chapter may be summarized as follows:

a. Of 108 public health organizations in ten states, in March, 1927, only 27 employed extra workers to help carry the spring load.

b. In the same month only 37 of the 108 had vacancies on their staffs. These 37 had 70 staff vacancies.

c. Of the 70 staff vacancies, 53 were filled and 17 were not. There were 289 applicants for the 53 positions, or an average of 5.5 applicants for each one.

d. That this excess of applicants over positions filled was not an accidental finding is indicated by the reports of directors, 69 per cent of whom stated that they usually had more applicants for staff positions than they needed, and another 14 per cent that this was true at certain seasons of the year. Only 17 per cent reported a regular shortage in applicants for staff appointments.

e. These facts hold true for large and small organizations alike.

f. The most frequent reasons for refusing applicants were usually because they lacked theoretical courses or practical experience in public health, or because they did not have the academic background needed.

g. In the larger organizations, lack of proper bedside technique seemed to be a more important problem in admitting new workers than in smaller organizations.

h. In the smaller organizations there was more difficulty about adjusting new workers to accept supervision than in the larger ones.

i. The three outstanding means for holding good workers, according to the directors, are: vacations on pay; regular hours; sympathetic supervision.

CHAPTER 7

WHAT PUBLIC HEALTH DIRECTORS SAY

The questions asked of public health organizations were confined rather strictly to questions of employment and supervision. The answers were typically as follows:

1. Shortage of Applicants?

Public health nursing is generally looked upon as a desirable field. There is no shortage of applicants.

MASSACHUSETTS.—No difficulty encountered in finding and keeping type of nurse desired.

NEW YORK.—We always have applicants.

MASSACHUSETTS.—It is not difficult to fill vacancies on the staff. But one cannot pick and choose. There is a scarcity of nurses with public health experience.

MASSACHUSETTS.—No difficulty in filling staff vacancies. Senior nurses at one of the local hospitals have opportunity to elect one month of "district." Are enthusiastic and interested and many of them apply for position.

ILLINOIS.—There is no shortage of nurses here. Our problem is to find nurses with sufficient academic background and with the necessary personality.

CALIFORNIA.—The reason we get more applicants for positions in the late summer is because a lot of nurses come to the University for summer session and then do not wish to go back to other states, so apply for positions here.

KANSAS.—If we employed additional married nurses, we could have applications of several splendid nurses.

CALIFORNIA.—There has never been a shortage of applications in this organization.

2. Education

If schools of nursing appreciated the tendency of public health organizations to require full high school preparation, it would doubtless influence their own entrance requirements.

MASSACHUSETTS.—I find very little trouble in securing nurses who can do good bedside work but they lack the public health point of view.

NEW YORK.—We are often obliged to take nurses with inadequate background of Public Health experience or training, because none are available at time vacancy occurs.

NEW YORK.—We find that the nurse with a fine background, good education, and dependable and desirable professional ability is the type to whom this place appeals. She is the type we want and we refuse to fill a vacancy permanently till we can get her. The finer the type, and the higher the educational background, the more eager the nurse is to learn from supervision without resentment.

MASSACHUSETTS.—We have the names of many nurses in our files who would be glad to come to us but they lack preliminary education as well as public health education. We cannot secure enough nurses who have had complete high school. Some few of the nurses who were with us before we had adequate supervision resent supervision as we have it today but the best nurses on our staff welcome supervision. Almost every new nurse who comes to us expects and is glad of supervision.

MASSACHUSETTS.—I have had great difficulty in securing applicants with full high school education. We always give them preference providing their character rating is good. We have no difficulty in keeping the type of worker we have. We closed the year with three nurses who had been on our staff five years.

New York.—We have a standard of high school graduates as fundamental. Many who would be applicants know this and therefore do not apply.

Massachusetts.—Fifty per cent of those admitted have public health training. Many of the others are ineligible for this training because they lack a high school course. When a nurse applies who is not a high school graduate, I always ask her what she would have done, if, when she applied for admission to her training school, she had been advised to finish her high school course and then re-apply. Nearly all say they would have done so—that their families wanted them to finish but they were eager to enter training school and when they found they could be admitted, they left school. Others say that they and their families would have made sacrifices to keep them in school if it had been explained to them that lack of a high school diploma might prove a handicap after they had finished training by preventing them from taking post-graduate work.

Massachusetts.—I have found that often the weakest part of a nurse's training in the smaller schools has been in obstetrical nursing. This, perhaps, shows up more in bedside work in the district when the nurse is left more or less to her own resources.

Georgia.—It is very difficult to make the nurses realize that, after taking a three-year training, they are still not fitted for Public Health Nursing. I have had to train all of my nurses except one in the very basic principles of public health.

Georgia.—There is a distinct feeling that only local nurses should be employed. The local schools of nursing are all small and clinical material limited. Also standards are none too high. It is only during the past two years that any high school training has been required. Only one or two nurses in this entire section have had any theoretical training in public health.

ILLINOIS.—Yes, we do have real difficulty in securing high type well educated nurses. They come from small training schools, so well satisfied with themselves, and with no ambition to learn any more.

ILLINOIS.—Nurses under twenty-five who have not had much home training and whose hospital training has been somewhat meager, no matter in what hospital they received it, rarely understand a sympathetic approach to a family in distress. Their own life experience has been too limited or too brief to permit them to understand that patients are usually people.

MASSACHUSETTS.—We have engaged nurses who have not had the special course but who are graduates from an accredited school, R.N., etc., and we have tried to train them in public health by attending conferences, institutes, staff conferences, etc. and have had no difficulty in securing good applicants and we believe we have a staff of good public health nurses.

CALIFORNIA.—There are many good private duty nurses who desire public health work but cannot spend the time in preparation. I have tried out some of these applicants but I find it is a loss to the Association. Much time is spent on them and so often they leave without much notice. The spirit of "seeing what it is like" seems to accompany these nurses, not the "student spirit." I believe the theoretical training is very important to create the point of view which we need in our public health nurses so badly. There are exceptions, of course. I have two splendid exceptions on my staff.

MASSACHUSETTS.—Public health nursing needs an

older nurse than is now being graduated from our schools of nursing—nurses from twenty-three to twenty-five at least. Educational background is most essential. Although supervised, a nurse is more or less on her own. Public health nursing demands a young woman who has family background and ideals, so that almost unknowingly she inculcates. Some institutions, as well as the state, are graduating many who are no credit to the nursing profession. (They still belong to the servant type, regardless of whether they pass state boards or not).

3. Salaries

Although the average annual salary in public health nursing is higher than that in private duty, there is plenty of evidence to indicate the need for a general increase.

NEW YORK.—There seem to be two main difficulties in finding and keeping enough nurses of the right type—namely, too low salaries, and inadequate concurrent education.

NEW YORK.—At the salaries paid, civil service is not able to demand public health experience or training, neither can it set educational standards higher than those of local hospitals.

NEW YORK.—One of the difficulties in keeping a permanent nursing staff has been that in engaging a nurse who has had previous public health experience and perhaps some theoretical training, as we should like to do, either she wants more salary at the end of a year (which, since she is paid by county taxes, she is not always able to get) or, more generally, she passes on to an executive position. She came to the county for a year's experience in rural work. All of which is very nice for the nurse, but not so nice for the county.

So we either have to take a nurse of training and experience with the expectation that she will leave in a year or so (and at that we can't always get such a one) or engage a local nurse without those prerequisites and hope to educate her gradually into being a good public health nurse. The latter course seems to be more satisfactory; continuity of service is more valuable than background in work of this kind in a rural district.

4. Staff Problems

Graduate nurses do not always take kindly to supervision, although it has proved a powerful, cohesive force in some organizations.

MASSACHUSETTS.—I have been in charge of the work here for the past three years and during this time have had six different nurses. Only one of these had had a special course in public health nursing. I find that every one of these nurses resents supervision and does not want to use a standard technique. Each one wants to do the work in her own way. Four were very poor in record-keeping and failed to see its importance. Some did not like the country. All of those six felt that they were entitled to the same privileges as I was in regard to time off, number of visits made, regardless of the fact that I have all the responsibility and clerical work to do. We have only one nurse besides myself in this town of 7,005 population.

GEORGIA.—The applicants for the supervisor or field director place were without previous experience in the majority of instances. The one with previous experience resented any supervision upsetting the staff and board to such an extent that a year later the harmful effects from it were still to be seen. How to get experienced workers with a mentality agreeable to supervision is one of our problems.

ILLINOIS.—I was on the staff of a large public health organization in another state. Among the staff members there seemed to be constant complaint of the supervision which was lacking in understanding, tact and sympathy. I often thought that we were treated as probationers rather than graduate nurses. In the same city was another organization whose superintendent is a most splendid one. Her nurses never complained although they worked hard. I asked a member of this group why she was always so very cheerful and never discouraged. She replied that it was because her superintendent was so sympathetic and understanding and seemed to have such great faith in the ability and judgment of her nurses.

LOUISIANA.—As the work is new in Louisiana, we have many applicants for positions. Our greatest difficulty in keeping the nurses is because the work is all field work in remote rural communities where living conditions are poor but we make frequent shifts and in this way keep the nurses satisfied.

PENNSYLVANIA.—The nurses prefer being busy and are much more content when their days are full.

MASSACHUSETTS.—The nurse's life in country districts has so few opportunities for interesting recreation that social problems are frequently involved. Another big problem is that of locating satisfactory board and room. We find it helps to allow the nurses to be given an extra week-end occasionally for a trip to the city for real recreation.

CHAPTER 8

ARE PHYSICIANS SATISFIED?

An attempt was made to reach physicians and, through them, their patients. Through the courtesy of the Journal of the American Medical Association questionnaires were sent to all subscribers to the Journal who were residents in the ten states where the special nursing studies were being conducted in March, 1927. It is impossible to judge with any accuracy how many of these questionnaires actually reached the hands of practising physicians, since many of the subscribers to the Journal are in executive or teaching positions which do not bring them in contact with patients, are lay people interested in medical problems, medical men and women who have retired from practice, and so on, through other classifications of people who would not ordinarily employ private duty nurses and would, therefore, not have been called upon to answer the questions in the report blank which was mailed them.

Returns were received from 1,459 physicians. Many expressed interest in the work but explained why their experience would not be helpful for the statistical studies contemplated. The material gathered through these 1,459 usable replies was so uniform in character and of such significance to the study that the need for gathering more material along approximately the same lines was strongly felt.

Accordingly, in November, 1927, a return postal was sent to every member of the American Medical Association. Of the 95,180 postals thus sent out, 23,500 have been returned at the time this report is being written, and more are being received daily. The postals asked, first, what the physician's special line of practice was; second, how often he needed private duty nurses in his practice; and third, whether he would be willing to cooperate with the Grading Committee by answering certain questions about his recent experience with private duty nurses. The results were extremely interesting.

1. Who the Physicians Are

The returns on the postal inquiry were compared with the total membership of the American Medical Association. As will be seen from the accompanying table, the returns are close to 22 per cent of the total A.M.A. membership. The per cent of returns in each geographical division is approximately the same as the corresponding per cent of American Medical Association members in that division.

TABLE 22. PER CENT OF PHYSICIANS ANSWERING THE QUESTIONNAIRE IN EACH GEOGRAPHICAL DIVISION, COMPARED WITH THE TOTAL MEMBERSHIP OF THE AMERICAN MEDICAL ASSOCIATION AND WITH THE MEMBERSHIP FOR THAT GEOGRAPHICAL DIVISION

Geographical division	Per cent of all A.M.A. members	Per cent of M.D.'s answering postal	Per cent of A.M.A. members in each section who answered postal
New England	8.2%	8.5%	22.2%
Middle Atlantic	22.6	23.0	21.9
East North Cent.	21.7	20.1	19.9
West North Cent.	12.1	11.5	20.6
South Atlantic	10.9	11.8	23.3
East South Cent.	6.6	6.7	21.7
West South Cent.	8.3	6.5	16.9
Mountain	3.0	4.2	30.4
Pacific	6.6	7.7	25.3
All	100%	100%	21.5%

Of the replies received, 51 per cent were from general practitioners, 9 per cent from general practitioners who also were beginning to specialize, and 40 per cent from specialists. These figures do not include the replies from physicians who had retired from service or were engaged in other than private practice. Upon examination of the detailed returns it was found that the group of "general practitioners with a specialty" voted on questions of nursing in such close agreement with other general practitioners that it was decided to include them all under the one heading. This has been done in the tables which follow.

2. Are Physicians Willing to Help?

When the physicians were asked whether they would be willing to answer questions concerning their experience with private duty nurses, 89 per cent said *Yes*, 3 per cent said *No*, and 8 per cent expressed their willingness to cooperate, but questioned whether their experience would be applicable. Some of these 8 per cent also suggested that they would prefer to read the questionnaire before deciding.

3. How Often Do They Need Special Nurses?

The physicians were asked how often they had occasion to utilize the services of private duty nurses. The replies may be summarized by saying that—

For general practitioners:

8% practically never need special nurses
5% need them occasionally
87% need them often

Among the specialists:

17% practically never need any special duty nurses
4% need them occasionally
79% need them often

Returns showing the physicians' judgments as to the relative frequency with which they need private duty nurses in the hospital and in the home were as follows:

General practitioners

8% never need any special nurses

13% never need them in the home
20% never need them in the hospital

7% sometimes need them in the home
4% sometimes need them in the hospital

80% often need them in the home
66% often need them in the hospital

Specialists

17% never need any special nurses

48% never need them in the home
20% never need them in the hospital

10% sometimes need them in the home
3% sometimes need them in the hospital

42% often need them in the home
77% often need them in the hospital

The two accompanying diagrams show the reports of physicians in each specialty as to the amounts of nursing service they need. Diagram 15 shows a series of bars for the different medical groups. Each bar is equal in length to 100 per cent. The white portion shows the per cent who report that they often need private duty nurses, and the black portion the per cent who rarely or never need them. At the top of the list come the surgeons, 98 per cent of whom frequently need private duty nurses; next come the obstetricians, with 94 per cent, and so on down to the physicians in the public health field, with only 9 per cent.

At the opposite end of the bars are figures showing, for the same medical groups, the percentage of physicians who have promised to answer the questions of the Grading Committee. The figures show that 96 per cent of all the surgeons who reply agree to answer questions, 95 per cent of the obstetricians, and so on down to 37 per cent of the physicians in the public health field. For all the physicians together, 84 per cent report that they frequently need private duty nurses on their cases, and 89 per cent promise to answer questions asked by the Grading Committee.

	% often need P.D.	% Ans.
Surgeons	98	96
Obstetrics	94	95
Internal med.	89	92
Gen. practice	87	92
Orth. surgery	86	91
Pediatrics	85	93
Urology	85	87
Opth. etc.	75	83
Neurology	57	68
Tuberculosis	47	67
Industrial	47	66
Dermatology	33	59
Roentgenology	25	45
Public health	9	37

Diagram 15.—Per cent of physicians in each specialty who often need private duty nurses ▭ and who rarely or never need them ■. (Figures at end of bars show per cents of physicians in each specialty who have agreed to answer questions for the Grading Committee.)

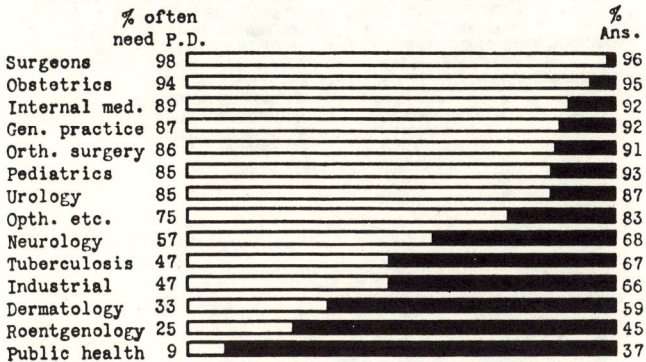

These are encouraging figures in themselves, and the returns are even more interesting when the two columns are compared; for it will be seen that the promises to answer decrease in very nearly the same order as the need for nurses. In other words, physicians who do not want to answer the questions of the Grading Committee about private duty are, in general, those who have least contact with that branch of the nursing profession. Many of them write: "I should like to be of help, but doubt whether my judgment would be of much value." Those, on the other hand, who write that they are constantly in touch with private duty are almost unanimous in their cordial willingness to cooperate in the studies now under way.

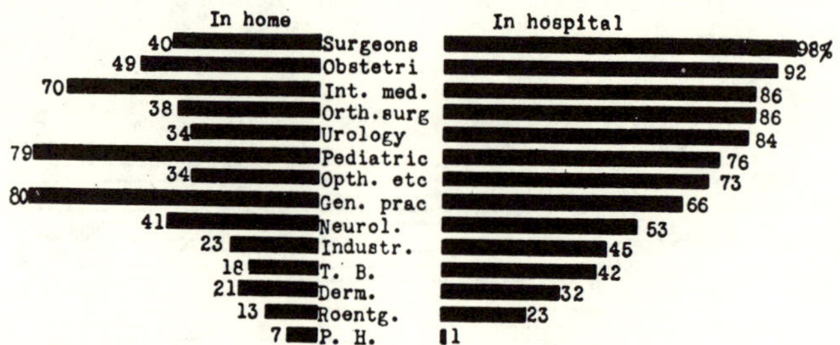

Diagram 16.—Per cent of physicians in each specialty who often need private duty nurses in the home or in the hospital

The second (or "bat wing") diagram shows, in its left wing, the per cent of physicians in each group who report that they often need private duty nurses in the home; and in its right wing the per cent who often need specials in the hospital. It will be seen at once that there are marked differences between the groups.

These two diagrams raise interesting implications. In the first place, it is cheering to note the hesitation to talk about private duty nursing on the part of physicians who do not know much about it, and the corresponding eagerness of those who do. Well over one-fourth of all the physicians to whom the preliminary inquiry was sent have already responded, and more returns are coming in every day. This is a much better return than the Committee dared expect. Every state in the Union is represented, and the returns from each geographical division are closely in proportion to the number of physicians resident there. Moreover, the returns are markedly cordial and cooperative. Many of the physicians write: "This looks like a valuable study. Please let me know more about it." Apparently many of them had never heard about the Grading Committee, and are just beginning to learn about it through this work.

In the second place, the two diagrams suggest reasons for the constant discussion of nursing problems in medical circles. In most of the specialty groups the percentage of physicians reporting that they frequently work with private duty nurses on their cases is surprisingly large. Such physicians must unquestionably be interested in problems of nursing education, supervision, and employment, because whatever happens along these lines in private duty has a direct and important bearing upon the success of the physician's work. The surprising thing is that there is not more medical discussion along these lines than less!

The "bat wing" diagram also shows that some of the specialties have much more frequent occasion than others to call on private duty nurses in the home; while other specialties seem to concentrate on hospital service. Remembering (as is shown in Chapter 4) that registries find it easier to supply good special nurses for the hospital than for the home, it is possible to pick out at once in the diagram several groups of physicians who must be suffering keenly from that condition, and will, therefore, in all likelihood, be particularly interested in the portions of this and other reports which have to do with suggestions for modernizing registries, and hourly nursing, and other experiments for solving the home nursing problem.

In the other wing are found certain groups of specialists

particularly apt to employ special duty nurses in hospitals; and, therefore, almost inevitably interested in the discussions of group nursing; or of the more general employment of competent and well-educated nurses on general duty.

The diagrams indicate, and the reports in the office show, that the members of the American Medical Association are interested in learning more about the work of the Grading Committee; they are glad to cooperate with it; and their cordial response is based upon a strong and apparently legitimate interest which they already have in the problems of private duty.

4. Further Medical Studies

Of the 23,500 physicians who volunteered to answer the grading questionnaires, 4,300 were engaged in types of practice which kept them rather out of touch with the private duty situation, and their cards were, therefore, laid aside for the purposes of the present study. A follow-up questionnaire was then sent to the remaining 19,200 physicians, from whom 2,882 returns have been received at the time this is being written, and additional returns are daily coming in. This second medical questionnaire, based upon the postal mailing list, was distributed early in January. It is unfortunate that this text must be written before all the questionnaires have been returned, but it is not believed that the additional numbers which are being received too late for tabulation would make any impressive change in the findings, since those already received seem to be showing a remarkably compact distribution.

Since these January returns are based on a forty-eight instead of a ten state list, they include a large number from physicians who had not been reached by the previous study. It was possible, therefore, in certain cases, to combine the returns from the March, 1927, study with those secured in January, 1928. Before combining these totals, the distributions were compared, and it was found that the types of answers were running so nearly in accord that the combination of the two sets would change the results in most cases by not more than one per cent. Although the percentage of returns is not as high as was hoped for, the reports show such close agreement among physicians on the questions asked that it is believed they furnish a reasonably safe guide for thinking. Most of the tables which follow are based upon more than 4,000 medical questionnaires.

The physicians who answered not only the postals, but the more lengthy questionnaires, are distributed according to the populations of the towns and cities in which they are practising. The following tables show for cities of different sizes the per cent of physicians belonging to each specialty; and for each specialty the per cent of physicians living in cities of different sizes.

TABLE 23. PER CENT OF PHYSICIANS RESIDENT IN CITIES OF EACH SIZE WHO PRACTISE EACH INDICATED SPECIALTY

Specialty	500,000 and over	100,000 to 500,000	25,000 to 100,000	10,000 to 25,000	Under 10,000	All
Gen. pract.	28%	28%	40%	49%	71%	47%
Surgical	22	25	20	23	14	19
Int. med.	13	14	10	5	3	9
Ophth., Otol., Laryn., Rhinol.	9	8	8	8	4	6
Obstetrics	13	11	9	4	2	8
Other	15	14	13	11	6	11
All	100%	100%	100%	100%	100%	100%

TABLE 24. PER CENT OF PHYSICIANS PRACTISING EACH SPECIALTY WHO LIVE IN CITIES OF THE INDICATED POPULATION

Population	G.P.	Surg.	I.M.	Ophth.	Obst.	Other	All
500,000+.......	13%	24%	33%	29%	40%	29%	22%
100,000 to 500,000	12	24	30	21	28	24	19
25,000 to 100,000	15	18	20	20	20	20	17
10,000 to 25,000	12	12	6	12	5	11	11
Under 10,000....	48	22	11	18	7	16	31
All...........	100%	100%	100%	100%	100%	100%	100%

5. Patients Needing and Securing Nurses

It should be remembered throughout the rest of this chapter that inevitably the physicians whose replies are given here belong to a selected group. They belong, that is, to those particular branches of the profession which are most interested in, and most closely in contact with, private duty nursing. The reasons for this are, first, that the Committee intentionally confined its distribution of the full page questionnaire to such physicians as reported that they frequently had occasion to use private duty nurses; and second, that people who are willing to be bothered by a questionnaire—to go to all the trouble of actually answering the questions and mailing it back—are naturally the people who realize through their own daily experience that the subject is important.

The fact, then, that the answers which follow represent not the whole medical profession, but rather such portion of it as is in closest touch with the private duty problem, implies two things. First, questions concerning quality of nursing service, types of service needed, etc., are answered by people who know, through repeated personal experience, what they are talking about. Second, questions concerning the numbers of nurses needed, the average nurses per patient, etc., represent not the general, nation-wide need for nursing service, but rather the demand in the group most frequently calling for specials.

January, 1928, was a period of relatively heavy sickness, so far as this winter is concerned, but probably relatively little sickness when compared with the Januarys of previous years. The reports from physicians answering the January questionnaire show that on the day they answered 51 per cent had some patients who needed private duty nurses but did not get them, 44 per cent had all their patients who really needed private duty nurses supplied, and 5 per cent had some patients who did not really need the private duty nurses they had. For the entire group and in cities of all sizes the average physician had three patients who needed special nurses and two who got them.

The March, 1927, study had yielded the same figures: that the typical physician had three patients who needed special nurses and only two who got them. In March, however, the question was followed up by another asking why the patient who *did not* have special nurses had failed to secure them.

The results were as follows (see Diagram 59, page 429):

45%	could not afford a nurse
29	were cared for by relatives or friends
13	did not want any nurse
7	were cared for by visiting nurse
Only 6	wanted a nurse but could not find one
100%	

The figures would seem to indicate that *under present conditions* the market for special nurses is close to the saturation point.

Physicians were asked: "Of the patients you had *during the past month* who did employ a private duty or special nurse—

a. How many were sick enough to need special skilled nursing care?
b. How many would not have needed to employ a nurse at all if a relative, friend, or competent servant had been available to take care of them in the home?
c. How many could have managed if a visiting nurse could have come into the home for, say, an hour or two each day?
d. How many could have been adequately cared for if they had been in a hospital on regular nursing service without a special nurse?"

The returns show that the typical physician in this study had had five patients during the space of the preceding month who were actually employing private duty nurses. Of these five, three needed especially skilled nursing care, and the other two could have been cared for by regular hospital nursing service. Of all the physicians whose patients were employing private duty nurses at the time the reports were filled—

92% reported patients who definitely needed some form of skilled nursing care.
72% said that some of their patients could have been adequately cared for by the regular hospital service.
26% reported that some of their patients could have been cared for by a visiting nurse or hourly service.
27% that some of their patients could have been cared for by relatives or competent servants.

It is evident from these figures that while in most cases physicians feel that their patients need the services of the special duty nurse, there is fairly general recognition of the possibilities for adequate care of certain types of cases through hourly nursing, group nursing, and enlarged and improved graduate nursing staffs in hospitals.

We do not know what per cent of the population, during months of heavy sickness rates, really needs skilled nursing care. If these physicians, whose practice represents so largely the nurse-employing class of patients, report that on the day they answered the question they had on the average three patients who needed skilled nursing care and two patients who were actually employing private duty nurses, three things seem probable.

First, it would seem that, for the profession as a whole, the daily average patients per physician actually needing skilled nursing care in January, 1928, must have been much less than three.

Second, since half of the physicians in this heavily nursed group report that every one of their patients who needed private duty nurses had them, there is reason to believe that the lack of a nurse may often be attributable not to a shortage of nurses, but rather to the patient's decision either that he did not want a nurse or that he could not afford to pay for one.

Third, according to these physicians reporting over a period of a month, of every five patients who had special nurses, at least two could have dispensed with the special if they could have been cared for on the floor service of an adequately staffed, well-run hospital. It seems reasonable to wonder whether, by extending the general nursing care of hospitals to include the really adequate care of private patients (even at a somewhat higher hospital charge to the patient), the result might not be a marked reduction in the employment of specials, and a marked increase in the employment of full time graduate nurses in hospitals.

6. Place, Hours, and Charges of Private Duty Nurses

The next few pages summarize the physicians' own reports upon private duty nurses working on their own cases. In order to simplify the questionnaire, each physician was asked to describe his "most recent case on which a private duty nurse was employed"; and where more than one nurse was employed on the case, to tell of the "one most recently employed."

Reporting upon these cases, the physicians were asked whether the patient was in the home, hospital, or both. The following table is an interesting contrast to the opinions of the physicians given in the postal study discussed in an earlier paragraph, concerning the frequent need of private duty nurses in the home and in the hospital. It should be remembered, however, that in the postal study they were talking about their experience in the long run, while in the study being reported upon here they were talking each one about a single case actually under his care in January, 1928.

TABLE 25. PER CENT OF PATIENTS IN THE HOME, IN THE HOSPITAL, OR IN BOTH, REPORTED BY PHYSICIANS PRACTISING EACH SPECIFIED SPECIALTY

Physician's specialty	Home	Hospital	Both	All
General practice	56%	35%	9%	100%
Surgery	9	81	10	100
Obstetrics, gynecology	24	56	20	100
Internal medicine	49	40	11	100
Ophthalmology, etc.	19	71	10	100
Pediatrics	63	22	15	100
Other	33	55	12	100
All	41%	50%	9%	100%

It was expected that there would be a marked difference between the amount of hospitalization in larger cities and in small ones. It was found, however, that except in towns of under 10,000 inhabitants there is no very great difference. (In the table which follows the "per cent in hospital" includes those who had special duty nurses both in the hospital and in the home, as well as those who had specials in the hospital only.)

TABLE 26. PER CENT OF PATIENTS WITH PRIVATE DUTY NURSES IN HOSPITALS, IN CITIES OF EACH SPECIFIED SIZE

Population	Per cent of patients who were in hospitals
500,000 and over	65%
100,000 to 500,000	70
25,000 to 100,000	70
10,000 to 25,000	68
Under 10,000	44
All	60%

Physicians were asked whether the nurse was on day, night, or twenty-four hour duty. The returns substantiate those received directly from private duty nurses by showing that twenty-four hour duty is very much more common in the home than in the hospital. The following table gives the results of this inquiry:

TABLE 27. PER CENT OF NURSES REPORTED BY PHYSICIANS AS BEING ON DAY, NIGHT, OR TWENTY-FOUR HOUR DUTY IN THE HOME AND IN THE HOSPITAL

Cases in	Day	Night	24-hour	All
Home	27%	12%	61%	100%
Hospital	44	21	35	100
Both	34	16	50	100
All	39%	17%	44%	100%

It also seems probable, from the figures given, that while the average of nurses per patient remains about the same whether the case is in the home or in the hospital, if the same patient is transferred from one location to the other, there is a distinct tendency to increase the number of nurses necessary. This may be because of the hesitation of certain nurses, accustomed to service in the hospital, to undertake home cases. A somewhat more probable explanation, however, is that patients sick enough to need nurses both in the hospital and in the home may also have required both day and night care, which in the hospital ordinarily means two nurses. The highest cases reported of change of nurses were one home case where there had been twenty different nurses, and one hospital case where there had been ten.

Twenty-four hour service is not only more frequent in the home than in the hospital, but it is also definitely more frequent in cities of smaller population. The per cent of twenty-four hour cases in cities of each size is given below:

TABLE 28. PER CENT OF NURSES ON TWENTY-FOUR HOUR DUTY IN CITIES OF EACH SPECIFIED POPULATION

Population	Nurses on 24-hour duty
500,000 and over	23%
100,000 to 500,000	40
25,000 to 100,000	44
10,000 to 25,000	55
Under 10,000	66
All	44%

There seems to be a distinct tendency for twenty-four hour duty to become a specialty of the practical nurse. The per cents of all R.N. cases and the per cents of all practical cases, giving each type of service, are as follows:

	R.N.	Practical
Day	39%	16%
Night	18	8
24-hour	43	76
	100%	100%

Physicians were asked how much the nurses had charged per day. R.N. charges so reported ranged from $1.00 to $15.00 a day; those of practicals from $1.00 to $10.00, and there is one case of a $20.00 a day charge in which the physician did not know whether the nurse was an R.N. or a practical.

7. What Kinds of Nursing Do Physicians Want?

In some ways the most stimulating and helpful of all the returns gathered in the medical study were those which came in response to the request: "Please check which of the types of nursing given in the list below were particularly needed for this case." The returns are as follows:

TABLE 29. WHAT PHYSICIANS WANT FOR THEIR OWN CASES. PER CENT CHECKING EACH TYPE OF CARE

Skill in giving general care and making patient comfortable	65%
Skill in observing and reporting symptoms	45
Care in following medical orders	43
Good breeding and attractive personality	34
Skill in handling people	30
Familiarity with hospital routine	27
Skill in asepsis	28
Experience and background	22
Skill in giving special treatments	22
Familiarity with your personal methods	21
Familiarity with particular disease	15
Ability to work under heavy strain	15
Responsible adult to take charge of family	3
Mother's helper and houseworker	3

Such agreement as this should furnish valuable guidance to nurse educators who are trying to select and teach students so that they will meet the real demands upon the profession *after* graduation.

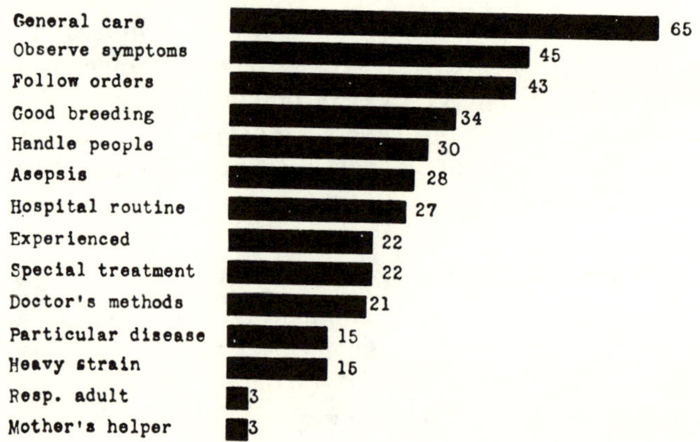

Diagram 17. —What M.D.'s want: "Which of these types of nursing were particularly needed?" For the patients whose cases they were reporting, 65% of all the physicians wanted "Skill in giving general care and making patient comfortable"; 45% wanted "Skill in observing and reporting symptoms accurately"; and so on, down to the 3% who wanted "Mother's helper and general houseworker"

While there is strong agreement among physicians in all specialties as to the relative importance of certain of these types of nursing care, and the relative unimportance of others, there is, nevertheless, considerable variation in the emphasis put upon each type, according to the specialty to which the physician belongs. The following table and diagram give the per cent of physicians belonging to each specialty who voted for each type of care.

TABLE 30. PER CENT OF PHYSICIANS IN EACH SPECIALTY WHO PARTICULARLY WANTED EACH TYPE OF NURSING CARE FOR THEIR PATIENTS

Types of care	Specialty of physician								
	1	2	3	4	5	6	7	8	All
	Gen. Prac.	Surg.	Obst. gyn.	Int. med.	Ophth. etc.	Ped.	Neu. psych.	Other	
General care	69%	59%	63%	70%	57%	60%	51%	60%	65%
Observe symptoms	42	50	46	44	41	46	55	45	45
Follow orders	45	39	38	53	35	57	45	36	43
Good breeding	28	33	49	41	34	43	56	32	34
Handle people	26	30	28	40	26	39	61	32	30
Hospital routine	19	47	40	21	26	15	20	27	27
Asepsis	24	42	50	10	28	11	11	21	27
General experience	20	23	26	22	18	31	41	23	22
Special treatment	19	22	24	21	35	33	25	23	22
Personal methods	15	30	35	16	28	19	23	29	21
Particular disease	12	12	21	13	24	18	33	22	15
Heavy strain	16	14	15	15	9	11	16	11	15
Resp. adult	4	1	5	3	2	4	5	3	3
Mother's helper	3	1	3	1	2	6	3	1	3

In the diagram the numbers in small circles stand for each of the main specialties, and by following the line across from circle to circle it is possible to trace how the votes of physicians in that specialty compare with those of physicians in other specialties. It will be seen, for example, that while all of the physicians emphasize the importance of general care, the surgeons (2), neurologists (7), pediatricians (6), and obstetricians and gynecologists (3) are particularly interested in the nurses' ability to observe symptoms. The pediatrician (6) and the neurologist (7)

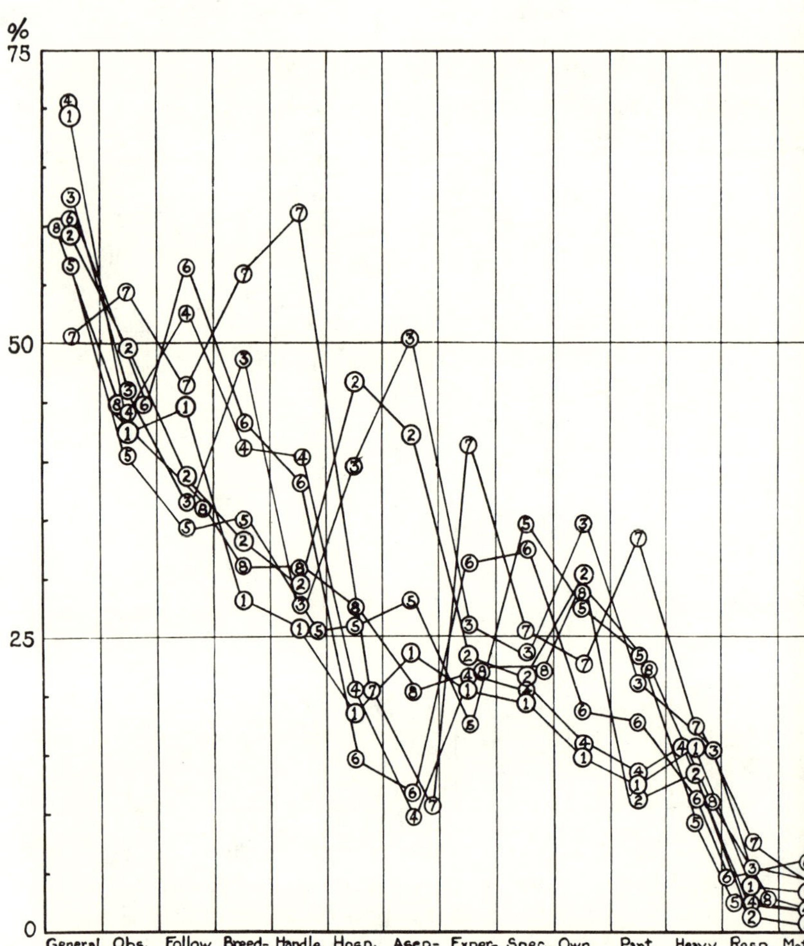

Diagram 18.—Per cent of physicians in each specialty checking each type of nursing care as especially important for their patients. Numbers in circles indicate specialties as follows:

(1) General practitioners.
(2) Surgeons.
(3) Obstetricians and gynecologists.
(4) Internists.
(5) Ophthalmologists, otologists, laryngologists, rhinologists.
(6) Pediatricians.
(7) Neurologists, psychiatrists.
(8) Other.

more than any other specialists emphasize good breeding. Skill in handling people is most desired by the neurologist (7) and least by the general practitioner (1), and the ophthalmologist (5) and others grouped under the same heading. Emphasis on asepsis is especially marked in the cases of the obstetricians (3) and the surgeons (2), but it is not particularly desired by the neurologists (7) or internists (4).

These shifting emphases may throw some light upon the lack of general agreement among physicians as to exactly what types of nursing education are needed if nurses are to handle their cases wisely. It will be seen, however, that practically all physicians are in general agreement upon the importance of those types of nursing which in the last analysis rest upon intelligence, good breeding, and a professional attitude towards work, combined with thorough nursing training in a high grade school and broad experience in the actual observation and care of patients.

8. What Were the Nurses Like?

Of all the material gathered from physicians, probably the most eagerly awaited was the answer to the question: "Would you like to have the same nurse again on a similar case?" The results are thoroughly encouraging. For the entire group, 89 per cent of the physicians say "Yes," only 10 per cent say "No," and 1 per cent hesitate. Physicians have serious criticisms to make of many aspects of nursing service, but when they speak of the nurses with whom they work day by day on their own cases, they are cordial in their approval and appreciation.

Eighty-eight per cent of all the nurses were R.N.'s, 11 per cent practicals, and in 1 per cent the physician did

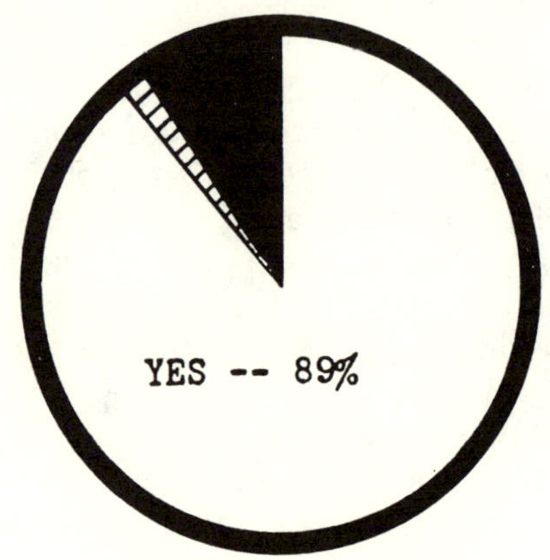

Diagram 19.—"Would you like to have the same nurse again on a similar case?" 89% of the physicians answered "Yes"; 1% were not sure; and only 10% said "No"

not know whether the nurse was an R.N. or a practical. The distribution of nurses of each kind between home and hospital cases was as follows:

TABLE 31. PER CENT OF NURSES WORKING IN HOMES, HOSPITALS, OR BOTH WHO WERE R.N.'S OR PRACTICALS

	R.N.	Practical	Not known	Total
Home	76%	23%	1%	100%
Hospital	97	2	1	100
Both	89	10	1	100
All	88%	11%	1%	100%

Forty per cent of the nurses were employed on home cases, 49 per cent on hospital cases, and 11 per cent on

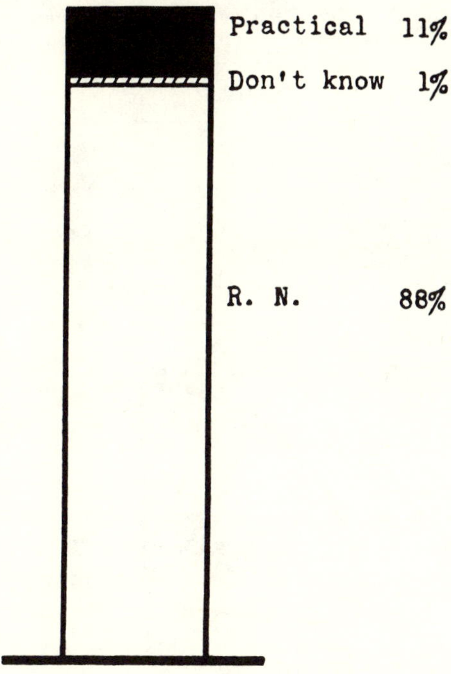

Diagram 20.—Some 88% of the physicians reported that the nurse employed was an R.N.; 11% reported practical; and only 1% did not know

cases which were both in the home and the hospital. There is a small but perhaps significant difference between the answers of physicians to the question, "Would you like the same nurse again?" since for home cases 88 per cent of the physicians want the same nurse again, while for hospital cases it is 91 per cent.

The votes were also classified according to the source from which the nurse was secured. Results are as follows:

TABLE 32. PER CENT OF ALL NURSES FROM EACH SOURCE WHOM PHYSICIANS SAY THEY WOULD LIKE TO EMPLOY AGAIN

Source	Per cent wanted again
Hospital registry	89
Central	86
Commercial	82
Physician's own list	95
From other physician	74
Other	73
Don't know	88
Total	89

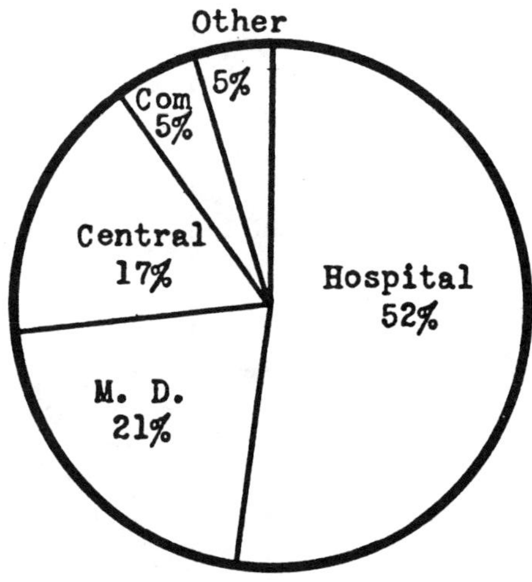

Source of Nurse

Diagram 21.—"Where did you get your nurse?" According to reports from physicians, the problem of the distribution of private duty service is, under present methods, primarily under hospital control

As might be expected, the physician finds nurses on his own list more satisfactory than those drawn from any other source. More than half of the nurses (52 per cent) were secured through the hospital registry, about one-fifth (21 per cent) from the physician's own list, 17 per cent from the central professional registry, 5 per cent from the commercial registry, and 5 per cent from other sources.

Physicians were asked to classify their nurses according to whether they were very good, good, fair, poor, or very poor. The votes under these headings were distributed according to the type of practice of the physician. The following table summarizes the findings:

TABLE 33. PER CENT OF PHYSICIANS IN EACH SPECIALTY WHO VOTED ON QUALITY OF NURSE AS SHOWN

Specialty	Very good	Good	Fair	Poor or very poor	Total
General practice	54%	33%	11%	2%	100%
Surgery	63	28	8	1	100
Internal medicine	58	27	12	3	100
Obstetrics, gynecology	59	29	8	4	100
Ophthalmology, etc.	59	25	13	3	100
Pediatrics	54	34	10	2	100
Other	54	26	18	2	100
All	57%	30%	11%	2%	100%

9. R.N.'s vs. Practicals

The same classification as to quality of nursing service was made for R.N.'s and for practicals separately. While there were a few R.N.'s reported as being "very poor," the number was less than half of one per cent, and does not, therefore, show in the table.

Physicians were asked: "For your own patients, which do you prefer, practical nurses or graduate nurses?" Of those who answered the question, 84 per cent said that they preferred graduate nurses, 8 per cent preferred practical, and 8 per cent said that the answer depended on the

TABLE 34. PER CENT OF ALL R.N.'S AND ALL PRACTICALS WHO WERE REPORTED BY PHYSICIANS AS GIVING EACH QUALITY OF NURSING SERVICE

Quality of service	R.N.	Practical
Very good	59%	35%
Good	29	40
Fair	10	21
Poor	2	3
Very poor	0	1
	100%	100%

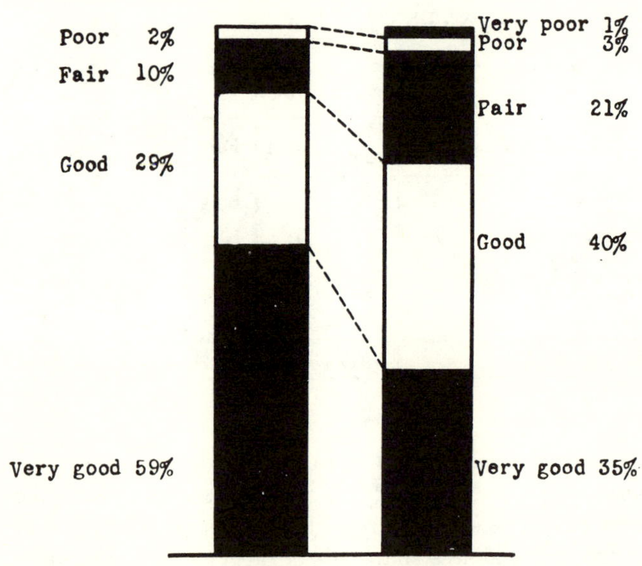

R. N. vs. Practical

Diagram 22.—"Doctor, in your opinion, was the nurse very good, good, fair, poor, or very poor?" 59% of the R.N.'s were reported as "Very good" while less than half of one per cent, too few to show in the diagram, were "very poor"

type of case. The answers, classified according to the specialties of doctors, are as follows:

TABLE 35. PER CENT OF PHYSICIANS IN EACH SPECIALTY WHO PREFER R.N.'S OR PRACTICALS FOR THEIR OWN PATIENTS

Specialty	Prefer R.N.	Prefer practical	That depends	All
General practice....	80%	10%	10%	100%
Surgery..........	93	3	4	100
Obstetrics........	82	8	10	100
Ophthalmology....	89	5	6	100
Internal medicine..	86	5	9	100
Other............	83	10	7	100
	84%	8%	8%	100%

Diagram 23.—Per cent of physicians answering question: "For your own patients which do you prefer, graduate nurses or practical nurses?"

Physicians were asked: "Is there a strong demand *among your own patients* for practical nurses? If so, which do you think they want the practicals for *most*, for bedside nursing or for taking charge of the housework?" Fifty-five per cent replied that there was a strong demand for practical nurses, 39 per cent said there was not, and 6 per cent said that there was some demand which they thought was not marked.

The demand for practicals is considerably stronger in cities of less than 10,000 than it is in larger places. While there seems to be comparatively little geographical difference, the demand for practicals is slightest in the South Central States, with a vote of only 48 per cent, and greatest in the North Atlantic States, where 59 per cent of the physicians gave an affirmative answer.

The difference between physicians in different specialties is more marked. Among surgeons and the group of specialists classified with ophthalmologists, about 30 per cent said that there was a strong demand for practicals among their own patients. Among obstetricians and internists there was a little less than 60 per cent, while among general practitioners it was 68 per cent.

Among the physicians who answered that there was a strong demand among their own patients for practical nurses, less than half said that these nurses were chiefly wanted in order to do bedside nursing and more than half that they were wanted either to do housework or to do a combination of housework and nursing.

In answer to the question: "If competent domestic servants could easily be hired at reasonable rates during sickness periods, do you think it would probably decrease or almost eliminate the demand for practicals, or would there probably be no change?" 56 per cent said that it would either decrease or eliminate the demand, and 44 per cent thought that an adequate supply of domestic service would make no difference. Population seems to have little effect upon this answer.

10. Which is Harder—Getting a Good Nurse or Paying Her Bill?

Physicians were also asked: "For most of your patients, which seems to be the more difficult problem—to pay the regular R.N. fee or to secure a really competent and cooperative nurse?" Seventy-three per cent agree that the chief difficulty for their patients is paying the R.N. fee. The vote becomes slightly less as the population units increase in size. There is very little difference in the votes of physicians in different specialties. Geographical conditions seem to have little effect, although the statement that the more difficult problem is the payment of the fee is slightly less emphatic in the North Atlantic States and more emphatic in the North Central and Western States than elsewhere.

11. Experience with Registries

The physicians were asked how many times during the past month they had called a registry and been told that no nurse was available for the case.

It should not be assumed that these calls actually went unfilled. Comments from physicians suggest that although for certain types of calls they frequently have to appeal to two or three registries, they rarely have to abandon the search. Apparently some kind of a nurse can always be secured. The physician's complaint is not usually that no nurse is available, but rather that he cannot get the kind of a nurse he feels is particularly needed for that case.

TABLE 36.—PER CENT OF ALL CALLS REFUSED ACCORDING TO TYPE, AND THE AVERAGE NUMBER OF CALLS REFUSED PER PHYSICIAN

Type of call refused	Per cent of all refused calls	Average calls refused per physician
Sunday or holiday	8	.15
Night service	15	.31
24-hour service	25	.50
Home calls	18	.36
Out of town	6	.12
Maternity	8	.17
Pediatric	3	.06
Contagious	3	.05
Male or G. U.	2	.05
Mental or nervous	3	.05
Alcoholic	1	.02
Other	8	.15
Total	100	1.99

12. SUMMARY

a. Three medical inquiries have been made—a ten state study in March, 1927; a nation-wide postal study in November, and a nation-wide, more detailed study in January, 1928. The returns indicate that physicians are interested, cooperative, and friendly to the nursing profession.

b. There is wide variation among the specialists in the amounts of nursing service they use and in the numbers of special or private duty nurses working with them on home cases and hospital cases. Consequently problems concerning the distribution, costs, and quality of nursing service in home and hospital affect the different specialties in different degrees.

c. On the day he answered the questionnaire the typical physician *in this study* had three patients who needed special nurses and two who got them.

d. During the entire month just ending he had had five

patients with special nurses. Two of these five could have been adequately cared for (in the physician's opinion) by the regular staff service of a good hospital. The study suggests:

(1) That for the entire profession the daily average of patients needing special nurses in a reasonably busy sickness period is probably well below three per physician.

(2) That when patients needing special nurses do not have them, the lack results not so much from a numerical shortage of nurses as from the patient's own decision either that he does not want a nurse, or that he cannot afford to pay for one.

(3) That there is some likelihood that the extension of general nursing care in hospitals to include the really adequate care of private patients (even at an increased hospital charge) might markedly reduce the employment of specials, and markedly increase the employment of full time graduate nurses in hospitals.

e. Twenty-four hour duty is more frequently found in homes than in hospitals, in small towns rather than in large, and with practical nurses rather than with graduate nurses.

f. While physicians differ in their emphasis, they are all in general agreement as to the types of nursing care most needed for their own patients. They all want:

skill in giving general care and making patient comfortable;

skill in observing and reporting symptoms;

care in following medical orders;

good breeding and attractive personality.

In other words they want young women of good social and intellectual background, of high professional principles, who have had thorough training and experience in the actual care of patients.

g. Nine out of every ten physicians like their nurses and want them back again.

h. Nine out of every ten physicians employed R.N.'s instead of practicals on their January cases.

i. Physicians are most enthusiastic about nurses on their own lists; but not at all enthusiastic about those from other physicians' lists.

j. Surgeons seem better satisfied with the special nursing available than do physicians in other fields.

k. Physicians find R.N.'s more satisfactory than practicals, and eight out of ten always prefer them.

l. A little over half the physicians report that there is a strong demand for practicals among their patients; and of these over half say that the demand comes because of the need for some one to do housework. Over half the physicians feel that an adequate supply of competent servants at reasonable rates would decrease or wipe out the demand for practicals.

m. Nearly three-fourths of all the physicians in all specialties report that it is harder for their patients to pay for a nurse than to get a good one.

n. Of all calls refused by registries about two-thirds consist of calls for 24 hour duty, night duty, home calls, or calls on Sundays and holidays.

o. There is evidence, however, that while these calls are unpopular, the physician can get some sort of nurse to accept them if he will call different registries. The difficulty is rather, for unpopular service, to get the kind of nurse he wants.

CHAPTER 9

WHAT THE PHYSICIANS SAY

The free comments written on the backs of their reports have shown how the rank and file of physicians are really thinking; and in some ways have been even more helpful than the facts given directly in answer to questions. It is of more than slight significance that the three most frequent statements made in these paragraphs, where the physician was free to say anything he chose, are:

"There is no shortage of nurses here." (37%)
"Most R.N.'s are competent." (35%)
"The cost of the R.N. is too heavy for my patients." (21%)

The following quotations are typical of the discussions on topics most frequently dealt with.

1. Good Nursing

There can be no doubt that physicians tend to appreciate good nursing.

OHIO.—My most recent extended experience with trained (R.N.) nurses was in the year 1926 when our village of 2,500 people was smitten with an epidemic —typhoid fever. There were in all about 160 patients of whom I had about 60 who were all in their own homes. The epidemic was due to the use of raw milk contaminated by a "carrier" employed in a dairy. Many of these patients were very sick and the illness lasted for from three weeks for the mildest cases to four months to the worst with complications. During that period I worked with about thirty-five nurses, some families having one, and one family, four of whose members were down at once, had four on duty at once, two day and two night. These nurses came from registries in Cleveland, Akron, Columbus, Lorain, Elyria (Ohio). The work for them was hard and sometimes discouraging, but I am happy to say that their services were always willing and intelligent. Really they saved the day. The points I want to emphasize are their:

1. Willingness to work.
2. Loyalty and cooperation.
3. Initiative and intelligence.
4. Resourcefulness.
5. Tact and general consideration for patient and friends.

This experience is sufficiently recent to make observations applicable, I think, and I am glad to share them with you.

ARIZONA.—This is a good nurse, good observer, gentle, thorough. She follows orders explicitly and reports changes promptly.

MONTANA.—My nurse had a sense of humor which helps a lot.

NEBRASKA.—She has stayed by a delirious pneumonia patient most faithfully during her twelve hour stay. In addition she has kept hordes of anxious relatives and friends out of the room, has been an adviser to a distracted wife, and has protected my interests for the benefit of family and patient many times, when demands were made to bring in other consultants and aids. In addition to this she has always been cheerful, has an optimistic point of view, and feels like I do, that if the doctor or the nurse gives up, then our usefulness is at an end.

MICHIGAN.—I called her for a bilateral pneumonia three miles out in the country. I didn't want to ask her to do 20-hour duty, but she saw the situation, offered voluntarily to do 20 hours until patient passed crisis, and has been very observant and efficient in every way.

RHODE ISLAND.—She combined a good technical training with common sense. She carried out orders, but modified them when the need was obvious. She had a proper sense of the dignity of the position without making undue demands on the family. She "fitted in" well.

WEST VIRGINIA.—I have not had a nurse for more than five years, that I could make one single complaint of. The nurses are getting more competent each year, and my patients always speak in the highest terms of treatment received.

KANSAS.—This particular nurse is intelligent, observing, not afraid to take a severe case twelve miles in the country with the responsibility attendant, well trained, pleasant but strict in following the doctor's orders in regard to patient, family and visits. I have had many nurses like this and some dismal failures. Financial conditions here are such that we have few trained nurses, but we have very little trouble getting one when required. My cxperience with practical nurses is not so pleasant. I wish every one of my seriously ill patients could have a Registered Nurse.

MASSACHUSETTS.—Any one who can feed a patient a half pound of cooked liver daily for four or five months, deserves credit for being a good cook and knowing how to handle people, as well as keeping a person cheerful in bed. It requires a reasonable amount of personality. This nurse has been at the game for over twenty years.

NEW YORK.—Case cited on front of this sheet was a gynecological case with distinct psychoneurosis of the melancholia type. The nurse engaged was an excellent surgical nurse of about twelve years' experience, who handled this rather difficult mental case and the family tactfully and well. The patient is most enthusiastic in her praise of the nurse as is the family—and there has been a very distinct improvement in the patient's mental condition during her stay in the hospital.

MASSACHUSETTS.—The nurse employed for my scarlet fever patient had the tremendous task of amusing a very greatly pampered ten year old child, living with her grandmother, who sees no need for special nursing at all, but who refused to send the child to the hospital. Then there are three aunts who try to run the house also, and the situation is often anything but pleasant. She is carrying out her nursing work very efficiently and manages to keep the child very happy. This often at a great effort, and sees to it that even the family are happy, though she has not been able to convince the grandmother that a special nurse is necessary in this case. Without her, the nurse, I fear that the neighbor's four children would have been exposed to the contagion of the grandmother's "brought my children through scarlet fever without any extra precautions . . ."

MASSACHUSETTS.—This case was one of diabetic coma. Patient's husband refused to have her sent to the hospital. He allowed me to get 12 hour nurses. The first nurse came within an hour, and when I got back to the house in an hour and a half she had the patient bathed, bed clean, ready to follow my orders. I watched her prepare for catheterizing and her asepsis was perfect. Then I watched her give the insulin. She was very competent. I asked same registry to send me a night nurse, and when she came and saw the house, she decided that she didn't want to remain. I could not call her a nurse. The third came at once and was very competent. The patient came out of the coma in 24 hours. I dispensed with the night nurse and kept the day nurse. You can see by the above that there are nurses who will only work when the surroundings are suitable. There are others who come in and go to work.

MISSOURI.—This nurse was pleasant, kind, a good observer, and of great value in preventing a psychosis from developing; a lady in every way, refined, absolutely impartial in her observations; skilful as well as surgically clean. She did not want to use narcotics or laxatives unless ordered by the physician—this was her first case for me. I cannot use any but graduate nurses on my private patients, and would rather not do major surgery if they are unobtainable.

NEW YORK.—The case was a poor family of seven. Of these, four had had the acute stage of scarlet fever and were convalescing. One was very ill with it, and the mother was developing a sore throat when I placed two specials at the home. These were procured through a registry which called another at Buffalo. The case was in a poorly equipped farm house, 2½ miles from an unincorporated village. Transportation was provided to and from this village where the nurses were quartered on their time off duty. Shifts were changed through blizzards and at zero temperatures by teams and bob sleds. One of the nurses was exceptionally good natured and tolerated these unpleasant conditions with the appearance of enjoying them, and the other, though she stuck to her job, repeatedly commented upon and complained of the difficulties encountered. The latter could not be blamed for not liking it, but the former found it easier to get along with the patient and the patient's family. We made life as pleasant as we could for both and got them relief after eleven days, during which the patient went through a septicemia. The relief nurses were easy to get, though the case was about fifty-five miles away from their registry. They remained on duty two days until the patient died and one stayed throughout the day, assisting about the place after the death of the patient. Their pay was advanced by the town and therefore was prompt. These are indeed conditions which test the quality of service of the nurses of the Buffalo registry.

2. Poor Nursing

If physicians could report such criticisms as the following to registries equipped to handle them in a thoroughly constructive and professional fashion, might not the general standard of nursing service be definitely advanced?

STATE UNKNOWN.—I would employ the same nurse because she is orderly, obedient, possesses a good knowledge of the transmission of infectious diseases (case is typhoid fever). One thing I don't like about her is that she is too ready to advise members of patient's family to take cathartics or other house remedies without consulting the physician. There is generally an abuse of cathartic remedies in this community, and there is no need that trained nurses shall contribute to this habit, not even mentioning the unfairness of meddling into the doctor's business. I cite the case because nurses are but too often inclined to act similarly.

NEW YORK.—Had two hypodermic abscesses in this particular pneumonia case. Do not get high class work we should from the commercial registry nurses.

ILLINOIS.—The one criticism that I might offer would be that I fear she did not realize quickly a rather sudden change for the worse in her patient's condition and notify the physician soon enough.

ILLINOIS.—I dislike very much to have nurses discuss medical topics with patients. Only lately a registered nurse told a patient that she would probably have a cancer because her mother had one, and the woman respected the comment because it came from a graduate nurse.

MICHIGAN.—One nurse, a fairly good one at that, changed her patient's bed throughout three times a day—not because it was soiled, but she liked nice clean linen.

NEW YORK.—The nurse in this case was very good as far as carrying out orders was concerned. She failed, however, to observe that the patient who was suffering from lobar pneumonia was becoming cyanotic and evidences of circulatory failure were impending. I feel that this nurse needed a little more schooling in observing and reporting symptoms.

NEBRASKA.—The first nurse called in this case was sent by a nurses' registry. She was in the home only about an hour. She had no tact. She seemed to think it was her duty to boss things generally. One of the first things she did was to tell the child's mother what she could or could not do if she expected her to nurse the child.

NEW YORK.—All night nurses without exception were found asleep on duty at bedside by me during the early hours of the morning. Patient complained many times that she had to wake nurse and nurse rebuked her. Patient was flighty at one time, and several nurses mentioned in her presence that she was demented.

CALIFORNIA.—The nurse was quite elderly and was somewhat weak on asepsis, as many of this type seem to become. She was deficient in urological knowledge.

NORTH CAROLINA.—Many times in the presence of the child's mother and other members of the family she made the observation time and again that the pulse was failing; that the child seemed to be turning black in the face; that the patient appeared to be dying.

3. General Criticisms

If it were possible to secure all the facts behind the following criticisms, it seems probable that the real difficulty would be found to lie in the unwise selection of students for training.

PENNSYLVANIA.—My chief objection to the older graduate nurse is that her ways of training are always the best, and she shudders at the idea of some method of treatment and technique other than she received in her course of training.

CALIFORNIA.—In my experience, there has not been such a great difficulty in procuring a nurse that is not busy; the great trouble in my experience has been: Is she willing to work. Will she take that kind of a case. Most usually, I am answered by the nurse (often unknown to me and I to her) by her asking what kind of a case it is, or that she does not take cases outside of hospitals, or that she does not take confinement cases, or, which is more reasonable, that she will go over to the patient's home and see them first before she can say. The latter, however, is not very satisfactory from my standpoint, of course.

MASSACHUSETTS.—While I admire the nurse I had last week, I swear every time I call her that I will never call her again. Once in an emergency when she could come, she would not because she had an appointment some hours later, which I afterward learned was a tea. She could have come and still been in time for her tea, because the baby died within an hour. It made no impression on her that I wanted a good nurse immediately and that the baby was dangerously ill. I called her again a few days later and she hesitated to come because she would have to begin night duty at once, and she did not take night work. She wanted to know how old the child was, and the diagnosis, and asked with trepidation if the case might not have diphtheria. We discussed the probable duration of the sickness, and how much care would be necessary, all of this while the mother, a very intelligent woman, was standing near me waiting for a decision. I like the nurse because she does her work well, but I wonder why she works at all, and if I could get another nurse equally as good, I never would think of dragging her out to nurse for a patient of mine.

VIRGINIA.—I dislike very much to have to say that nurses are disappointing in the general run of cases—that is, the ones we get here—so much so that people well able to pay them do not employ them if a practical nurse can be used, though they would much prefer a graduate nurse.

ALABAMA.—The graduates of many nursing schools are not very competent—they are usually girls from poorer homes—little preliminary education, little culture and acquire it slowly if at all, and many of them are not very interested in their work and marry at first opportunity and frequently make very unfortunate marriages. The men they marry are usually of lower social class and not earning good wages, so the nurses return to nursing, avoid raising families, and on the whole the nursing situation is unsettled and unsatisfactory. The women who enter nursing at later years of life—25 to 35—usually are steadier and more satisfactory.

IOWA.—In calling nurses for duty in homes, the family very frequently object, or at least express the fear, that if a nurse is called, the nurse will require special attention in a home more or less disorganized by illness, and that such special attention cannot consistently be given. That this is unfair to the majority is unquestionably true, but I am convinced that such a common view is based on something tangible.

TEXAS.—Those that are tactless, inattentive and indolent make poor nurses, regardless of their training.

This latter type is paid the same fees as are the tactful, attentive, and industrious nurses.

Perhaps the "weeding-out" process should begin in the training schools. During a training of three years it should be possible to pick out the worthy ones, and let the others drop out. This problem is not peculiar to the nursing profession, of course, and in the final analysis the responsibility rests upon the doctor, who can obtain first class nursing assistance, if he demands it, just as the bank executive does.

MINNESOTA.—Some nurses have a personal preference for a certain doctor, which is natural, but they let it be known by remarks to patient which come back to doctor or even by direct comments to doctor or to patient while doctor is in patient's room. That is rare, but it happens here in this smaller hospital and locality where there are always more gossip and rivalry among and in regard to physicians.

MICHIGAN.—More often than not graduate nurses have caused me embarrassment or worse when on cases by criticizing my methods, recommending other doctors, ignoring orders, antagonizing the family, personal uncleanliness, or doing things for the patients that were not ordered. The best nurses are not taking anything but hospital cases or else are regularly employed. The poorest nurses use a registry.

WEST VIRGINIA.—Registered nurses are entirely too careful about preserving their professional dignity and absolutely refuse even to do the simple things, such as sweeping out and caring for the patient's room in the home. Refuse to do anything they choose to call "menial."

WISCONSIN.—My only criticism is that in practically every case except two or three I have had to suggest and insist on nurses keeping clinical charts. They seldom keep a bedside record unless requested to do so.

MASSACHUSETTS.—The graduates of our local hospitals have had no real training for children's work—cannot take pulse of an infant—cannot get sample of urine from female infant, do not know how to put up formulas, etc.

MASSACHUSETTS.—I feel that the nurses from some of our famous hospitals are far ahead of those trained in small hospitals away from medical teaching centers and deserve a different classification. The instruction of nurses is the weak point in our local hospitals.

NEVADA.—Nurses are rapidly changing the profession of nursing into a trade. They have no idea of service and no ideals. They simply put in the time giving routine service with more or less skill. They quit at quitting time whether relieved or not, and regardless of the patient's need. But if they come on in the middle of the day or night, they quit at 7 p. m. and charge for a full shift. They will not take out of town cases unless assured of an easy case with comfort and service for themselves.

MAINE.—I think that the whole question comes up to the fact that since the physician in the case requires the nurse to assume a heavy responsibility, it is distinctly *up to him* to see to it that girls he *knows* to be competent and faithful are employed. This may be difficult in the extremely large cities, but not an insurmountable problem, but in the smaller cities many of the nurses doing private work are graduates from the local hospitals and men can easily know about them in all ways. I have had lazy nurses, incompetent nurses, disloyal nurses. The first time that such occurs the nurse is at fault, but the second time it is mine.

IDAHO.—Most R.N. and graduate nurses refuse to do so many little things about the home that it causes dissatisfaction with the patient especially if she be the mother of the household.

ARKANSAS.—I think more care has to be exercised in selection of nurses for pediatrics than in any other branch of nursing. I do believe that the nursing association should allow pediatricians the same courtesies of 24 hour duty as they allow obstetricians, because often we have difficult feeding cases that require prolonged nursing care, and the parents are not able to keep a day and night nurse and at the same time should have just one nurse in charge because she learns the peculiarities of the case. Another nurse comes on at night and the child has to be won over again. The changing of nurses upsets the child for a few hours each day.

DELAWARE.—Many of the younger nurses are too much interested in having a good time and are not in love with their work.

WYOMING.—The city nurses will not come to the small towns and if they do are always quite superior.

Nurses suffer from that strange pathological malady, "Itching foot," and are ready to pack and leave in an instant. Although given more responsibility in a small place, they still keep the psychology and attitude of hired hands.

4. Education

The excerpts in this section are typical of a considerable body of very thoughtful opinions. An impressive number of physicians answering the questionnaire evidently believe that only women of good social and educational background should be permitted to enter schools of nursing.

KANSAS.—The best educated nurses have proven most satisfactory to my need. My disappointment has almost always been the lack of preliminary education. The case here referred to is an old man who had a ruptured gall-bladder. One nurse is a college girl. The other only two years of high school. There is no comparison!

OREGON.—The greatest complaint among people having a registered nurse in a private home is that they must hire some one to take care of the nurse and unless they are seriously ill they put it off as long as possible. Believe a great deal of this is due to poor training in the nurses. Really need the best home training before taking their nursing course.

NEW YORK.—The trouble is that the nurses of the day seem to be of the same mental and social strata as our chambermaids of twenty-five years ago.

ILLINOIS.—I have long observed the lack of preliminary education among nurses. They take orders and execute them fairly well under instructions and sometimes supervision but seem to lack initiative and technical training.

MICHIGAN.—The morale of the profession is not as high as it might be. I think this is due largely to the small schools with low entrance requirements.

NEW YORK.—There are few graduates of today that equal the graduates of 20 years ago. The hospital has never concerned itself with the moral standard and family history or the motive for studying nursing as has Canada, hence we find a different type of nurse graduated in this country from that of our neighbor.

When a girl of good family and pleasing personality studies nursing because she is desirous of helping the sick, she is a better and finer nurse than the woman of poor family history, poor early environment, who goes in for nursing because she has to do something and nursing offers a comfortable income, easy work, and the possibility of chance leading to a better marriage than she otherwise might make. I have little respect for the manner in which the R.N. qualifications are derived.

CALIFORNIA.—I am entirely opposed to the lowering of the standards of nursing or to shortening the period of training.

Kansas.—The ability and character of work as shown by nurses after they graduate is dependent entirely on their superintendent during student days. Some of the best nurses we have had locally came from one of our smaller hospitals when it was in charge of a good superintendent.

New York.—I always ask nurses for their R.N. cards. Many nurses are sent out from registries as supposed R.N.'s but are not. Some nurses need cultivation in tact. I find that I get good results when I hire nurses whom I have watched at work during my rounds at various hospitals. Personal intelligence goes hand in hand with the skill and efficiency of the nurses. I believe that adequate preliminary training and graduation from high school are necessary prerequisites to training.

California.—Girls of good personality and with an education such as is needed to become an efficient nurse seem to be going into other occupations.

California.—Selection of material for entrance and from which to train the nurse-to-be is entirely too lax. Young women who have no powers of observation or no nucleus for training in this special field are readily admitted. We cannot hope to develop Easter lilies from onion slips. Burbank is no longer with us.

North Carolina.—Ignorance due to a lack of cultural contacts is the cause of many failures. The nurses from the best families are the best.

5. Training

The returns indicate in many ways that specialists have considerable difficulty in securing nurses. This is particularly true of the psychiatrists.

Colorado.—Many nurses are incompetent on the subject of dietetics. They scorn the preparation of food. It seems to be beneath their dignity. This usually occurs in those who are poorly trained in dietetics.

North Dakota.—Often a male patient does not get a private bath.

Massachusetts.—Nurses trained in smaller hospitals appear in my estimation to possess the better qualities for a graduate nurse than those from larger institutions. I am inclined to believe that the nurse in general hospitals is obliged to care for too many patients and acquires her attitude from overwork and being driven by a force of matrons, whereas, in the smaller private hospitals the nurse in training cares for on the average three or four patients.

Ohio.—Very few nurses are really competent in handling orthopedic apparatus.

Oklahoma.—In this section of country most nurses have excellent "operating room training" but poor bedside training.

Maryland.—For the care of patients suffering with diseases of the eye, the training of nurses in even the best general hospital is most inadequate. For this reason I use, so far as possible, only those nurses with whom I have already had some experience and whom I know to be proficient. This small group gives services which are entirely satisfactory. Whenever I have to use a nurse outside this group I find that I have to spend a great deal of time explaining how the case should be cared for and that I am, even then, a good deal concerned as to whether my orders are properly executed. I do not believe that practical nurses can, in general, be trusted with eye cases, but I prefer a practical nurse who has had one year's experience in an eye hospital to a graduate nurse who has had long experience in a general hospital but no special training in the care of eye cases.

North Carolina.—The problem I am most often baffled by is competent registered graduate nurses willing and wanting to do tuberculosis work and having, beside the proper training, the social and educational background to remain with the case long enough to really help the patient over such an acute complication as a hemorrhage, etc.

Massachusetts.—The nursing problem in obstetrics is very acute. It is hard work, confining work, requiring unusual tact. No nurse will do it who does not like it. There is so much hospital nursing with its short hours and lack of real responsibility that nurses need do no home nursing, in this vicinity, if they do not so desire. Many nurses refuse home cases in obstetrics. Many will not take obstetrics even in the hospitals, so I say, the nurse must really enjoy it to do it. And those who enjoy it are good nurses.

California.—The training of an average graduate nurse is lacking in how to care for or handle patients wearing plaster casts, especially body casts. Therefore it is necessary for one doing plaster work to be extremely careful in selecting nurses from sources other than one's own private list.

Massachusetts.—The attitude of a disciplinarian which many nurses acquire in general hospitals is disadvantageous when taking care of mental cases.

Massachusetts.—I practise psychiatry in a small town and find it fairly difficult to secure a well trained mature nurse, professionally and personally competent to handle cultured, psychoneurotic patients. We are faced with the necessity of finding more nurses for this work. We usually secure a nurse when we need one but we often have to comb the east and even go to Canada to find them.

Illinois.—Psychiatric post-graduate training of graduate R.N's. is too rare and there are not enough really well trained psychiatric nurses for private duty. There are not enough nurses for institutional work either. There are too many half trained nurses and attendants posing as nurses.

NEW YORK.—Probably the most difficult type of case to handle is the mental or nervous one. It requires vigilance, intelligence, resourcefulness not learned in nursing schools, great elasticity and adaptability. Nine out of ten nurses prefer physical to mental activity. They prefer surgical cases where a dressing is done once a day and they are left more or less to their own devices thereafter. Such care is easily learned. It requires special interest and great mental effort to learn to care for nervous cases. Most nurses are unwilling to make the effort or find the work too difficult or distasteful. When a physician finds one of superior type, he or she is a jewel.

MICHIGAN.—My commonest quarrel with the nursing profession is to have them refuse to take cases that are in dire need of nursing care because they are in the home or of a contagious nature. I was utterly unable to secure a nurse for my last case of diphtheria when I desperately needed one. To my knowledge there is only one "private duty" nurse in town who will nurse diphtheria.

6. Registry

The physicians and the registrars are in substantial agreement on problems of placing private duty nursing. The question arises, "Are they due to the pattern of the training or to the fact that registries demand relatively little of the nurses on their lists?"

MISSISSIPPI.—The greatest difficulty is to get a good nurse when needed. There is no compulsory or rotating rule here and nurses are very independent, taking a case if they think they would like to and refusing or giving all kinds of excuses if not. To get one nurse last month, I called 18 nurses and found only one who did not make excuses.

IOWA.—I have had much trouble to get trained nurses when needed. They were tired or had just come in from a case or they wanted a rest, etc. Had to beg and coax, usually.

CALIFORNIA.—A few weeks ago I spent $8.00 on telephone calls and about two hours' time trying to locate a special nurse for an acute surgical case. Finally found one only by a happy coincidence. (Signed) "Country M.D. residing within two hours' ride of several wide-awake towns of 3,000 population."

MASSACHUSETTS.—One month ago I treated a patient for cerebral hemorrhage, a man of wealth and influence in the community. None of the 18 nurses on the registry was willing to take a night duty case.

CALIFORNIA.—It is difficult to secure well trained reliable nurses for home work. If a doctor can't get one he knows, it is almost better not to call one as those from registries sent out to home cases are usually way below par. For hospital cases there is no difficulty whatever.

PENNSYLVANIA.—There is no nursing shortage but a number of women with below the average education are charging higher rates for second and third rate services. The hospital gets the pick of the nurses and often it is difficult to secure a first class nurse for private patients. I rarely have difficulty in securing good nurses for my hospital patients.

ILLINOIS.—I believe we should have nurses following certain specialties the same as physicians, i. e., surgical nursing, medical nursing, pediatric nursing, and general nursing so that the physician or surgeon may choose the nurse for the particular kind of case.

IOWA.—I well realize that there are many graduate nurses in this city whom I would not care to have on cases because of their lack of skill, personal appearance, and inability to please the family. These I am able to avoid, but the physicians in the towns about are not so fortunately situated and have to take what is sent them by the central registry.

MICHIGAN.—We have a small private hospital in a small town but have to depend on nurses from the city. There are lots of good nurses there but we get lots of poor ones. We call the registry where there are a few poor nurses who are almost always there. They will send these if we don't ask who they are and object to the lame ducks.

7. Shortage

Physicians are in substantial agreement with registrars on the question of "Shortage." The registrars are quite as aware as the medical profession of the difficulty of securing nurses over week-ends, but have as yet developed no mechanism for handling the problem.

NEW YORK.—Nursing shortage is all nonsense. It is the same as hospital bed shortage. If there were enough nurses to do all the work at times of epidemics, there would be too many at all other times. On the other hand, the nursing profession is never over-crowded for the exceptionally good nurse. Same as doctors. There are never too many good doctors and never too many good nurses. Always, everywhere, too many poor, careless, unskilful or dishonest doctors and same with nurses except that fewer nurses are dishonest than doctors. That's some of what thirty years' experience has put in my mind.

KANSAS.—I do not feel that there is a shortage of nurses in this locality but there are still a number of hospitals turning out nurses who have not been properly trained.

NEW YORK.—It is not a shortage of nurses that bothers the great number of doctors in this city. It is the fact that the great mass of people cannot afford the luxury of the present day graduate nurse. I use the word "luxury" correctly. All of my interest is obstetrical. It is an unnecessary luxury for the normal case to have a private duty nurse while in the hospital.

MASSACHUSETTS.—I am surprised to hear that there is any question on the shortage of nurses. Certainly I have never had any difficulty in securing nurses here in this city or in its vicinity. In fact various registries are continually reminding me that they have nurses on hand.

MASSACHUSETTS.—This winter past has seen a long list of nurses without cases. It is ridiculous economically to expect to have such a supply of nurses that there is not enough work for them. Such a state of affairs would utterly demoralize the profession because of poverty.

NEW YORK.—From my experience during the past year I believe that instead of a shortage of nurses we have on the contrary more nurses than needed; whether those nurses are in reality R.N. or not I am not prepared to say.

PENNSYLVANIA.—It is impossible for me to answer your questions for there has not been a graduate nurse available in this community for over two years. This is a small mining community and rather isolated, so the nurses are reluctant about making calls here. We have a state nurse who holds a baby clinic here once a week but she is unable to go from house to house should the occasion arise. Nursing is usually done by members of the family or the neighbors.

PENNSYLVANIA.—I cannot admire nurses for leaving the physician and patients high and dry over the week ends and holidays.

CALIFORNIA.—A shortage of nurses in my own work relates only to the times when holidays and vacations are in order. Many of the nurses agree in not taking cases for example at Christmas and during the summer.

UTAH.—The greatest need in this community is distribution of nurses during vacation periods. During early summer, Thanksgiving, and especially all of the Christmas holidays, so many R.N.'s go on vacation that it is often impossible to get enough care for really sick surgical cases. Yet many months during fall, late winter, and summer there is an overabundance of nursing supply on the registry.

LOUISIANA.—The only shortage of nurses that I have met with is due to their distaste to go on duty just before Sunday or holidays. There is no shortage of nurses existing in New Orleans.

8. Hospital Care

Apparently the hospitals could avert many misunderstandings if they would make a definite statement of the amount of nursing care patients may expect to have included in the regular hospital charge, and would give this amount in all cases even though it might need to be supplemented on occasion with special duty nursing.

TEXAS.—All hospitals in town which I attend have an insufficient number of nurses and most of them lack a graduate nurse in charge of the floor.

OREGON.—The local hospitals can not give a really serious case the attention necessary with regular hospital nurses. A patient suffering or uncomfortable must hire a special.

PENNSYLVANIA.—In many hospitals in Philadelphia it is necessary for a private patient to have a private nurse, even though there is hardly anything for her to do.

CONNECTICUT.—The chief difficulty we find is the care of the patients in the hospital wards and at least a part of the difficulty I feel is due to youth and lack of experience of the head nurses and their lack of control of the pupil nurses under them.

California.—I do not believe the general care at any hospital adequate for any serious case and always employ a special whenever I can.

Washington.—The greatest difficulty I meet is not attributable to nurses. It is the great cost of hospitalization and special nursing, an economic condition that is especially pressing in this community.

Illinois.—Many of my patients need special nurses but cannot afford same and naturally they are gotten on floor duty in the hospital. Some hospitals render to these patients who have no special nurse excellent care, in fact almost the same as a special, whereas other hospitals take the attitude that if they have no special, the floor nurses can give only ordinary care. This, in my opinion, is a great problem for these people that cannot afford a nurse.

California.—It is most important, to my way of thinking, that when patients enter a hospital with the understanding that they are paying a given rate per day for hospitalization and nursing, *that they receive efficient and adequate nursing.* Few patients can afford $6.00 per day for room, $12.00 per day for nursing 12 hour duty, besides laboratory and board for nurses, charged extra. Consequently most patients leave hospital one to many weeks before they should.

Kansas.—We rarely have need for a private duty nurse. We have an affiliation with the Kansas State Agricultural College with a five year course. Our ladies in training are mature and usually very efficient. Our patients are satisfied and we rarely have a call for a special nurse.

South Dakota.—The great problem is, at least in this portion of South Dakota, the care for the finances. There are some people who can afford to pay a special nurse, but this type of patient is usually willing and anxious to go to the hospital if the doctor in charge of the case mentions that they are sick enough to need a special nurse.

In addition to this, the usual charge in this state is something like $6.00 a day, and the average room in our best hospital is $4.50 to $5.00, so that from a financial point of view they find it cheaper to go to a first class hospital and there secure the best of care under ideal surroundings, at a cheaper rate than they could hire a nurse to come into the home and work with makeshift equipment in most cases.

New Hampshire.—In almost all instances where a nurse is needed, I strongly advise going to a hospital instead because (a) it is cheaper (if an R.N. is employed); (b) Supervision and care are more satisfactory; (c) The family gets along better in the absence of the sick one; (d) Accommodations are lacking or unsatisfactory for caring for a nurse in many instances.

South Carolina.—Patients have developed the hospital habit as it is cheaper than two nurses at $35 per week each.

New Jersey.—In hospitals, in relation to my own work, the real need for special duty nurses is almost negligible.

Kentucky.—I use my own nurses in the hospital for all cases. Don't use any special nurses if I can help it. I think all hospitals should take care of their own cases as far as possible without calling in specials. Specials cause friction.

Vermont.—I preach to the hospital authorities that nursing must be so good that only exceptional cases will require specials.

9. Practicals

Physicians were at obvious pains to express their distaste for undergraduate and practical nurses.

California.—The worst curse I have to contend with is the practical nurse. The mother of a family can be relied on to do what she is able for the patient but the practical nurse is always a headstrong fool who does not hesitate to criticize the physician and to make a diagnosis and make herself generally useful in outlining the treatment.

California.—Two days before the patient died, this practical nurse suggested to a friend accompanying the patient that they employ a certain undertaker!

California.—The reason why I will not have another practical "correspondence course nurse" is that their theory is all right but their practical work is *no good*, and another point is that they "know too much" and don't observe enough and report symptoms.

New Mexico.—I get much better service out of the practical nurses and at about one-half the cost. Of course, the practical nurses I use have worked for me in my private hospital and I have trained them to suit me and do my nursing as I wish to have it done. The R.N. nurse has always been very unsatisfactory to me.

Pennsylvania.—I use R.N.'s only. I find the practical nurse worthless for the care of the sick. I advocate employing a domestic servant to relieve a member of the family who can care for the patient rather than employ a so-called practical nurse when finances or other reasons make it impossible to secure a graduate registered nurse. I think that the nurses should be required to have as high standard of education and training as physicians have in their profession.

GEORGIA.—In the average case I would rather use an untrained woman than a practical nurse for they cause me more worry than any problem I have in the nursing question.

ILLINOIS.—This community has more practical nurses than patients. We never had difficulty in getting nurses from the nearby cities. Those we get occasionally are fine nurses but our practical nurses do more harm than good. They are ignorant and know nothing about cleanliness. Many people seem unable to differentiate between good and poor nurses.

NEW YORK.—Too many nurses are being sent out by the registries who are not graduate nurses although they charge $8.00 per day. They don't know their business and they give the people a bad impression of the nurses and the nursing profession.

NEW YORK.—This town is full of cottages for tuberculosis and boarding houses. The nurses available are generally a most questionable lot and relatively few are graduate nurses. However, they all charge as much as possible, often really more than a well-trained nurse would charge from a New York hospital.

TEXAS.—In my opinion there is no place for the so-called practical nurses. In my locality she is employed mostly for obstetrical patients in the home, for which she receives three to four dollars a day. She has had no training but thinks she knows all about obstetrics because she has had 6 children herself or has nursed a number of cases. Sterile goods mean nothing to her.

I believe both mother and baby are safer in the hands of an intelligent relative who can be given minute directions and who will usually do just as she is told.

TEXAS.—I have a graduate nurse at this time on duty with a diphtheria patient who has a tracheotomy tube. She is *very satisfactory* and saves me much trouble.

I have a practical nurse on a puerperal infection case. She is very unsatisfactory and causes me to have to make a number of unnecessary calls.

MICHIGAN.—I have tried to train several women to do practical nursing when particular training was not needed. As soon as they learned to take a pulse, read a thermometer, and give an enema, they boosted their prices beyond their worth and almost as high as the R.N.

NEBRASKA.—My only objection to a practical nurse is the lack of discipline. After they have nursed for a short while they get the notion that they could write a book on treatment. I have three practical nurses on my list that are as good as any R.N. but they charge $35 per week so we are not helped a bit on charges.

NEW JERSEY.—In homes 24-hour service is greatly needed and can be met as a rule only by "domestic" nurses as the expense of registered nurses is inordinate for most of my clientele. The absolute lack of grading or control of "domestic" nurses is a serious situation. Development of a community system of hourly or visiting nursing service would partly meet the difficulty of present conditions. In conjunction with greater availability of good domestics, it would go far toward doing so.

OHIO.—I personally believe I have had hundreds of patients sick enough to require the services of an R.N. but there are very few R.N.'s who will do 24 hour duty and I do not blame them one bit. I am not in favor of a girl working this hard as all the nurses who try it are soon under par physically. It is difficult to find a family in the average working class who can afford to pay $12 a day for two twelve-hour duty registered nurses.

Our practical nurses are absolutely useless. They

do 24 hour duty and all the housework for $5 per day but as far as carrying out instructions is concerned and recognizing symptoms, they are a detriment rather than an assistance.

NORTH CAROLINA.—I never know the outcome in a case handled by a practical nurse.

SOUTH DAKOTA.—I practise in a large, sparsely settled territory, and maintain a 10 bed hospital. In my experience practical nurses have proven generally unsatisfactory because of their lack of poise and tact, inability to understand and carry out orders, and occasional disregard of orders, so I employ only registered nurses.

INDIANA.—I think a registered nurse should always be used in all surgical cases (including severe infections), obstetrical cases, and some contagious cases, providing the family can pay for services rendered. If unable to pay, a practical nurse is of course, the next choice. It has been my experience, however, that a great many people class themselves as practical nurses. In fact they are servants who have a "smattering" of a few medical facts. Many times, I find, they assume the rôle of doctor, and carry out the doctor's orders if they wish, change orders without consulting doctor, or begin some "quack" practice of their own that is "guaranteed to cure."

MISSOURI.—I feel comfortable when a graduate nurse is in charge of any sick patient. Many practical nurses are satisfactory in most cases but I am always uneasy in case the patient has some sudden change for fear that they will not notice it and let me know.

MAINE.—My experience with nurses is that the R.N.'s have been very good on the whole. Our practical or domestic nurses have sadly deteriorated in this section.

WEST VIRGINIA.—My objections to practical nurses

are that they don't know what to do in an emergency if the physician is not in reach and also they attempt to do things they have not had training to accomplish.

NEBRASKA.—Working in the country as I do, I meet with much ignorance and interference from meddling neighbors who criticize nurses and think they should do everything from caring for the sick to washing the family car. They think the R.N. gets too much for what she does—not seeing her trained skill. Most of my patients want practical nurses and I find they are capable of ordinary cases, but no good for anything serious.

IOWA.—It is very rare to find a practical nurse who is not obnoxious to family and every one else. They expect to be treated with the same or more respect than a trained R.N. I like either a trained servant or a *competent* R.N.

FLORIDA.—Practical nurses, in my experience, talk too much and know too little. The physician can always trust the graduate nurse to do exactly as he says. Knowledge, coupled with a sunny disposition and a pleasing personality, are essential in the sick room.

MASSACHUSETTS.—This nurse is a high grade practical nurse. The patient was a primipara, only her husband and self in the family. I feel that the best practical nurse is not good enough to give mother and child the proper care and to keep the house running. The patient doesn't begin to do as well as when in the hospital or with a trained nurse. No doubt I will employ this practical nurse but will always feel that the hospital or trained nurse would be much better.

KANSAS.—(Town with less than 10,000 people) I do surgery mostly. Have no public hospital facilities so have a woman who has given her home up to hospital work for eight years, she managing it altogether. She hires from one to three practical nurses (usually widows) who live in the community and need work. The same force is employed and trained for long periods of time until they know my methods and what I require of them. They generally give good service or quit soon.

ILLINOIS.—I had a case of scarlet fever, three down. The R.N. demanded $10 per day. They could not pay it. They secured a farm hand and he assumed the responsibility and saved the family at least $140 and they couldn't have had better attention.

ARKANSAS.—All the doctors here much prefer graduate nurses and use them. They discourage patients using practical nurses. We think if patient needs a nurse, she needs a capable one.

10. Costs

Physicians give serious thought to the cost of nursing service but none has suggested a subsidized service of any sort.

TENNESSEE.—We have about discontinued using graduate nurses unless it is a surgical or very desperate case of sickness, for after they pay the nurse there is nothing left for the doctor. People who live in New York and practise among people of wealth do not know what a hardship it is on ordinary country people when you put a couple of nurses in their home at $14.00 a day. It looks like a lot of money to them, and is. Can't you people turn out some nurse that won't be so highly educated that they can go to the country and help us on these cases? The same thing has taken place with our young graduates in medicine. They won't go back to the little towns or to the country, and in a way I don't blame them, or the nurses. It is a hard life, even when you don't weaken. I don't want you to get the impression that I think graduate nurses charge too high for their service. Lord knows, I know a good one earns what she gets. The question is, couldn't we get along on less training for ordinary cases so they could work cheaper?

MICHIGAN.—There is only one drawback to R.N. service, and that is the ability of the family to pay.

ILLINOIS.—The trained nurse has been a wonderful help to me in my work, and I wish that I could use more nurses than I do. The unfortunate part is that not many of my patrons can afford the nurse. For instance, recently a bank clerk had a trained nurse when his first born arrived and paid the nurse $7.00 per day and her traveling expenses, and he was earning but $5.00 per day. However, I am for the nurse.

MINNESOTA.—My experience with private duty R.N.'s has been very satisfactory—the only trouble is that in doing a pediatric practice so many of the people who have children have not much money and that with some of them it has been a real hardship to pay an R.N. for any great length of time.

MICHIGAN.—In my work the large majority of patients require two twelve-hour nurses for the first three to five days. Then as improvement takes place they dispense with the night nurse and keep the day nurse as long as they feel able. The difficulty with this is that of expense—two nurses at $7.00 per day each and their board of $1.50 to $2.00 each makes $17.00 to $18.00, plus price of room ($4.50 to $8.00) daily almost exorbitant for the average pocket book. We are trying out small groups of from two to six beds in a room and trying to arrange for one nurse to care for two or four, depending on the amount of attention required.

NEBRASKA.—The cooperative nurse in the hospital (1 to 3 patients) and the visiting nurse in the home seems to me to be the solution of the nursing problem for the majority of my patients. Seventy-five per cent of my patients who are confined in the hospital (and most of mine go to the hospital) would be crippled financially for many months if they hired nurses at the current rates ($7.00 per 24-hour duty—four hours off—all maternity cases) besides paying the hospital bill. Hourly or group or cooperative nursing must be developed in order to give proper nursing service to the middle class.

11. Suggested Remedies

Running through most of the suggested remedies for the high cost of nursing service is the thought of a graded service—graded according to preparation and competence as well as to financial returns.

RHODE ISLAND.—Good practical nurses are very valuable and equally rare. A hospital course of one year (practical) and a regulation to hold their prices well below those of the R.N. would be most valuable.

ILLINOIS.—I often feel the need of a nurse who perhaps does not need to possess the skill of the regular graduate and have often felt that if girls might be given a short course it would help the situation. Yet I feel there is a great deal of danger in this, much as there would be in cutting down the requirements for medical graduates. It would turn out a great many incompetent people, and Heaven knows enough of the regulars fall by the wayside to fill the demand after all.

ILLINOIS.—There is a need for practical women to care for obstetrical and chronic cases outside of hospital. There should be a way for bright young women with a fair education to take training in obstetrical nursing and be registered as such. There should be a standard for practical nurses established and a registration for the same. We must always have the well-trained graduate, registered nurse.

West Virginia.—There is a field for the practical nurse who could be employed at a smaller rate of pay but I am afraid that if this was advocated it would take away from the trained graduate who now in many cases finds it hard enough to get employment. We are turning out these women as trained nurses for the public and it is our duty to try to see that they have a decent living.

Michigan.—We must have two classes of nurses. First, a minority of R.N.'s trained well for special cases, and a majority of nurses, trained better than our "practical nurses" but not so trained as to need over $5 a day, or to feel themselves too superior to common cases, to house help, and to the attending physician.

Nebraska.—A nurse who has a ruptured appendix patient with general peritonitis is worth all we can pay her if she knows the game, while one on a clean case who does about an hour's work a day is not worth so much and should not be paid as much as the skilled woman of experience. Our worst trouble is that they all want six dollars a day whether they earn it or not. Now if you can grade them according to ability, experience, and willingness to work, you will have done the public a great service.

Michigan.—My experience with so-called practical nursing is not at all satisfactory. They are usually uneducated, undiplomatic, talk too much, etc., and as a rule upset the patient by their chatter.

Illinois.—In my opinion there is very real need for hourly nursing and for the care of two or three patients by one nurse in hospitals.

District of Columbia.—I very freely employ instructive visiting nurses. Otherwise I usually employ registered nurses for my patients. Of course sometimes patients would do much better had they available such specialized skill at practical nursing rates. And were all nurses to be regarded as servants some patients would benefit (financially). I do not desire a nurse to act as a servant. Also I would not approve of a plan by which three or four patients would share the cost and services of the same nurse in a hospital. We have that now in the floor girls. The most insistent—not the most needful patient—would secure the special for the greater time, and none would be pleased, perhaps not even the physician.

MASSACHUSETTS.—There is no shortage of nurses in Boston. People in moderate circumstances and others resent the cost of nursing. We are turning to hourly nursing more and more to save expense.

INDIANA.—I think some way ought to be devised to try out group nursing. It would require especial cooperative effort in hospital to group the patients advantageously. Probably the nurses would not like it.

VERMONT.—I think there is a field for group and hourly nursing in the hospital and I also think that hourly nursing in the home would be a great help, especially for patients discharged from the hospital, but not fully recovered.

CALIFORNIA.—Hourly nursing is solving many problems, especially chronic cases that need a limited amount of professional care daily.

NEW YORK.—The trained nurses for the most part do their work well, and while the fee seems higher to many than it should be, in my opinion it is not higher than it should be. My own proposals for the solution of the nursing problem are two—hourly nursing outside of the hospital and group nursing in the hospital. I believe that the latter plan would prove valuable although I have never seen it tried.

ILLINOIS.—In my city the visiting nurse association does a wonderful work and I frequently use them in lieu of the needed hourly nursing.

12. Visiting Nursing

There is conflicting evidence as to the value of the visiting nurse. Evidently, the services vary considerably in type.

INDIANA.—This community is unfortunate in having a Visiting Nurses' Association which is attempting to give a fair sized hospital force all the experience in outside or home nursing. There does not appear to be enough demand from the sick to keep all students busy, so the daily papers are scanned for births, accidents, and reported illness, and like the "ambulance chasing" lawyer, a nurse arrives on the scene and insists on being allowed to administer to the need (?) of the patient whether she be wanted in the home or not. She continues to repeat her daily visits so long as she is tolerated and the fee forthcoming. Sometimes she calls the physician that evening or the next day and tells what she has done. More often the physician has no knowledge of her intrusion until he makes his next call on his patient.

This is *not* the *whole* situation. A life insurance company maintains a staff of nurses who not only seek, but *demand*, access to every policy holder who may be sick, no matter whether the physician or patient or both prefer that this pest attend to her own affairs.

MAINE.—Our particular problem is in supplying nursing care to patients who cannot afford to pay a graduate nurse. This need is supplied in part by a visiting district nurse, and in part by practical nurses who are worse than useless.

KENTUCKY.—Visiting public health and practical nurses are of no use to me in my work. They cause confusion and loss of confidence in the attending doctor and only too often are salesmen for some favorite specialists.

MICHIGAN.—The visiting nurse is the solution of this problem, and the one I am using now drives her own car and can wash and dress eight babies and change and care for the mothers in one forenoon, and they don't all live in the same ward either. She had a lot of practice after she was an R.N. before she could do it, however.

13. Miscellaneous

Often the incidental comment proves illuminating.

IOWA.—Many good nurses work too hard.

ILLINOIS.—I sometimes wonder how we can get private duty nurses at all when there are so many institutional positions open which require only ten-hour duty daily. Nurses are only human and naturally seek the positions which give them more leisure hours during the day.

ILLINOIS.—My worst trouble is that I never know a nurse's name. She is a part of the machine and usually fills the bill.

PENNSYLVANIA.—The outlook for the nurse is gloomy—she needs more encouragement and should be paid better for her services.

CALIFORNIA.—I have found it better to have nurses on eight or twelve hour duty only, and not living in the home. The professional character is better sustained, service is better, and friction is less.

STATE NOT KNOWN.—The nurses under my observation "during the past week" have been fairly satisfactory. I seldom have difficulty in obtaining nurses even during the busy season. The shortage, as far as I can observe, is "alleged" and not real. I believe the standard rate of wages is fair for the service rendered. Their ethics is surprisingly good considering the prevailing lowering of ethical standards throughout the professions now. They are no better or no worse than the doctors, lawyers, clergymen, etc. Not many have a true vocation—they are accepted without adequate inquiry into their fitness (physical, moral, temperamental, or mental). They are "trained" by selfish people for selfish reasons, and it is not surprising that they become actuated by selfish motives when they graduate. They are the product of their training and environment. To try to make them idealistic is futile until they are reared in such an atmosphere from the beginning. There has been too much destructive and not enough constructive criticism. The doctors who are responsible for their training are their severest critics. We must all lend a hand toward correcting the public's attitude toward the R.N. and making the training schools what they should be.

CHAPTER 10

ARE PATIENTS SATISFIED?

First-hand reports from patients were felt to be important, but it was realized that care must be taken in approaching them, so that they would not misinterpret the attitude of the Committee. The safest way in which to secure a frank discussion of the experience of the patient with the nurse seemed to be to approach each patient through his own physician and ask the physician to explain to the patient why the material was needed and how it would probably be used. Accordingly, every questionnaire sent to a physician was accompanied by another to be given to one of his patients who had recently employed a private duty nurse. In the earlier study a second questionnaire was included for patients who had been in hospitals, but this was not followed up later, since it was decided that the study of experiences of patients in hospitals might well be left for a later inquiry.

The returns from patients who have had private duty or special nurses now total 1,892, and more are being received every day. If we assume that only those physicians who themselves answered questionnaires took the trouble to pass questionnaires on to their own patients, which seems a reasonable assumption, we then have a 44 per cent return on these questionnaires. While the patient reports are not extremely numerous, they are very frank and appear to have been written by intelligent and thoughtful people, who were genuinely interested in the nursing problem. The comments written on the backs of the questionnaires are highly illuminating.

1. Location and Type of Case

Reports were secured from patients in all parts of the United States.

32% of the patients came from the North Atlantic States
39% of the patients came from the North Central States
9% of the patients came from the South Atlantic States
8% of the patients came from the South Central States, and
12% of the patients came from the Western States

Of the total, 43 per cent were in the hospital, 41 per cent in the home, and 16 per cent both in the hospital and in the home. Hospitalization seems highest in the Western States and lowest in the North Atlantic.

Before giving the questionnaire to the patient, each physician was asked to note upon it the type of patient and the type of illness on which the report was based. According to these reports, 53 per cent of the patients were women, 25 per cent men, 12 per cent adolescents, and 10 per cent children. The types of illness were classified as follows:

Surgical	50%
Medical	37
Obstetric	5
Pediatric	3
Contagious	3
Mental and nervous	2

About three-fourths of the surgical, medical, and pediatric cases were considered "severe" by the physician in charge of the case, and about two-thirds of the contagious and mental cases. Only about one-third of the obstetrical cases, however, were reported as "severe" by the physician in charge. The question as to whether the case was "long" or "short" showed that about four-fifths of all the mental and nervous cases were long time cases, about half of the medical and contagious, two-fifths of the surgical, one-fourth of the pediatric, and one-fifth of the obstetric cases.

2. R.N.'s and Practicals

Patients reported that 88 per cent of all their nurses were Registered, 11 per cent practical, and 1 per cent did not know what kind of a nurse had been on the case. There was marked difference between the per cents of R.N.'s and practicals, depending upon whether the case was in the hospital, in the home, or both.

TABLE 37. PER CENT OF PATIENTS WITH R.N.'S, AND WITH PRACTICAL NURSES IN THE HOSPITAL, HOME, OR BOTH

	R.N.	Practical	Total
Hospital	46%	19%	47%
Home	37	72	38
Both*	17	9	15
All	100%	100%	100%

Patients were asked how they secured their nurses. Those who employed R.N.'s reported as follows:

46% secured nurses through a hospital registry
29% secured nurses from their own physicians
15% secured nurses from the central registry
3% secured nurses through friends
2% secured nurses through the commercial registry
5% secured nurses from other sources

When the question was asked for practicals only, it was found that of all the practicals reported:

51% were secured through patient's own physician
15% were secured through hospital registry
14% were secured through central professional registry
13% were secured through friends
3% were secured through commercial registries
4% were secured through other sources

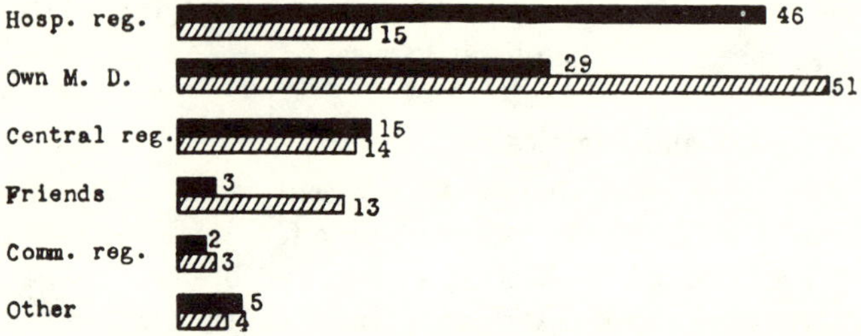

Hosp. reg. 46 15

Own M. D. 29 51

Central reg. 15 14

Friends 3 13

Comm. reg. 2 3

Other 5 4

Diagram 24.—Per cent of patients with registered nurses ▬ and per cent of patients with practical nurses ▨ who secured their nurses from each source

3. Days, Hours, Costs

One-fourth of all the patients reported that they had had the nurse for eight days or less, one-half for fourteen days or less, and three-fourths for twenty-eight days or less. In half the cases where an R.N. was employed, she remained on the case for fourteen days, and in half the cases where the practical nurse was employed she remained on the case for sixteen days.

Of all the patients, 37 per cent reported that the nurse had been on day duty, 14 per cent on night duty, 49 per cent on twenty-four hour duty.

The charges of Registered Nurses ranged from no charge at all in several cases to one nurse who charged $20.00 a day. Among practicals there were no cases of free service reported, but the charges per day ran from $1.00 to $12.00. If all the nurses are placed in order from those who charged least to those who charged most, it is found that the R.N. one-fourth of the way up and the R.N. one-half of the way up both charge $6.00 a day, while the R.N. three-fourths of the way up charges $7.00. Similar figures for the practical nurses showed that the practical one-fourth of the way up charged $3.00, one-half the way up charged $5.00, and three-fourths the way up charged $6.00. The reports seem to indicate, in other words, that Registered Nurses are more apt to give charity service than do practical nurses. The extreme charges for Registered Nurses are higher than for practicals; but the extreme charge of the practical nurse is well above the ordinary charge of the R.N. The R.N.'s are much more uniform in their rates of charge, and there are only a few R.N.'s who charge less than $6.00 or more than $7.00. There is much greater variety among practicals. In general, however, the patient who employs a practical nurse saves about a dollar a day.

It was found that when all cases were reported together, the typical or median day case, night case, and twenty-four hour case cost the same—$6.00. Nurses seem to make no difference in their charge to fit the type of daily service required.

As is the case in most of these computations, the median or middle charge is slightly below the average, which in this case is $6.26. The average is always affected by the extreme charge at the top of the list. The following table shows the per cent of all nurses—R.N.'s and practicals combined—who charge each amount per day.

The tabulation of charge per day combined with the number of days the nurse was on service is impressive in the illustration of the fact that there seems to be little attempt to adjust salaries in the light of whether or not the case is long or short. In most professions, short time is paid for at a definitely higher rate than long time, since short time employment implies a corresponding period of unemployment before the worker can locate again. In nursing, however, the charge for a single day

TABLE 38. PER CENT OF ALL NURSES (R.N.'S AND PRACTICALS COMBINED) WHO CHARGED EACH AMOUNT PER DAY

Charge per day	Per cent of all nurses
0	.2
$1.00	1.0
2.00	.8
3.00	3.5
4.00	1.7
5.00	15.1
6.00	39.7
7.00	28.9
8.00	6.7
9.00	.9
10.00	1.0
12.00	.2
15.00	.1
18.00	.1
20.00	.1
	100

is in many cases no larger than the charge per day for the case which lasts for a year or more. The long time cases are, of course, in many ways unattractive, yet from the economic standpoint they do provide many advantages. On the long time case the nurse actually receives the maintenance which in theory she receives but does not often get on short time cases. She is not obliged to maintain a room of her own; she does not have heavy charges for carfare, taxis, extra meals, extra laundry, and the like, and practically everything she earns on the long time case is over and above the cost of maintenance. In the light of these facts, therefore, it is interesting to note that

One patient who employed a nurse for 1,095 days paid $5.00 a day plus maintenance.
One patient who had a nurse for 730 days paid $6.00 a day.
Another who employed a nurse for 607 days paid $7.00.
One who employed a nurse for 548 days paid $8.00.
One who employed a nurse for 321 days paid $9.00 a day.

Shorter cases are often also very expensive, as with the patient who employed a nurse for 32 days at $20.00 a day. It should, of course, be remembered that some of the charges which look excessively heavy were made for mental and nervous cases or for other cases where the strain upon the nurse was exceedingly great. Full details are lacking on this point, but it seems entirely possible that some of the heavier charges were well justified because of the nature of the nursing service called for. The longest case on record was one in which the patient reported having employed a nurse for 1,460 days, but in this case the nurse charged only $3.00 a day, plus maintenance.

In the earlier patient study the question was asked as to whether a tip or money gift was given to the nurse in addition to her charge. A little less than three-fourths of the patients reported that no such gift was given, and a little more than one-fourth that there was. Practically all of those who gave tips did so because they genuinely wanted to, and only 9 per cent of those who gave felt that the nurse expected some sort of extra reward. These figures are cheering in the light of the frequent allegation that in so far as money is concerned many nurses are unprofessional in their attitude. It would seem from the reports of patients that while there are in the profession a few nurses who tacitly regard themselves as on the social level of servants, these cases are actually rare.

4. Patient's Attitude towards Nurse

In answer to the question, "Would you like to have the same nurse again?" 86 per cent of all the patients answered "Yes," 12 per cent "No," and 2 per cent would hesitate. Practicals seem as popular with the patients as do the R.N.'s, which is definitely untrue when similar reports are secured from physicians. Men patients were slightly more enthusiastic about their nurses than were women, but the difference is not marked. Difference in size of city where the patient lived had apparently no effect upon the popularity of the nurse.

Patients in the first study were asked, "Were you yourself an easy or a difficult patient to take care of?" About one-third of all the patients reported that they were difficult to take care of. Child patients, however, were reported as difficult in more than half of the cases. When the patient's own report as to whether he was easy or difficult to care for is combined with the physician's statement as to the type of case, it is found that about two-thirds of the mental and pediatric cases regarded themselves as difficult to take care of, two-fifths of the medical cases, and about one-fourth of the surgical, contagious, and obstetric cases.

Patients were asked, "Which seems to you the more difficult problem, to meet the cost of nursing care or to get the right kind of nurse?" Among the patients the difference is not nearly so marked as among physicians. It will be remembered that when physicians were asked this question 73 per cent reported that it was more difficult to meet the nurse's fee than to get the right kind of nurse. Among patients, however, instead of 73 per cent, only 54 per cent say that cost is the more difficult problem, and 46 per cent say that getting the right kind of nurse is more difficult. Whether the patient had an R.N. or a practical seems to make little difference in this judgment. The daily charge of the nurse did not seem to have any effect upon this decision; neither did the patient's experiences as portrayed in his statement as to whether or not he would like the same nurse again.

5. Why Patients Employ Special Nurses

Patients were asked why they employed a nurse in the home, or why they employed one in the hospital. For patients who had a private duty nurse in the home the reasons given are as follows. The table shows the per cents replying under each heading where the patient was a woman, where the patient was a man, and for all patients.

TABLE 39. PER CENT OF PATIENTS GIVING EACH TYPE OF REASON FOR EMPLOYING SPECIAL NURSES IN THE HOME

	Men	Women	All patients
No one in the family had time to take care of the patient	21%	22%	19%
The members of the family were too tired to take care of the patient	6	6	6
Some one was needed to take charge of the housework, or children, or both	4	6	6
Patient wanted to be relieved of all responsibility	7	2	11
Patient was so ill that special nursing service was necessary	62	64	58
	100%	100%	100%

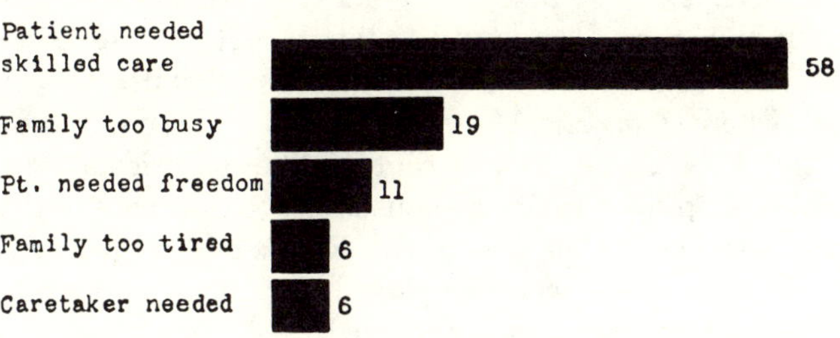

Diagram 25.—Per cent of all patients having special nurses in the *home* for each reason

Just why men patients seem to feel the need of being relieved of responsibility by having a nurse in the home to a greater extent than women patients is something which the reports do not explain. The outstanding fact in the table, however, is that only 58 per cent of all the patients had nurses because they needed special nursing care, and 42 per cent employed nurses in the home chiefly because a capable, unworried, reasonably intelligent worker was needed to take charge at a time of family crisis.

It was interesting, in reading the questionnaires, to note that the response, "family had no time to take care of the patient," was higher in the largest cities and in the smallest towns than in cities of moderate size. The per cents run as follows:

In cities of		
500,000 and over	21%	report family had no time
100,000 to 500,000	15%	report family had no time
25,000 to 100,000	17%	report family had no time
10,000 to 25,000	24%	report family had no time
Under 10,000	20%	report family had no time
Total	19%	report family had no time

The reasons given for employing a nurse in the home were tabulated according to whether the nurse secured was a Registered Nurse or a practical. Where a Registered Nurse was employed, 63 per cent of the cases needed special nursing care, as compared with 38 per cent where a practical was employed. Three per cent of the R.N.'s and 15 per cent of the practicals were frankly employed to do the housework or take care of the children; and 23 per cent of the R.N.'s and 36 per cent of the practicals were employed because the family either had no time or was too tired.

Patients who had had nurses in the hospital were also

asked why they had special nurses instead of depending upon the regular nursing care furnished by the hospital. The returns were as follows:

TABLE 40. PER CENT OF PATIENTS GIVING EACH TYPE OF REASON FOR EMPLOYING SPECIAL NURSES IN THE HOSPITAL

	Men	Women	All patients
Because most of the patient's friends have special nurses when in hospitals	2%	2%	2%
Because hospital suggested that private patients usually have special nurses	3	2	3
Because the patient felt that the regular nursing service furnished by the hospital would not be sufficient	22	22	22
Because the members of the family wanted to be sure the patient had the best possible care	31	33	33
Because the physician felt the patient was so ill that special nursing care was necessary	42	41	40

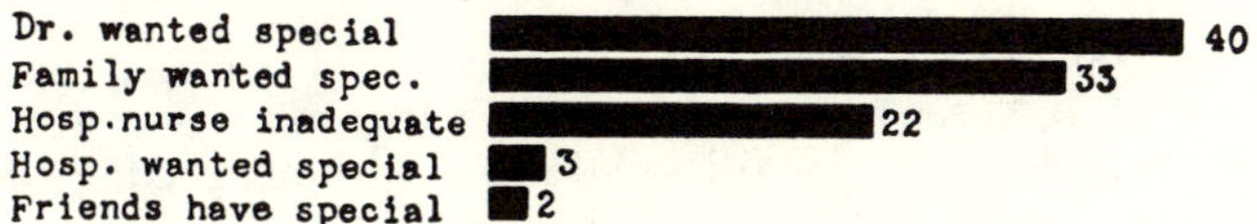

Diagram 26.—Per cent of all patients having special nurses in the *hospital* for each reason

It will be noted that among hospital patients there is practically no difference between men and women. The three chief reasons for having a special in the hospital are, first, that the physician urged it; second, the family felt that having a special would mean that the patient received better care; and third, the patient himself felt that the regular hospital service would be inadequate.

There seems to be very little difference in this point of

view among the patients living in cities of different sizes, but there is a marked difference in the per cent of physicians who urge the employment of special duty nurses for each different type of case.

Surgical cases........	41% of the physicians urged special nurses
Medical cases........	47% of the physicians urged special nurses
Obstetrical...........	22% of the physicians urged special nurses
Pediatric............	47% of the physicians urged special nurses
Contagious...........	69% of the physicians urged special nurses
Mental or nervous.....	53% of the physicians urged special nurses
Other...............	50% of the physicians urged special nurses
Total................	40% of the physicians urged special nurses

6. Hourly and Group Nursing

Some attempt was made to discover to what extent patients were thinking in terms of hourly and group nursing. The questions were:

"If you had a nurse in the home, would you be interested in a plan by which you could arrange to have her come in for an hour or two each day, charging only for the time she gave?"

"When you had a nurse at home, would you have welcomed an opportunity to talk over her work with a nurse supervisor if you could have done so without getting the nurse into trouble, or do you feel that a visit from a nurse supervisor would not have been of any particular help to the nurse or the patient?"

Some 59 per cent of the patients felt that they would have been interested in some plan for hourly service. In general, the per cent increases as the size of the city in which the patient lives grows smaller, but the difference is not marked. In answering the question about opportunities for talking with a visiting nurse supervisor, 30 per cent of the patients felt that it would have been an advantage to have had some opportunity of that kind.

Patients were also asked:

"If you had a special nurse in the hospital, would you be interested in a plan by which three or four patients shared the cost and services of the same nurse?"

Just as was the case with hourly nursing, 59 per cent of all the patients said that they would be definitely interested in some plan for group nursing. There was greater interest expressed in group nursing by patients living in rural communities than by patients in the larger cities.

7. SUMMARY

a. The reports from patients agree closely with those from physicians as to the ratio of R.N.'s to practical nurses; the location of cases; nurses' hours; pay, and the like.

b. Most patients secure practical nurses through their own physicians, but R.N.'s through hospital registries.

c. The typical R.N. charges $6.00 a day, and the typical practical $5.00. R.N.'s sometimes give free service, but practicals almost never do.

d. Charges are practically uniform regardless of hours, location, type of case, or length of case.

e. Patients usually like their nurses, although they are not quite so satisfied as physicians. Eighty-six per cent of the patients (as against 89 per cent of the physicians) would like to have the same nurse again.

f. When asked "Which seems to be the more difficult problem, for the patient to pay the cost of nursing care or to get the right kind of a nurse?"

    73 per cent of the physicians, but only 54 per cent of the patients, say that the hardest problem is to pay the nurse.

27 per cent of the physicians, but 46 per cent of the patients, say that the hardest problem is to get the right kind of a nurse.

g. Of all patients having nurses in the home, only 58 per cent had them because they were ill enough to need special nursing care. The other 42 per cent employed nurses in the home chiefly because a capable, unworried, reasonably intelligent worker was needed to take charge at a time of family crisis.

h. Of all patients having special nurses in the hospital, 40 per cent did so because the physician felt the patient was ill enough to need a special nurse, 33 per cent because the patient's family wanted to be sure that the patient had the best possible care, and 22 per cent because the patient believed that the regular nursing care furnished by the hospital would not be adequate.

i. There are marked differences according to the type of case in the per cents of physicians urging special rather than staff nursing.

j. About three-fifths of the patients were definitely interested in the possibilities of group and hourly nursing.

CHAPTER 11

WHAT THE PATIENTS SAY

The better the nursing, the less the ordinary patient thinks about it. This should be remembered in reading the quotations which follow, for, except where patients are unusually observant, the methods by which the skilful nurse succeeds in keeping the patient steadily moving along the path towards recovery are imperceptible to him. The good nurse may say to the mother, "See how nice and pink your finger-nails are!" But she does not say, "See how by manicuring your nails I have made you stop worrying about your baby!" The traditions of the profession even inhibit the nurse (and this is probably unwise) from discussing her psychological technique with the physician in charge, for fear that she may appear to be overly proud of her own tact and insight. The result is that patients, and sometimes doctors, fail to realize that the "stubborn" or "charming"; "brusk" or "wonderfully kind"; "silent" or "interesting" nurse may be playing a part called for by the condition of the particular patient. She may not have been born that way; she may simply be practising the art of nursing.

The second thing to realize in reading the reports of patients (and this applies particularly to those who have had nurses in the home) is that hospitals call back for their own specialing those among their graduates who are particularly good nurses; and keep these nurses so busy on hospital work that comparatively few of them spend much of their time on home cases. Some of the stories in the section on home nursing give a black picture. It is not believed that they represent nurses who are typical of the rank and file of the profession, or even of the best of the home duty nurses. There is ample evidence at hand, however, to indicate that high grade private duty nurses taking home cases are obliged to compete with altogether too many low grade nurses, actually licensed under lenient state laws to practise nursing, but totally unfit to be called nurses. While these women are occasionally found in the hospital (witness a few of the hospital stories!) they cannot usually find hospital employment even by the hospitals which put them into the profession. They make most of their living from patients in the home. There are probably many hundreds of patients (and unfortunately many hundreds of physicians) whose whole idea of the nursing profession is based upon their experience with the "servant girl type" of nurse such as is described by some of these patients.

1. Good Nursing in Home and Hospital

Patients tend to be appreciative of good nursing. The frequency with which *adaptability* is mentioned is quite striking.

> MARYLAND.—She was neat and particular with me and my baby. She kept her eye on the boys for me through the day. Both baby and I got on wonderfully. I surely would like her again.
>
> RHODE ISLAND.—We were particularly pleased with the nurse we had because of two outstanding characteristics she possessed to the extreme: first, unqualified willingness to help in any way she could; second, her cheerfulness. It should be mentioned that the case was not a trying one and although on 24-hour duty she managed to get a fairly good night's rest all the time. My wife is not well or

strong (her father was the patient) and the nurse volunteered to wash dishes for occasional meals, etc. In one sentence, we like her because she tried to fit herself into our particular needs—accommodated us as her employers and endeavored to make herself worth $6.00 a day to us. This she did and more. (And she got a little more because we appreciated it and it was Christmas!)

State Unknown.—The whole household, including the servants, liked this nurse. She was always tactful, quiet, and refined in her manner, often doing work which could not usually be asked of a nurse, when there was illness or absence of servants. She was at all times professional in an unobtrusive way. She was loyal to doctors and patient and discreet regarding the personal affairs of the family. We especially trusted her because she did not gossip about previous patients or narrate her professional experiences. She was always cheerful and quietly optimistic. I know this all sounds "too good to be true," yet it is true, nevertheless. Would that there were more like her!

California.—Tips? No. We wanted to but she told us that we had paid her for service rendered and quality of service would not be affected by tip or no tip.

North Dakota.—She did not expect to be waited upon. For anything we didn't have she soon found something that would do. To be able to fit in any home is the greatest asset a nurse can have.

Illinois.—One immediately felt she knew her business and there was that delightful sense of peace that comes with perfect understanding between friends and she had a decided sense of humor. You know what a wonderful gift that is. I have my very kind and capable doctor to thank for getting this splendid nurse.

KANSAS.—Mine was a very serious case, my baby being an instrument case. I required so much attention as I was torn so badly and if she had not used every caution and care I might have been infected. She was always in the best of humor and had a sunny disposition. She fixed my trays all of the time. In the home she did not go ahead as she did in the hospital. She was not as thoughtful of me as she should have been in my home and I suggest that the nurses be trained to be more self-reliant and more thoughtful in the home.

KANSAS.—The case under observation was lobar pneumonia following five weeks of a severe attack of whooping-cough. The patient was a delicate 2 year old baby girl. The nurse we employed was entirely competent, conscientious, kindly but firm, considering above all else the welfare of her patient but at the same time using all consideration for others. She was constant and tireless in her service and was a Christian. Fair in her reports to us concerning the case, giving neither false hope nor despair. She kept the patient clean but was most careful not to use more linen than was necessary. She was careful to cause just as little added work as was possible. We would indeed employ her again if occasion demanded because we feel she was the greatest factor in saving our baby and because her services were entirely satisfactory. Another thing we appreciated was that when her experience told her the case had reached the point where we could handle it as well as she, she told us and did not stay on with added expense to us.

ILLINOIS.—I will always feel that if it was not for the excellent care my nurse gave me my babies and myself would not have been here. So, of course, if there is anything I can do in my small way to help the nursing cause along, I will be more than glad to do so.

RHODE ISLAND.—This was a very severe mastoid case with complicating anæmia from the type of infection. Patient was severely ill for a long time. I can truthfully say that had it not been for the type of nursing given the child, she would not have been the healthy, robust child she is today.

CONNECTICUT.—For ten months we had the same two nurses on a case of encephalitis. The patient needed constant care and was not left alone ten minutes at a time, day or night. I was thankful that I could afford the best and give my time to their care. "God bless trained nurses!" I often say.

CALIFORNIA.—She put in over-time several days in order to see that the child was doing what he should do. She was continually thinking of things to amuse him. He loved her very much and she gave me confidence during the critical days.

PENNSYLVANIA.—I could begin today and talk for a month of the wonderful nurse I had. I am sorry that you don't have the opportunity of knowing her—she was one of the sweetest and best nurses a patient could have. A mighty fine nurse as I was seriously ill and to her goes a great deal of credit for my recovery.

NEW MEXICO.—She was ready at all times to do her duty and was loyal to the physician and family. She was neat in appearance, kept everything in the sick room neat and tidy, and carried out orders as given.

COLORADO.—She was on duty twenty hours every day and some days more. She worked hard and did everything possible for my comfort and well-being. Even after she was discharged and her pay stopped, she came in every day for several days and waited upon me.

KENTUCKY.—She was like a mother to me although I was older than she.

VIRGINIA.—I liked my private nurse because of her gentleness, her patience, her sympathy and her ladylike manners. Of course she was efficient, but efficiency does not always carry with it popularity—not the ability to make one's self indispensable to a patient.

MAINE.—My nurse was quiet and very willing and would always get up in the night with a smile.

ILLINOIS.—She was a red-headed old maid. Very pleasing and on the job all of the time. She was thinking of her work all of the time. I would want her again.

NEW YORK.—She was a lady and a nurse. She was one who made you feel that you were safe in her care.

MISSOURI.—I count her among my most valued friends now, and we had never met prior to my illness.

CALIFORNIA.—As mother of child this nurse cared for, can say that nurse handled child much better than I ever could.

MISSISSIPPI.—They were not arbitrary in enforcing the doctor's orders but gave me time and encouragement. They managed to move and change me without causing pain.

CALIFORNIA.—She had the ability to have me do the thing that I did not want to do and make me feel that that was what I really wanted. She was a joy to have near you although she was not young or good looking.

IDAHO.—I appreciated the service of my nurse as she was so quiet and efficient and followed doctor's instructions regardless of my whims or wishes. I suffered greatly and often did not wish to take the treatment she was instructed to give me but she was firm in her determination to do as instructed and I know now that that is what saved my life.

North Carolina.—If I objected to something the doctor had ordered on the ground of pain, or because I felt it unwise, she did not attempt to order me about herself, but was willing to consult the doctor and then stood by what he said. We always adjusted everything with perfect satisfaction to all. She did not seem to feel as some do, that the doctor was an august person not to be disturbed by any questions from the patient, but was ready and willing to ask him anything I wanted to know at any time.

South Dakota.—Tactful, considerate, alert to every need, firm in seeing that the doctor's orders were carried out to the letter—I fail to see where this particular nurse could be improved upon.

Michigan.—She was very thoughtful, especially proficient, it seemed to me, and very careful. She was powerful and stern without it becoming annoying and to me her ability to carry on an intelligent and interesting conversation was most helpful. She enjoyed nursing and certainly showed it in her work.

New Jersey.—She did things at times that annoyed me and I thought a bit hard, but since, and consider ing that my nerves were a great part of the trouble, I have come to the conclusion that it was probably just what I needed *and she knew it.*

Virginia.—The three hospital nurses who looked after me were all lovely too. I especially admired them because of their good dispositions and their friendliness. They were all entire strangers to me, yet I now feel that I have a friend in each of them. Furthermore they always had time to look in with a smile, no matter how rushed they were.

South Carolina.—After I had dismissed these ladies, I found out by comparison that they made my bed a little better, bathed me a little better and with less effort, than the nurses in attendance. Remember that the attendant nurses were girls in training having completed about one and one-half years of a three-year course.

MASSACHUSETTS.—In all of the time that I was in the hospital I was never spoken to crossly by any of my nurses. The nature of my illness and my age (68 years) made me a very hard patient to take care of.

ILLINOIS.—I think the patience and kindness shown in this hospital by all connected with it are wonderful. I am a paralytic case and have been on my back all the time and have had no bed-sores or trouble of any kind.

CALIFORNIA.—Nurses made me feel as though they were interested in me personally. Although that wasn't necessary it made one feel at home and not hemmed in by four bare walls.

KANSAS.—The reason I would go back to the same hospital was because I received such good care from the doctor and the nurse. They make one feel as though she was on a visit instead of in a hospital. They were always so jolly and happy it made you feel happy too and you forgot your own trouble, and then the operation was such a success.

MASSACHUSETTS.—She has been an eye-opener to me to realize the deep-rooted genuine interest taken in the technique of her calling. I don't believe anything short of a storm would make her forget even the most minor detail in treatments.

FLORIDA.—This nurse was pleasing to look at, neat and clean and quiet, a cultured and educated woman from a fine training school, where the entrance requirements are high. She did not talk, but could, if it was desired. To me, a sick patient, this was a great virtue.

Missouri.—Seemed to possess an understanding of scientific principles underlying her work.

Wisconsin.—When it was necessary that I have the services of a private nurse over a period of nine weeks, I noted a marked difference between the work of a nurse who received her training in the county hospital compared with the work of the nurse who was trained in a private institution. The county trained nurse, substituting for a period of ten days, was very dictatorial and very careless in her technique, while the other nurse was always courteous, careful in her work, and always solicitous of my personal comfort.

Missouri.—Nurse is a Canadian. To her nursing is a profession in which she takes pride. I think we should try to raise the standard of nursing in the U. S. A. by raising the requirements for admission to our training schools which should work with a university and give a degree to graduate nurses.

California.—She is well educated, proficient in her work, and a delightful personality. She anticipated my every want and I felt perfectly confident that she would do the best possible for my new baby. Should it be necessary again, I should be greatly pleased to have the same nurse. She is the daughter of a doctor and to my mind a very splendid example of what a woman in her profession should be.

2. Poor Nursing

Although the paragraphs which follow will present to many nurses a painful and well-nigh incredible picture, it is necessary to include them because they are truly representative of a large body of testimony from patients in all parts of the country.

Note: The following quotation is given at length because it is of especial significance. The patient, who signed her name, is personally known to a member of the Committee as a woman of sanity and essential fairness, with a broad professional background. She is the wife of a clergyman and the mother of several children. She told a member of the Committee that she had been in the hospital previously (it is a famous hospital in a large city) and received such excellent care that she had been eager to return. She remarked, however, "I knew that the former superintendent of nurses had resigned, but I had no idea that that could have such an effect on the quality of nursing service!" Extracts from her report follow:

No nursing care provided during labor. The night nurse on the floor went off for a rest period; the only nurse left was the one in charge of the babies, and since there were about twelve of these to be taken out for feedings she had no time to watch antepartum cases and had never seen a woman in labor.

This doubtless was partly my own fault, since I should have demanded my own doctor early in labor. I had not the faintest idea, however, that there wouldn't be any one to answer my calls when real need arose.

It was interesting, afterwards to note the attitude of the nurses. All the student nurses knew that I had narrowly escaped being "a precipitate"—a disgrace to the nurse who was responsible, and they took turns in reproving me because I didn't begin screaming early.

Inconsiderate attitude. Some 5 or 6 hours after delivery the nurse brought bowl, cloth, etc., and instructed me to take a bath. I remarked that I wasn't sure I could; I was still pretty dopey with morphine, whereupon the nurse waxed pretty tart. As a matter of fact, I had had a hemorrhage, and the doctor had given the morphine and urged especial quiet, and watched some time by my bed to make sure I got it; after his departure the nurse swung into her routine adapted to cases a little more fit.

The nurses grumbled openly, "This is nothing but an enema shop" and "they make me sick," referring to other patients, etc.

Poor training for the baby's feeding habits. The time at which baby was brought to me to nurse varied as much as 90 minutes, contrasting with the clinic doctor's advice to "nurse the baby on the hour, not 5 minutes before and not 5 minutes after."

(The patient then described an appalling lack of decent bed-pan technique.)

On the whole I felt sorry for the nurses; I felt so sure that conditions could not be good or such a wholesale attitude of dejection and irritability could not have prevailed. I feel this especially as I had had two highly satisfactory experiences in the same hospital, same grade of room, etc. I felt

(a) Nurses had too much to do. One nurse, with the assistance of the floor maid, had 10 to 14 patients to care for, according to the nurses' accounts.

(b) Supervision—real supervision—seemed almost totally lacking. An assistant supervisor came once a day to collect the napkins; neither the supervisor nor assistant supervisor made any inquiry as to patient's condition nor the kind of care she was getting, etc. They never accompanied student nurses to see how they were doing their work. The nurses seemed left to their own devices.

There may have been arrangements for supervision of which I knew nothing—doubtless there were—but surely something was lacking or those girls would not have grumbled so much, and might have displayed more pride in their jobs.

Of some 14 different nurses, only 3 seemed to have ideals of helping the patient. One said, "Wouldn't it be lovely to have only one patient—you could make her so comfortable?" But she was tired and worried. Most of the others grumbled openly or shrugged and were apathetic. Surely some spark of enthusiasm and hopefulness and pride of work could have been infused by a good supervisor. The floor maid was as hurried as the nurses in point of time, but she carried a different atmosphere. She was older and had developed her own point of view.

New Jersey.—Nurse came on duty with smell of cigarettes on fingers to a patient with temperature of 105 who did not smoke.

Kansas.—When nurse was giving my bath she rolled me out of bed. I hit a commode and stayed in hospital longer, due to three broken ribs.

California.—Smoked in room as soon as I emerged from ether.

State not Known.—I was seriously and painfully burned with paraffin on both my arms, from shoulder down to tips of my fingers on the left arm, and from my elbow to my fingers on my right arm, and of course I was unable to help myself at all. I am a nurse myself, and I had some ideas about the way patients as sick as I was should be treated.

In the first place, I was unable to get a private room, because of the usual crowded condition of a hospital in the winter. I had to take a four-bed ward. She did not like this at all, and kept me smothered with screens. I did not tell her I was a nurse, as I was interested in making a test.

The first three or four days were terrible suffering for me, and I think I must have been delirious one night, for I woke up, and I was completely uncovered, and being near an open window I began to shiver. I groaned and the patient across from me asked me if I wanted my nurse. She had just left for midnight lunch. I was unable to even ring the bell. So I told her to wait a bit, perhaps I could stand it, but she said as long as I was paying for special services to call her. So she did. And in a few moments my special came in. She snapped on the lights and said, "Well, I can't even eat without you calling me." She covered me again, and marched out. The other patient said, "You poor little dear, why do you keep her, when she is so impudent?" But I said that perhaps she was hungry.

But the rest of the nights were really nightmares to me. The pain was intense, and my doctor had left order for narcotics p.r.n. The ward nurses were lovely to me, and gave me one when I could not stand it any longer, but my night nurse would argue me out of it, because she would be sound asleep before I had to disturb her, and I guess she did not want to get up to get it.

On the whole, there were innumerable incidents that make me grind my teeth when I think of her.

California.—Probationer on night duty, no night superintendent, attempted a catheterization, and failed. Another who was on a private case next door came to her rescue.

The night nurse gave my baby to another mother to nurse, the mother recognized that it was my baby (the practice in this hospital seemed to be to take the babies from room to room on exhibition). On her refusal the nurse (student) insisted that it was her baby. After much discussion pro and con, the baby was brought to me for decision. The one thing that was the determining factor in the case was the fact that my baby was a girl and the other was a boy. This fact was recorded on the chart.

I liked the food and the manner in which it was served.

I think that nurses should receive some instruction and should be supervised until they are acquainted with the nursing care a patient requires, especially since the hospitals accept such young, inexperienced, uneducated girls in training.

California.—I think the nursing care of the baby would have been improved by a larger number of pupil nurses on duty at a time and by smaller nurseries. The baby was sometimes wet and cold when brought in because she had to be changed *in her turn* instead of just before leaving the nursery. The nurse in charge of the ward was one of the loveliest women I have ever met and altogether my experience at this hospital, without special nurse, but with careful, cheerful service of student nurses and occasional visits from the head nurse, remains a pleasant memory.

MINNESOTA.—Our little son was in a large hospital last spring as a feeding case and was on general care. He had never been sore before, but became raw while there. I do not consider general care in large hospitals adequate.

CALIFORNIA.—She never left me alone with my husband or callers for any length of time. If she left the room she returned within a few minutes to join in the conversation if she liked the person calling. She took an intense dislike to my mother, and when she called she would sit, silent but always present, in the corner of the room. As my parents had come from a great distance because of my illness and I had not seen them for over a year, it was very difficult to handle without hurting her feelings and still manage to have a private visit. They were not able to remain in the city after I returned home, and this made every minute especially precious to me.

STATE NOT KNOWN.—I had a fractured femur and hip. The night nurse used to leave a small pus basin for me to urinate in—when this was full I had nothing to use, and the nurse would not answer my bell. One night I got to crying, and she came in and scolded me for making a noise and went out slamming the door, but without emptying the pan. I was obliged to pour the urine on the floor.

OHIO.—I was in a small hospital where five nurses

were in charge, with only one patient there when I went for surgical work. But somehow before I was out of the ether they gave me a third degree burn with a hot-water bag. After that happened I ordered a special nurse, as I didn't think the hospital was giving me proper attention and care.

Massachusetts.—Night nurse very efficient, but one objection to her was her habit of constantly praising a certain surgeon (a very popular one in this city, especially this hospital) and speaking slightingly in comparison of the surgeon I had. To me it was very objectionable, as I had utmost confidence in mine, but had I been as nervous as I have been in past years, it would actually have worried me; as it was, however, it merely "riled" me.

Illinois.—The night nurse had to be awakened by the patient for any service needed at all. They manifested no interest in the patient at all, permitted constipation to exist too long and to such an extent that a rectal fissure developed, all the time recording on the chart—patient fine. Doctor read the chart and paid no attention to the patient's story. Night nurse left patient alone one hour at midnight every night when she went to her supper. One night patient in delirium got out on floor and lay there until nurse came back.

California.—One of the worst things about general care, and I found this a common thing in *all* of the mentioned hospitals, was that the nurses were not instructed to give a patient a basin of water to cleanse herself after a bowel movement. Not a single nurse ever gave me water to cleanse the genitalia and hands *without being asked* to do so, and then it was often done grudgingly. Surely, they wouldn't want to be left in such a condition!

Another horrible thing to me is the system of awakening sick people at five and six o'clock in the morning for early care. Often one has just fallen asleep after a restless night. Surely sick people need all of the rest that they can get.

While at . . . . . this practice was discontinued, the patients being awakened at seven, and I know one thing, and that was that the patients were better pleased.

Most hospitals serve their meals too close together, and the patient is not allowed to get hungry. . . . . was the only exception, serving at eight, one, and six o'clock.

Bells are not answered promptly in any of the hospitals where I have been a patient. Everywhere the nurses have too much to do, and have no time to devote to the ART of nursing.

ARIZONA.—The nurse looked upon her doctor as a deity, and the patient as a mere instrument to be handled according to directions. She tried to force the doctor's orders instead of putting patient's objections up to him. Patients are treated too much like automatons both by doctors and nurses; you would actually think from the superior airs adopted by both that they were infallible and that the patient never had any experience in the treatment of disease or the care of his own health. Knowing the experiments that doctors are continually making in order to find proper remedies, and knowing something about the mistakes made by some doctors, I do not believe any one should be foolish enough to resign his body to a nurse and doctor to do anything they like with it.

PENNSYLVANIA.—Perhaps she knew her stuff, but she treated a human being like a piece of metallic crockery. I felt better after she was gone.

GEORGIA.—This nurse was fine if you didn't want her to do something. Then she would get out of patience. She liked to sit around and gossip about her boy friends, uninteresting and painful to me in my condition. I needed quiet. The first night after my delivery I didn't call her all night. I guess she expected this to continue. The next night I was very uncomfortable, and I called her several times, and she called me down, saying that it was all in my head. I told my husband that my nerves would be a wreck if she stayed on much longer, so I let her go and had the students take care of me. They knew their profession. This other nurse couldn't even catheterize.

NEW YORK.—After giving painstaking and efficient care during most serious part of illness, she wore an air of boredom during my convalescence which irritated me. Since I had been sick for a year and was pretty well bored myself, my own boredom was about all I could stand.

DELAWARE.—My nurse's only fault was that she sometimes talked too much.

NEW YORK.—I was never given a clean bed-pan in four months. Other patients said the same thing.

NEW JERSEY.—She cleansed the rectum with cotton and with the same piece wiped the inside of the thighs, which felt unclean even if the cotton looked clean.

INDIANA.—She forgot to wash the baby's mouth, was more concerned about charting how many times he urinated in a day than in keeping his little legs from chafing, and she did not remove the bands around my breasts and abdomen in giving an alcohol rub.

ILLINOIS.—The night I went to the hospital I wasn't feeling the best, and the nurse that got me ready was very rough and careless. Everything she did was work, but she was only on night duty two nights while I was there. She was rough about shaving me. She got the bed wet. She would never be a good nurse, for she acted disagreeable all of the time. I was very much relieved when she left.

I was very much opposed to going to the hospital. I never had been ill or sick before. But now I know that it is the only place to go in such a case. I shall go to the same hospital and have the same doctor if I am taken ill again.

ALABAMA.—She wasn't as sanitary in her methods as the patient thought necessary, except when the doctor was present.

ILLINOIS.—My nurse handled dressings with her bare hands and then handled my baby. She did not seem to know what my doctor wanted done.

NEW YORK.—Not competent in emergency, failed to recognize severe bleeding after cæsarean section. I almost died.

PENNSYLVANIA.—My husband was no trouble, not sick, that is, no fever. He had endocarditis, and sat up in chair most of the time, and sometimes at night had gas on stomach and needed relief. I always got up at night because the nurses, except the first one, stayed in bed. The night before he died at 11.40 he had some trouble with gas. I got up and in few minutes called the nurse, who had been very pert and disagreeable to him for the week and a half she was here. She got up and gave him some medicine and went right back to bed again. I worked with him until 2.30, and she never coming near, when I called up the doctor and told him. He told me what to do and promised another nurse in the morning. The nurse, when she heard me phone the doctor, was very angry and called him up, I do not know what she said, but she talked dreadfully to me and my husband, and banged doors. I finally ordered her out of the room and to bed, and she said she would do as she pleased. I said she had to be quiet and go to bed or leave the house. It was about 3.00 or

3.30 A.M. So she went to bed. I stayed with my husband all night. Was afraid to leave him alone. The doctor and another nurse arrived about 7.00 A.M., and the nurse causing all this trouble informed the new nurse that he was dying. I asked her before the doctor and new nurse arrived if she could not give him anything to relieve him. She answered very pert "No, nothing more can be done for him," in his presence. He was perfectly conscious and told her she had no heart and it would come back to her some day. She acted all the time as if she were mad—never smiled.

The last one the doctor brought that morning looked like a little girl and very anemic looking, very white lips, and she told me afterwards she had a spot on her lung. She was very nice, but head full of boys. The nurses all were so very young, 20, 21, 22, and seemed very much younger and did not seem to be nursing for anything but for money, and to do as little as possible. It has decided me against trained nurses, practical ones having far more common sense and judgment. Two nurses I did not like took three and four hours off every afternoon. My husband died that evening at 7.20. Can you wonder I am bitter against trained nurses?

NEW YORK.—Treated patients roughly, had no idea of technique of contagion, did not realize the seriousness of condition of the patient, did not obey orders.

MASSACHUSETTS.—I think that nurses should not be so touchy about taking suggestions from the patients. For instance, in the care of the baby, not so on their dignity that the patient is afraid to ask for what she wants. That is a common fault and makes the patient nervous and uncomfortable. If the nurse feels she knows best, she should be willing to talk it over with the patient, and not be omnipotent and mysterious in her power and annoyed if her discretion is questioned.

NEW YORK.—The first nurse was very undesirable, although I kept her for fear of hurting the doctor's feelings. She gave my boy his powders wrong twice, and what my family did not like about her was that she heated the same flaxseed poultice all night and refused to make a fresh one during the five nights she was there. She never saw the doctor once, for she got to the house at 8.30 P.M. or 9.00 P.M., after he had made his call.

But I certainly cannot say enough in gratitude for the other nurses whom I had for fourteen nights. They were really a pleasure to have in the home and were so devoted to the patients. They well earned their money and were worth more if I could have afforded it.

OHIO.—I liked my nurse because she was good company and would smoke and drink high balls with me in addition to rendering me any little services and comforts. One day my husband came home and found us both a little drunk. He immediately discharged the nurse, and I made a rapid recovery.

I cannot recommend temperance too strongly to nurses and other women—especially against drinking with other women in the day-time and at other times without one's husband present.

WISCONSIN.—I have had eight graduate nurses in my home at different times. Of this number, there were only two I would have called again.

Of the other six I would say that they had two faults which were outstanding. Either they were lazy or careless as regards cleanliness, or both. Three of the nurses were so dirty in the care of the patient as to be a positive menace.

NEW JERSEY.—I liked her because she was kind and patient and mixed well with my family and servants, and because of her attitude toward my husband

and the other men of the household. I did not like her management—she gave me no time to rest or sleep. She was so slow getting me ready for bed and so slow during the day with her work that I was alone to rest only about seven hours out of twenty-four.

MARYLAND.—The second one was competent, but was harsh, disagreeable and dictatorial. She interfered with and was rude to the household servants, broke up china, mislaid various articles, and was a nuisance in the home. At the hospital she was disagreeable and dissatisfied, and was inclined to avoid carrying out orders which required exaction or unusual services.

WEST VIRGINIA.—The nurse I had shirked every duty she could put on my maid or my laundress. She continually found fault, although we have a comfortable home, and things were arranged for her convenience. She quarreled with my maid and my children.

KENTUCKY.—She was a woman with a family. During her hours off in the afternoon she went home, cleaned the house and cooked and prepared meals for the family, and came back to her patient worn out and unloaded family troubles to a patient too weak to scarcely live, without knowing the burdens of a nurse.

CALIFORNIA.—She was very unpleasant to my housekeeper, who is a very refined woman, and if I had kept the nurse longer I am sure it would have necessitated my finding new help, so we had no regrets in letting her go.

CALIFORNIA.—Personal appearance very unattractive, untidy. Never remembered to give medicine on time. Couldn't prepare the simplest sick-room diet properly. Entertained her husband two evenings at patient's house. In short, she was the poorest excuse for a registered nurse it has ever been my misfortune to meet.

New York.—She had dancing, booze parties and in general good time on the brain all of the time. Would appear many times as tired and lazy the next day after a booze party. Spent too much time talking over the phone making dates with her gentlemen friends.

(Doctor's note—added as postscript: This nurse was the exception, not the rule. There are a few of these nurses, but not many.)

3. Education and Breeding

The few quotations that follow tally with statements made by physicians as to the somewhat shocking lack of breeding displayed by *some* nurses.

California.—The nurse was not strict enough and deferred to my desires too much for various things. This was probably due to the fact that she had just graduated and was very young—21 years of age.

Oklahoma.—Would have liked her better if she had had a more pleasing personality, and a more general education. I like to think of a nurse as being more than a servant or someone just to carry out orders. Certainly they should be psychologists.

Texas.—It seems to me that the nurses (I have had experience with several recently) I have had dealings with are poorly educated, with mediocre training, temperamental, demanding high salaries for small services—expecting much in the way of equipment, food, service, without regard to cost.

Massachusetts.—My criticism is that applicants for training should be considered more carefully before being taken into training. Some of them are sadly lacking in education and this helps a great deal in all walks of life. Some of them are unfitted for the profession.

NEW YORK.—The majority of student nurses on the hospital staff, in my opinion, are so very young as to make them insensible to the real duty of a nurse.

MINNESOTA.—She talked so much as to be exhausting, even keeping me awake to talk.

PENNSYLVANIA.—One nurse in particular worked only with the thought of a gift in her mind, and she was particularly below the other nurses in every way, *i. e.*, her grammar, her conversation, her moral character and general demeanor were those of a girl who has recently come from a mill, which I believe is true. Her desire to finish her work, to shirk duty, and to worry about her gift was very pronounced, but I must say that this does not apply to any other girl at that hospital with whom I have come in contact.

ILLINOIS.—My nurse was well educated and capable of a more pleasing companionability than the general run of younger girls at the hospital, many of whom were not only frightfully ignorant, but just plain dumb.

NEBRASKA.—She could not carry on an intelligent conversation.

4. General Comments on Hospital Care

The patients' comments will remind hospital administrators of facts the good ones already know, i. e., a good nursing service requires an adequate number of workers, adequate equipment, and careful supervision. There is no more frequent comment than that stressing the constant pressure on the nursing service.

NEW YORK.—I am a registered nurse and during my stay at the hospital I found that the regular hospital nurse was superior to the private duty nurse I had obtained from a registry. She was very busy, having at least eight patients to care for, but she did the very best she could to make all of her patients most comfortable.

WISCONSIN.—If one is really sick or needs much attention, the regular nurse service given in hospitals where the work is done by student nurses does not amount to much, as these girls have entirely too much to do and do not have enough supervision by really capable nurses.

CALIFORNIA.—The floor nurse who was nicest and most interested in her patients and really tried to make them comfortable had her cap taken away during the patient's stay in the hospital because she had stayed out a little longer than the hours allowed for student nurses at night.

IOWA.—Patients are sometimes neglected when depending on general nursing because in some cases the nurses are given too many to look after.

PENNSYLVANIA.—Without a special nurse I would not go to the hospital again. The regular staff did all they could but, with so many to care for, especially when they had operations, there would be a long time that a nurse was not available when needed.

NEW YORK.—The hurried way in which you were done up for the night. For a rub, you get a few passes up the back, rolled back into the same nest from which you came, bedding not even straightened, pillows not shaken up or adjusted, and there you are left. Now these are exceptional cases, but it occurred to me that a nurse's duty was to make the patient at least as comfortable as possible for the night. With a few exceptions I have had excellent care and would return if ill. The exceptions, when reported, have been jacked up by the head nurse, who was very delightful.

NEW YORK.—The night nurse had to help in the operating room when there was a delivery, leaving the floor without any one. They were the best nurses but overworked.

New York.—They did their work conscientiously and pleasantly, but there was too much work for them to do satisfactorily to the patient. In other words, there were too few nurses.

Massachusetts.—During the morning there were three or four nurses on the floor so I could get one quickly, but during the afternoon and night we had only one nurse and she was kept very busy. They were supposed to go off at 7 P.M., but they often worked until 8 P.M. and I could see that they were very tired. They were very sweet and always tried to do everything possible for our comfort.

Massachusetts.—One nurse in training is insufficient to take care of 20 patients on two floors after 7 P.M. The nurse was given more than was humanly possible for one person to do. It took her one hour in the evening to remove the patients' flowers from the rooms to the corridors. She not only acted as nurse but as flower girl too.

Pennsylvania.—There were only two nurses on duty at night and if any extra cases came in one of the nurses had to go to the delivery room and it left us with only one nurse. It was too much for one nurse to do to answer all of the bells, etc.

Pennsylvania.—I know it would have been a great relief to our night nurse if she had had some help. She had about 21 mothers and 24 babies to take care of. She told us in particular of having gone to bed at 10 A.M., couldn't sleep because they were house-cleaning, and then getting up at 2 P.M. for class until 6 P.M. She certainly was almost run off of her feet.

Pennsylvania.—Does not rinse utensils after use, such as those used for washing and cleaning the teeth. After all, it is the little cheerful offerings of service that mean so much to the patient in bed for some time. In justice to this nurse, must say that she has 14 patients, 7 of whom are bed patients and perhaps, after all, she does all she can for us.

ILLINOIS.—In the two hospitals that I have been in, there has been a shortage of nurses, for at times the baby would be left with me for as long as two hours. They had inexperienced nurses on the floor to give us our baths, etc., who were only in training a week or two.

NEW YORK.—I have come to recognize nurses, as a class, as the most self-sacrificing, considerate body of people I know. But I have yet to see one on duty who wasn't in a hurry. They always seem to have every minute provided for, either in duties or in class. It is from this fact, I would say, that perhaps there is a shortage.

STATE UNKNOWN.—Tips for nurses? Yes, but they were not expected. Got the same service tip or no tip. The orderly service could be improved. The men expected tips and plainly indicated it. I gave each a stated amount each week, and got good treatment.

LOUISIANA.—The head nurse was entirely too personal and her speech with the doctors, while attending to patients, was too vulgar, so much so that it would not bear repetition, and I'm neither narrow nor old.

ILLINOIS.—If this doctor in this case was not so familiar with the nurses, the latter could give better service. What they need is discipline.

ILLINOIS.—Some nurses act too gushy and a bit too frivolous when patients are sick. Overheard crude remarks—"No. 120 croaking" and others, which made me realize how hard folks get when it's some one else. Also heard "crab" applied to the patients. I was near the desk, so that I got a poor impression of the nurses and the doctor's remarks. They don't seem to mean so much by it but it sounds very bad. Lots of them could stand a little more refinement and love of mankind and a little more appreciation of the fact that a sick body means a sick mind too, which will clear up when better health comes back.

KENTUCKY.—A good surgical nurse is not a good bedside nurse and training schools in hospitals whose cases are largely surgical specialize too much for the comfort of the patient.

NEW YORK.—Awakened at 5 A.M.—too early—and sometimes lights not out until 9 or 10 P.M. Difficult to obtain bed-pan and bottle promptly.

NEW YORK.—Why is it necessary to be awakened at 5.30 A.M. to be washed, when at 7 A.M. you are bathed, and then you are not washed for meals at any time?

WASHINGTON.—Waking me up at such an ungodly hour. I was in bad need of sleep when I left.

PENNSYLVANIA.—Not answering the bells, leaving you on a bed-pan for 20 minutes to one hour. Leaving the bed-pans around until asked to remove them.

GEORGIA.—Why couldn't there be a bed-pan provided for each room? On the floor where I was there seemed to be only 3 or 4 bed-pans. They were not sterilized after use but merely rinsed out and placed under the next one that needed it. I could not help but wonder if I could catch some contagious disease from some of the other patients.

VIRGINIA.—The diet patients on special diets, I find, often have to be the judges as to what they can eat from the tray as it is brought to them. Foods not on their list are put on their trays quite often.

NEW YORK.—My case demanded special diet and I received it as planned in quantity and food value by my doctor, but there was not the least attention given to consistency in choice of foods. Eggs three times a day for three days cease to be palatable. Receiving one's nutrition at mid-day with the flimsiest kind of supper served from 4:30 to 5:45, as best suited the special diet kitchen, does not produce the sweetest disposition. I am afraid I vented my spleen on the poor student nurse who had nothing to do with it. I know she reported it, for the intern promised to rectify it and the nurse said she had been bawled out by the dietitian. I write this that perhaps there might be some consideration given to the fact that the hospital might be to blame for the trouble and not the nurses.

California.—It seemed impossible to fit the treatment to the patient's needs. For instance, when improper food caused digestive disturbance, a requisition for hot milk instead required so many signatures that the order would be lost in the way. (I never did get the milk.)

Massachusetts.—Too much efficiency by hospital nurse and superintendent regardless of patient's welfare.

5. Costs

Here again the question of an inflexible salary schedule for private duty nurses whether good, bad, or indifferent is discussed from first-hand observation and experience.

Virginia.—Hospitals do not exercise enough supervision over nurses on private cases. Also when one pays a stiff price for a room, they should receive a little attention from a hospital nurse. As a matter of business they should receive more than a ward or charity case would receive.

Colorado.—I was forced by Hospital Management to have both a day and a night nurse, which cost me $6.00 per day each plus board for both nurses, or

$12.00 per day for both nurses plus $20.00 per week board for both nurses. This condition worked a great hardship on me.

OREGON.—I feel that the expense of a private nurse either in hospital or home is a great financial problem for the average person. I think the 24-hour duty plan would be the best for the average patient.

Besides my own case I had a mother sick in bed at home for three years, and during that time we have had to keep one registered nurse and one practical nurse all the time. Now, one with 24-hour duty and help of the three daughters would have done very nicely.

MICHIGAN.—The question of paying nurses is such a tremendous problem—people can't be ill or have operations.

ARKANSAS.—We are not able to pay either the R.N. or M.D. bills, but by borrowing on the future we were able to pay both, and I have been incapacitated for six or eight weeks.

MASSACHUSETTS.—The nurse attending me performed all duties conducive to my general comfort and did nothing to aggravate my disability. But, do nurses earn the price demanded?

NEW YORK.—$9.00 a day for seven days. Tipped her $10.00 for the week, as she seemed to expect it.

NEW YORK.—They charge too much for what they give in return and are cold and mercenary, as well as inefficient.

WISCONSIN.—It is hard to pay the nurses the high wages they command, but it is much harder to get a nurse who is skilled and conscientious in the performance of her duties.

IOWA.—The $7.00 per day charge was the greatest criticism. If a longer period of nursing than fourteen days had been necessary, it would have been impossible, from financial point of view, to have kept a registered nurse. Was well pleased with the services rendered. Had been nursed by a practical nurse on another occasion, and she was impossible.

VERMONT.—The nurse wanted $70 because he was a man. Surely it was not his fault that he appeared in the world as a male. I thought nursing was sexless.

NEW YORK.—The first day in the hospital I had a young nurse who was very irresponsible, and she was discharged. The next one was a nurse with years of experience and a priceless nurse. It seemed utterly ridiculous and all wrong to think that the first mentioned was able to demand the same salary.

TENNESSEE.—My day nurse was excellent and drew the same pay as night nurse which did not seem quite right, as night nurse was very inefficient—the young flapper type. Seems that there should be some way to compensate a thoroughly capable and interested nurse more than those that are there for the money they get and not the service they render.

CALIFORNIA.—Have had several nurses, but this one in particular I like to think of—she was quiet, refined, pleasant and above all an efficient nurse. She did not tire me out by doing too much, but knew what was to be done and made me feel free to always ask her for anything that I wanted otherwise. Such a nurse is underpaid. She is worth more than $6.00 a day.

The other kind who is unrefined and doesn't have that understanding, who taps foot of bed when standing there holding conversation, or brings *hot food*, luke warm, etc., is not worth $6.00 per day.

I believe the fault in not turning out more of the desirable kind (from my observation while in hospital) is due to the superintendent of nurses in retaining the wrong type of girl when through with probation period. An unrefined girl should be frankly told she will never make a *much wanted nurse*. We all like pleasant, tolerant, refined folks at all times and to be sure more so when indisposed.

6. Shortage

It seems probable that the matter of seasonal shortage of private duty nurses is one calling for a reorganization of registry practice.

NEW YORK.—I was in the hospital six weeks and had two day nurses and four different night nurses. Two nights when I needed a nurse the most, none could be found. We exhausted every available list. Many were taking their vacations.

MASSACHUSETTS.—This nurse was engaged for July 12, 1926. The baby came July 9, 1926, and the nurse could not get here until eight hours post-partum. In spite of phoning to various hospitals and six registries, no nurse could be obtained to assist during the delivery. Reasons given: (1) Nurses on vacations. (2) Nurses available would not take obstetrical cases.

NEW YORK.—Recently one of children had pneumonia, and our regular nurse was ill, and I was worn out for want of sleep. With seven nurses off duty I was unable to have one agree to come.

7. Hours and Duties

"Circumstances alter cases" could well be said of nurses' hours.

NEBRASKA.—In many cases a twelve hour duty nurse is the most satisfactory, as you get much more service for your money. A day nurse is on from seven to seven, and you have her when you need her. If a patient has good nights, a day nurse is all that is needed. Otherwise your patient sleeps all night and needs no extra care, and your nurse is gone half of the day—usually at a time when you need her.

MASSACHUSETTS.—On twenty-four hour duty with only the care of a perfectly well infant, she expected an average of four free hours a day, but instead of taking that amount of time every twenty-four hours, felt it her privilege to stay at home one day and take seven or eight hours the next, which did not seem at all as it should be to the patient.

NEW YORK.—If nurses' hours only overlapped a little while, say a half hour, it would help a lot.

NORTH DAKOTA.—The biggest problem arising about the nurse is where her work starts and begins. I mean, is she supposed to do the housework if there is no one else? Is she supposed to do her patient's washing and the infant's?

I believe every woman should have a nurse in a confinement case, especially in the country where you cannot go to the hospital. And in that case she should be able to do and meet with conditions of a farm home. Most of us don't have modern conveniences. Therefore, it would be better for her to know before she comes whether it is in the country or town.

GEORGIA.—I live in a country town, and in this instance and other cases I find that well-equipped, competent nurses, who are accustomed to modern conveniences, are unwilling to go into the country in their work. I do not blame them for this, for in the country proper they have a great many inconveniences to meet with and usually large crowds of visitors in the patient's room. People expect a nurse to have superhuman powers, such as doing without sleep. I find if they can be informed of the condition in the home, they will not hesitate to go into the country.

8. Practicals

Patients corroborate many of the things physicians say of practical nurses.

NEBRASKA.—By having both a practical and a registered nurse at the same time, we learned the benefits derived from three or four years of professional training.

OHIO.—We had a practical nurse the first three days and found her absolutely worthless. We think a practical nurse, because of lack of training, is more likely to be detrimental than helpful, although as a rule in this locality they charge around $35 per week.

ILLINOIS.—Unable to get graduate nurses to come out into the country. Best practical nurses charge as much as the graduate nurses.

CALIFORNIA.—I was run down, nervous, and had skin trouble which lasted a long time. I paid her graduate nurse's wages, and when I got suspicious of her, I wrote the registry and found out that she was misrepresenting herself and was not entitled to those wages. She cried all of the time and told me that her child was dying from lack ot proper housing and lack of food and that if she had $400 she could get a home, etc. I loaned her the $400, and she never gave me any security. However, I made her pay me back out of her wages. She stole over a $100 worth of sheets and pillow-cases, etc., from me. I was so nervous that I kept her rather than make a change. I did not report her to the registry, for I felt sorry for her child.

NEW YORK.—She was a practical nurse and only charged $5.00 per day. Did the housework also, but was too old and had no patience with the children.

NEW HAMPSHIRE.—Nurse lacked refinement, and

while signing herself "R.N." was not graduate of first class school with full period of training.

New York.—She was a practical nurse, but her personality was bad, irritating patient. As a matter of fact, she was disagreeable about everything.

New York.—Would have under no conditions employed a practical nurse if I could have gotten a graduate nurse.

9. Miscellaneous

Nurses have their own troubles with patients. These three comments make one understand why nurses sometimes hesitate to take home cases.

Oregon.—My biggest problem was what I could do with her if she went home with me. We were living in rather cramped quarters at the time and where room could be found for an extra member of the household was more than I could imagine. But the matter was taken out of my hands by the competent manner in which my nurse arranged things. It was hard on her because she had to sleep on a cot too short for her and her dressing room was a tiny corner behind the dresser in my room. I could not but appreciate the cheerful spirit with which she met such hardships and added to the fact that she took such good care of me is reason enough for wanting her again.

Kentucky.—When I was ready to dismiss my nurse and pay her the amount in full, a lawyer stepped in and demanded we do not pay her—there were unpaid grocery bills twice the amount of her wages and also a note (unpaid and overdue) at bank twice above amount. This worried me too. A patient so sick and weak as I was just can't have these worries.

Kansas.—Our nurse was handicapped by the fact that the doctors could not agree. Neither doctor would admit that any complications that had developed were serious. The nurse finally felt that she had to inform my parents that things were really serious. My parents brought me to the hospital and also the same nurse. The doctors here feel that the nurse realized the danger and really saved my life by being prompt and insisting on a drastic change in the way things were going. I am to return to the hospital in several months for repair work and shall certainly have the same nurse.

CHAPTER 12

WHAT ARE NURSES LIKE?

Individual reports from nurses in different branches of the profession constituted the first material collected. At that time no one had any clear idea of how many nurses were actually in active service, nor what types of work they were doing. It was not even possible to secure a single list either of nurses registered by the different states or of the members belonging to the American Nurses' Association, since in this latter case membership lists are kept not by the central office, but by the individual states.

It was soon clear that a nation-wide survey of nurses would not be practicable, partly because it would cost heavily, but primarily because it would take too long to secure mailing lists of nurses from forty-eight or more different sources. Accordingly, after many consultations, the Committee selected ten states which had signified their eagerness to cooperate in the study, were representative of different parts of the country and of different sorts of economic and nursing conditions, and had readily available lists of nurses in their own areas. These states were as follows:

Massachusetts	Illinois
New York	Kansas
Pennsylvania	Wyoming
Georgia	California
Louisiana	Washington

It will be noted that whereas in the cases of physicians and patients the inquiries of the Grading Committee cover the entire United States, the material which follows is based mainly upon returns from these ten states only. It is believed, however, that these returns are reasonably typical, since the ten states studied include 39 per cent of all the nursing schools in the country and, according to the United States Census of 1920, 50.1 per cent of all nurses actively practising the profession. It would seem, therefore, that a rather large proportion of all the nurses are probably covered in this study, and that the returns for the group may be taken as reasonably representative of conditions for the profession at large.

The cooperating organization in each state was supplied with return postals to be sent to the nurses in that state, asking certain questions concerning her professional status and history, and also asking in each case what kind of nursing, if any, the recipient expected to be doing during 1927. Some 59,000 of these cards were distributed, of which 24,389, or 41 per cent, were returned, properly filled out, to this office. This is an exceptionally high return when it is remembered that many of the cards sent to the states were in excess of the real needs and were, therefore, unused. The returned postals furnished a classified list, so that appropriately worded questionnaires could be sent to the nurses in different branches of the profession. The totals sent out and returned in this part of the study are as follows:

TABLE 41. QUESTIONNAIRES SENT OUT AND RETURNED, AND PER CENT RETURNED

Questionnaires	Sent	Returned	Per cent returned
Nurses' postals	59,000	24,389	41
Private duty nurses (March)	9,666	3,392	35
Hourly nurses	154	49	32
Public health nurses	3,422	1,456	43
Institutional nurses	4,296	1,908	44
Unclassified nurses	700	313	45
Private duty nurses (August)	9,666	2,213	23
Total	86,904	33,720	39

The findings of these studies are presented in this and the following chapter.

1. Where Was Her Father Born?

The nurses were asked in what countries their fathers were born; and the returns were compared with those for males resident in the United States, over twenty-one years of age in 1900, since this would seem to be the group most nearly comparable to present-day fathers of adult women.

TABLE 42. PER CENT OF NURSES' FATHERS WHO WERE BORN IN EACH COUNTRY, COMPARED WITH CENSUS FIGURES FOR WHITE MALES OF VOTING AGE, IN THE UNITED STATES IN 1900

Birthplace	Private duty	Public health	Institutional	All	1900 Census
United States	56%	59%	57%	57%	74%
Other Americas	12	10	12	12	3
British Isles	16	17	18	17	7
France	1	..	1	1	..
Northwestern Europe	6	6	5	6	4
Germany	6	5	5	5	7
Central Europe	1	1	1	1	2
Other	2	2	1	1	3
	100%	100%	100%	100%	100%

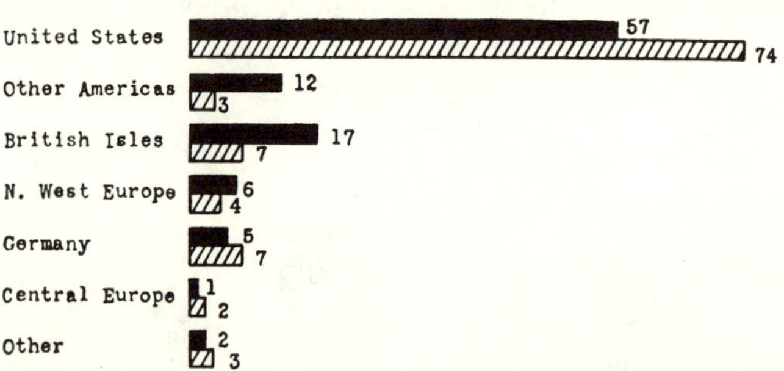

Diagram 27.—Per cent of nurses whose fathers were born in each country ▬, and per cent of male residents in the U. S., in 1900, over voting age who were born in those countries ▨

The interesting figures in this table and its accompanying diagram are for the per cents of fathers born in the United States, in "Other Americas," which probably means largely Canada, and in the British Isles. The figures would seem to furnish some support to the frequent statement that rather large numbers of Canadian and British nurses have come to the United States to practise nursing.

2. What Does Her Father Do?

The following table and diagram show the occupations of the fathers of nurses, compared with the 1920 census figures for males from forty-five to sixty-five years of age.

TABLE 43. KINDS OF WORK IN WHICH NURSES' FATHERS HAVE BEEN EMPLOYED

Occupation	Private duty	Public health	Institutional	All	1920 census
Agriculture	33%	24%	30%	30%	33%
Mining	2	1	1	1	3
Manufacturing	25	31	25	26	31
Transportation	6	7	6	6	8
Trade	18	19	18	19	12
Public service	3	3	3	3	2
Professional service	9	11	11	10	4
Domestic service	2	2	3	2	4
Clerical	2	2	3	3	3
Total	100%	100%	100%	100%	100%

It will be noted that while the gross number of nurses whose fathers are in agriculture is large, nevertheless the per cent is smaller than might reasonably be expected, considering the large per cent of all United States males of the ages given who are employed in agricultural pursuits. In general, it may be said that nurses are less apt to come from the agricultural, mining, manufacturing, transportation, domestic service, and clerical groups than might be expected, and are more apt to come from the groups engaged in trade and professional pursuits. The professional fathers, especially, are far in excess of the per cent for males in general.

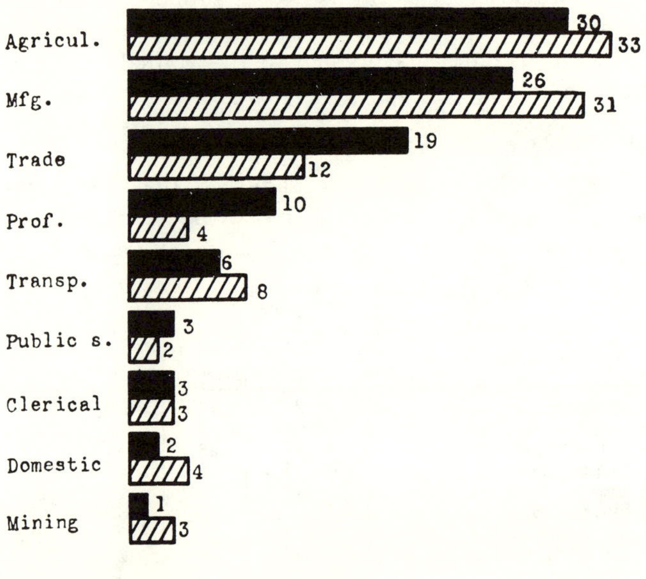

Diagram 28.—Per cent of nurses' fathers working in each occupation compared with per cent of all males between 45 and 65 years of age, in that occupation (1920 census). Merchants, professional men, and men in public life seem to be more than ordinarily interested in nursing as careers for their daughters; while fathers engaged in farming, manufacture, transportation, mining, or domestic service, are apparently more than ordinarily uninterested

3. How Many Active Nurses are Married?

At the same time that the records were being studied of graduates from nursing schools (as reported in Chapters 2 and 3), additional tables were compiled for the 71,561 nurse graduates of whom the marriage and work records were known. The results may be summarized as follows: (It should be remembered that these are all based upon what the heads of schools were able to report about their graduates. They are not based upon direct reports from the graduates themselves.)

Still nursing		55.7%
Not nursing—at home	38.1%	
Gone into other work	1.1	
Dead	5.1	
Total not nursing		44.3
Grand total		100%

A special study was also made of the marriage records as given by the schools. For the 40,115 actively nursing graduates, 8.9 per cent were reported by the school principals as married. The detailed figures are as follows:

TABLE 44. PER CENT OF ALL ACTIVELY NURSING GRADUATES EACH NUMBER OF YEARS OUT FROM TRAINING SCHOOL WHO ARE MARRIED

Years out of school	Per cent of actives who are married
Under 1	3.2
1	5.6
2	8.0
3	9.3
4	9.6
5	9.1
6	9.4
7	10.9
8	12.7
9	10.9
10–14	12.1
15–19	10.4
20–24	9.6
25–29	8.9
30–34	8.0
35–39	10.0
40 plus	23.1
Total	8.9

These figures offer what was at first a perplexing contrast to reports of nurses themselves on this same question. The figures just cited are based upon individual records of 40,115 active nurse graduates as compiled by their superintendents of nurses. In March, 1927, however, the Grading Committee received individual replies from 24,389 nurses who were then out in the field. From these replies the following figures were secured for married and unmarried women, all of whom were actively engaged in the practice of nursing.

	Mrs.	Miss
Private duty	22%	78%
Institutional	16	84
Public health	18	82
All	20%	80%

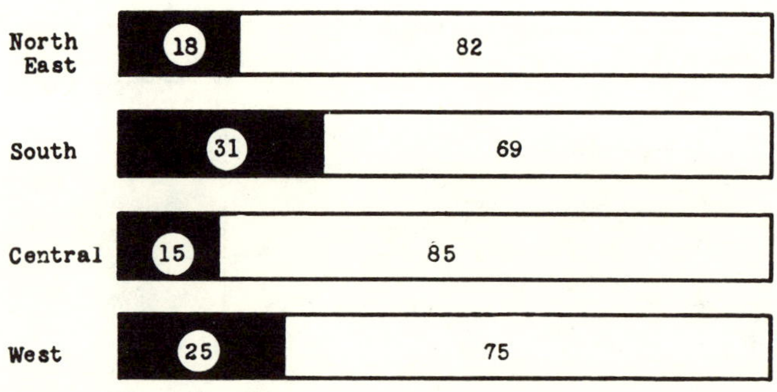

Diagram 29.—Of 24,389 nurses actively engaged in private duty, public health, or institutional nursing, 20% write *Mrs.* in front of their names. The per cent for each geographical division is shown above in black

As will be seen, these per cents for married nurses in active practice are very much higher than the returns on the same point from the superintendents of nurses. The probable explanation for this difference is that apparently many nurses marry and leave the profession for a short time, only to return to it later. The chances are large that the superintendent of nurses, knowing that the student has married and not knowing that she has come back into the active nursing group, has reported her to the Grading Committee as married and out of the profession. Moreover, in tabulating the data from the schools, where the nurse was checked as "Mrs." but with no additional information, her name was placed in the "Married, not nursing," group. It would seem probable that many of the names in this group properly belong under Active. The Committee is still inclined to accept its earlier findings, that "One out of every five active nurses is married."

4. How Many Married Nurses are Working?

A different, and from some points of view even more significant figure is that which answers the question: "Of all the girls who marry, how many keep on in active nursing?" The figures which are available, however, are only those which were reported by the superintendents of nurses; and as has already been indicated, there is reason to believe that considerably less than half of the "married and working" cases have been known as such by the heads of the schools. For the entire profession, the Committee believes that, although the schools report only about 9 out of each 100 *active* nurses as married, the true figure is more nearly 20 out of 100. Similarly for the table which follows the figures as given by the schools would seem to be definitely lower than the true figures. What the actual difference is the Committee is not prepared to state. It seems probable, however, that readers will not go very far wrong if they multiply the per cents as given in the following table by two.

TABLE 45. PER CENT OF ALL MARRIED NURSES, OUT EACH NUMBER OF YEARS FROM TRAINING SCHOOL, WHO ARE ACTIVELY NURSING. (Reports based on 71,561 records of graduates from 420 schools of nursing. The total as given here is probably less than half of the true total for the profession.)

Years out of school	Per cent of all married who keep on nursing
Under 1	43
1	30
2	24
3	20
4	17
5	14
6	12
7	12
8	12
9	10
10–14	10
15–19	9
20–24	8
25–29	7
30–34	6
35–39	6
40 and over	7
Total	12

5. Mrs. R.N. vs. Mrs. College Graduate

The Committee compared the records from nursing schools, as to the total number of graduates (whether working or not) who were married, with similar reports from the registrars of women's colleges. Reports were accordingly secured for 46,830 women college graduates extending over the same fifty year period which the nursing records cover. For the two groups it was found that 45 per cent of the college graduates and 41 per cent of the nursing school graduates are married. It should be noted, however, that marriage rates are low in both groups for students graduated within very recent years and that the proportion of recent graduates in the total nurse graduate body is larger than in the college graduate body. The following table gives the per cent of married graduates each number of years out of school, in the nursing and college graduate groups.

TABLE 46. PER CENT OF GRADUATES WHO ARE KNOWN TO BE MARRIED EACH NUMBER OF YEARS AFTER GRADUATION FROM A NURSING SCHOOL OR A WOMAN'S COLLEGE

Years out	Nursing school	College
Under 1	7%	4%
1	16	11
2	26	20
3	32	27
4	37	34
5	40	43
6	44	45
7	48	52
8	52	54
9	51	54
10–14	53	57
15–19	51	59
20–24	48	58
25–29	46	56
30–34	42	55
35–39	37	51
40 and over	37	57
Total	41%	45%

It is interesting to note that nurses in the earlier days were apparently less apt to marry than those in more recent years, and that while the same tendency is visible for the college graduate group, it is much less marked. During the first four years after graduation a higher per cent of nurses are married than of college graduates, but from the fifth year on the per cent of marriages seems to be higher in the college group.

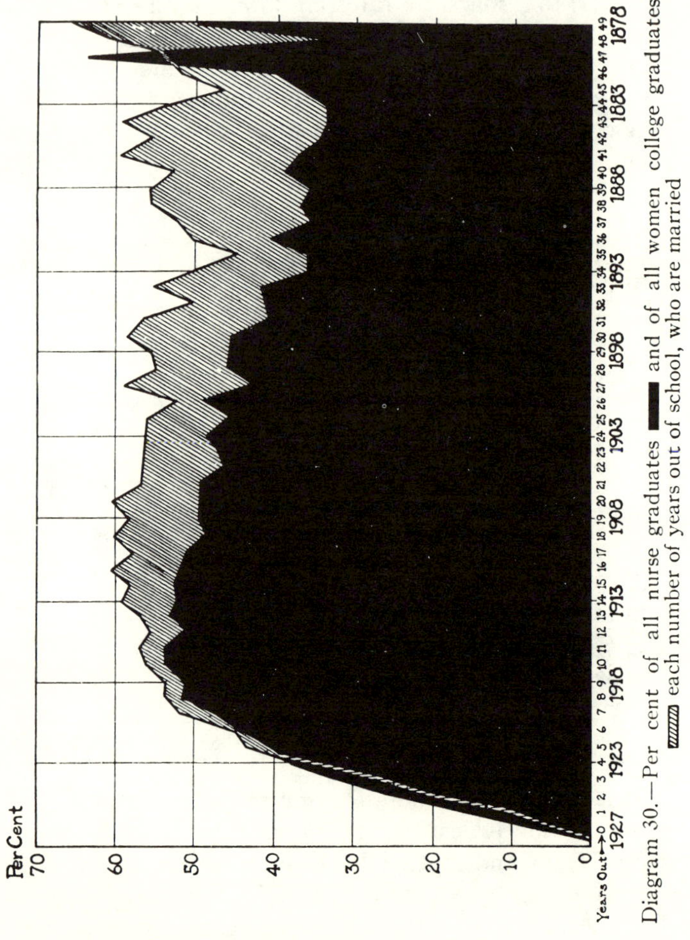

Diagram 30.—Per cent of all nurse graduates ▬ and of all women college graduates ▨ each number of years out of school, who are married

6. Into What Fields Does She Go?

It is difficult to ascertain what the true proportions are for nurses in the different branches of the profession. The returns received by the Grading Committee indicate that of all the nurses who answered—

54% are in private duty
19% are in public health
23% are in institutional work
4% are in unclassified activities

It should be remembered, however, that many nurses did not answer the questionnaire, and there is no easy way in which to discover whether the questionnaires appealed more directly to nurses in one group than in another.

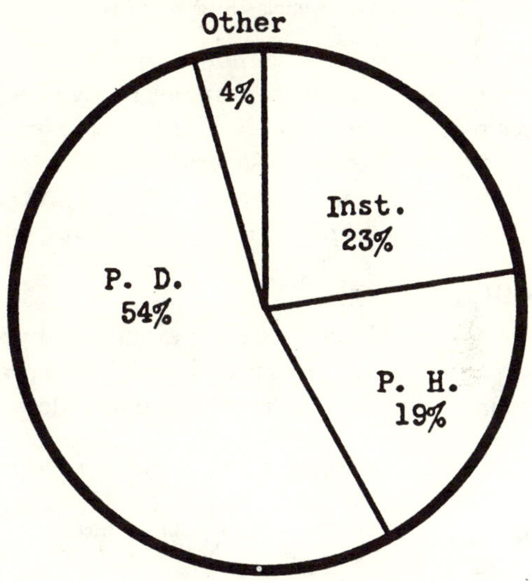

Where Do Grads Go?

Diagram 31.—Per cent of 24,389 graduate nurses actively at work in 10 states, who belong to each nursing field

We have some light on the problem of distribution from New York and from Wisconsin. In the Report for 1926, issued by the New York State Education Department, registrations of graduate nurses for that year are classified according to type of position. These seem to indicate that of the graduate registered nurses—

57% are in private duty
14% are in public health
29% are in institutional work

A similar report for the state of Wisconsin for 1927 indicates that—

40% are in private duty
18% are in public health
37% are in institutional work
5% are in unclassified activities

These three reports are close enough to each other to suggest that the Grading returns are not badly skewed, but do in fact represent reasonably well all three branches of the profession. They also suggest that the frequently quoted "70 per cent in private duty" and "12 per cent in public health" are rather far from being safe estimates.

7. How Old is She?

We did not ask the nurses their exact age, but we did ask how many years it was since they had been graduated from training school. The returns are as follows:

TABLE 47. PER CENT OF NURSES WHO HAVE BEEN OUT OF TRAINING SCHOOL EACH NUMBER OF YEARS

Years out	Private duty	Public health	Institutional	All
0– 5	40%	24%	35%	35%
6–10	21	25	22	22
11–15	15	21	16	17
16–20	12	15	14	13
21–25	6	9	7	7
26–30	4	4	4	4
31+	2	2	2	2
	100%	100%	100%	100%

If we assume that most nurses now are about twenty-one years old when they are graduated (and this is probably somewhere in the neighborhood of the truth), then we see that a third of the nurses in the country are probably twenty-six years old or less, and probably about half are under thirty. Private duty nurses are younger than those in other fields. This may partly be because there is a tradition in the profession that nurses do well to try private duty before going into public health or institutional work, and partly because the young nurses enjoy the freedom and lack of responsibility which private duty affords, whereas most mature nurses begin to realize the advantages of belonging to the more organized branches of the profession.

8. What is her Educational Background?

Each nurse was asked to give an account of her academic schooling. The following table shows the results for all the nurses in each group.

TABLE 48. PER CENT OF NURSES WHO HAVE HAD EACH INDICATED AMOUNT OF SCHOOLING

Years of school	Private duty	Public health	Institutional	All
8th grade or less	14%	9%	9%	11%
1 year high school	14	10	12	13
2 years high school	17	16	12	15
3 years high school	13	11	12	12
4 years high school	33	34	33	34
1 or more years college	9	20	22	15
Total	100%	100%	100%	100%

It will be noted in this table that over one-fourth of all the private duty nurses and about one-fifth of all the others have never gone beyond the first year of high school. It is encouraging, however, to note that almost half of the nurses have had more than three years of high school. Moreover, while the condition is rather slowly improving, there is, nevertheless, evidence of a real advance in the emphasis upon academic education as a prerequisite to nursing. The following table shows the per cent of nurses who have had one year of high school or less, according to the numbers of years out from training school. It indicates that while there are still large numbers of nurses being graduated every year with nothing beyond one year of high school, the per cents of such under-educated women are considerably smaller than they were ten or fifteen years ago.

TABLE 49. PER CENT OF NURSES WHO HAVE HAD ONE YEAR OF HIGH SCHOOL OR LESS

Years out	Private duty	Public health	Institutional	All
0– 5	19%	13%	16%	17%
6–10	27	17	20	22
11–15	36	25	22	29
16–20	32	22	29	29
21–25	35	24	23	28
26–30	49	24	34	39
31+	47	39	34	42
Total	28%	20%	21%	24%

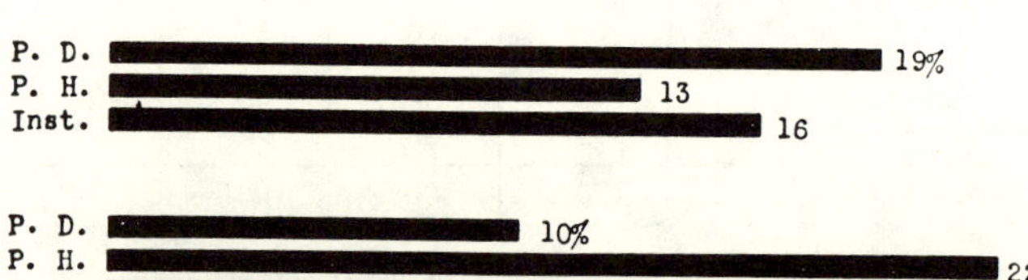

Diagram 32.—Per cent of all nurses graduated *within the past five years* who have had 1 year of high school or less (top bars) and 1 year of college or more (lower bars)

In this connection it should be remembered that lack of proper academic schooling among recent graduates is probably far more serious than a similar lack among graduates of many years ago. It is only within the past twenty or thirty years that high school education has become generally available to intelligent students who want to secure it. Many of the ablest members of the older nursing groups have had very little formal education, because in the days when they were of high school age there were few high schools within reach. Women of excellent family background and professional traditions, if belonging to the older group, might easily be included in the table just given and yet might be among the most valuable members of the profession.

Today, however, conditions have changed. High school education has become not only within the reach of almost any intelligent and ambitious boy or girl, no matter what his economic background, but the social pressure for education has become so great that it is hardly respectable for young people at present not to have at least several years of high school education. While there are still exceptions, it is in general true that applicants for admission to nursing schools who have failed to complete their high school courses should be viewed with grave suspicion, since there is probably more than an even chance that they are mentally unable to carry work of high school grade, that they are repelled by the orderly and controlled discipline of the educational life, or that they come from families to which professional traditions are unfamiliar. It would seem a matter for serious concern that one-sixth of all the students who have been graduated within the past five years have never gone beyond the first year in high school.

While nurses with low academic preparation are rather more numerous in private duty than in public health or institutional nursing, conditions are serious in all three fields. The following table shows the per cent of nurses in public health work occupying each type of position, who have had the indicated amounts of education.

TABLE 50. PER CENT OF NURSES IN PUBLIC HEALTH WHO HAVE HAD EACH SPECIFIED AMOUNT OF EDUCATION

Nurses	8th grade or less	1 year high school	2 or 3 years high school	4 years high school	1 or more years college
Staff nurses	12%	10%	27%	37%	14%
Floating nurses	20	10	20	35	15
Supervisors	5	10	30	37	18
Directors	1	7	21	28	43
Other	10	10	26	35	19
Total	10%	10%	26%	35%	19%

A similar table for institutional nurses follows.

TABLE 51. PER CENT OF INSTITUTIONAL NURSES WHO HAVE HAD EACH SPECIFIED AMOUNT OF EDUCATION

Nurses	8th grade or less	1 year high school	2 or 3 years high school	4 years high school	1 or more years college	Total
Supt. of hospitals	8%	12%	20%	37%	23%	100%
Supt. of nurses	3	4	18	40	35	100
Supt. both hospitals and nurses	7	6	20	41	26	100
Asst. supt.	9	9	21	35	26	100
Instructors, super.	4	10	22	37	27	100
Staff nurses	16	18	26	30	10	100
Head nurses	13	15	29	29	14	100
Nurses on sp. service	13	18	24	37	8	100
Administrative, clerical	6	22	16	28	28	100
Other	14	13	29	35	9	100
Total	9%	12%	24%	33%	22%	100%

9. Where Did She Receive Her Training?

Note was made of the daily average patients in the hospital where the nurse received her training at the time when she was a student there. The following table shows that over one-fourth of the nurses were trained in hospitals with less than 100 patients, and that well over half were trained in hospitals with less than 200 patients. The per cents are as follows:

TABLE 52. PER CENT OF NURSES WHO WERE TRAINED IN HOSPITALS WITH A DAILY AVERAGE OF PATIENTS AS INDICATED

Daily average patients	Private duty	Public health	Institutional	All
0 to 50	9%	6%	9%	8%
50 to 100	22	18	20	21
100 to 200	28	32	26	28
200 to 300	15	15	13	14
300 to 400	9	8	10	9
400 to 500	4	4	4	5
500+	13	17	18	15
	100%	100%	100%	100%

There seems to be some connection between the size of the school and the academic education of the students. In general, half of the nurses who go into private duty from schools with a daily average of less than 100 patients will have had two years or less of high school, and half of the nurses going into public health and institutional work will have had three years or less. For schools with a daily average of 100 patients or more, the corresponding figures are three years for private duty and four for public health and institutional nursing. The larger hospitals are evidently laying more stress upon academic preparation.

10. Where Does She Live?

Nurses were classified according to the populations of the towns and cities in which they are now working.

TABLE 53. PER CENT OF NURSES COMPARED WITH PER CENT OF UNITED STATES POPULATION LIVING IN CITIES OF EACH SPECIFIED SIZE

Population	Private duty	Public health	Institutional	All	U. S. population 1920 census
500,000 and over.	46%	37%	43%	43%	15%
100,000 to 500,000	16	17	14	16	10
25,000 to 100,000	17	17	16	17	10
10,000 to 25,000	10	11	10	10	7
Under 10,000.	11	18	17	14	58
	100%	100%	100%	100%	100%

It will be seen that private duty nurses are apt to be found in the larger cities, and that the proportion of nurses to population must be very small in rural areas.

11. How Many Different States Has She Worked In?

There seems to be a distinct tendency for public health nurses to travel more than nurses in either of the other fields. Contrary to general belief, almost half of the private duty nurses are now working in the states where they were trained, but only a little over one-fifth of the public health nurses have remained in their own states. The following table gives the figures for all three groups.

TABLE 54. PER CENT OF NURSES WHO HAVE WORKED IN EACH SPECIFIED NUMBER OF DIFFERENT STATES

States	Private duty	Public health	Institutional	All
1.	45%	22%	45%	45%
2.	25	23	25	25
3.	14	18	15	14
4.	8	17	7	8
5.	4	8	4	4
6.	2	5	2	2
7+.	2	7	2	2
	100%	100%	100%	100%

While it is true that public health nurses are apt to travel more than nurses in the other groups, there is a distinct difference between the public health nurses holding different sorts of positions. Some 82 per cent of the staff nurses have worked in only one state, 65 per cent of the floating nurses, 75 per cent of the supervisors, 59 per cent of the directors, and 78 per cent of all other members of the group.

12. What Does She Know about Other Nurses' Work?

It is a striking fact that nurses shift from one field to another with great frequency. The following table gives the per cents of nurses who have tried private duty, public health, and institutional work.

TABLE 55. PER CENT OF NURSES NOW IN PRIVATE DUTY, PUBLIC HEALTH, AND INSTITUTIONAL WORK WHO HAVE AT SOME TIME DONE EACH SPECIFIED TYPE OF WORK

Of the nurses now in			
Private duty	Public health	Institutional	
100%	88%	74%	have done Private duty
50	45	37	Nursing a relative free of charge
43	47	80	Hospital nursing staff
41	33	37	Hospital floor duty
17	15	7	Hourly nursing
14	62	11	Visiting nursing
9	59	11	Other public health
9	9	8	Physician's office
7	20	5	Industrial
8	9	9	Sanitarium staff
6	7	14	Anesthetist
5	13	23	Nursing school teacher
4	5	5	Resident in school, orphanage, etc.
2	2	1	Dentist's office
1	..	..	Demonstrator of drugs, appliances, etc.
6	13	11	Other

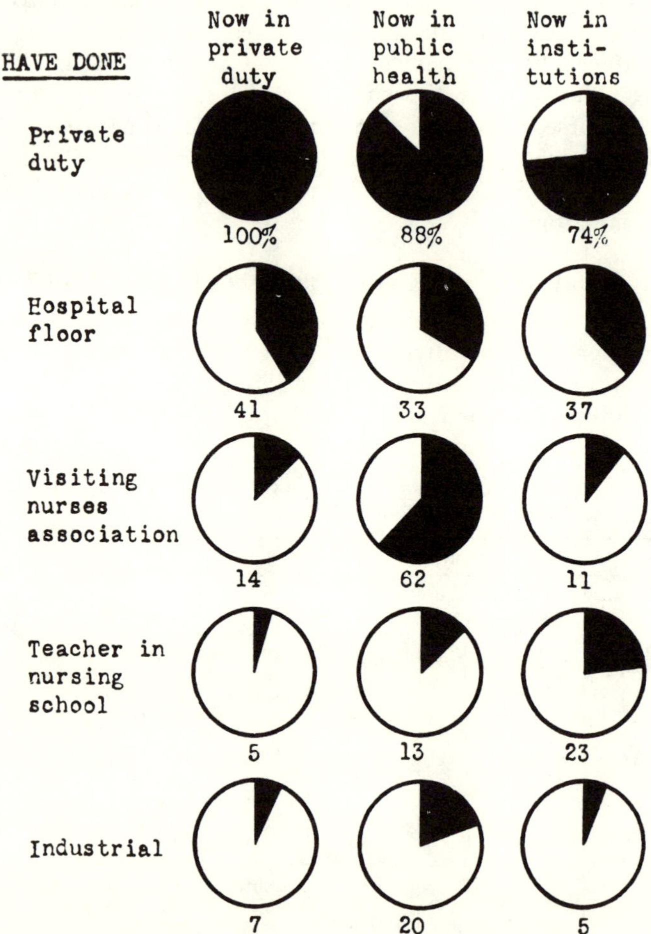

Diagram 33.—Black portion shows per cent of nurses now in private duty, public health, and institutional nursing who have previously done nursing of each specified type

The table shows that 100 per cent of all the nurses now in private duty, 88 per cent of the nurses now in public health, and 74 per cent of the nurses now in institutional work have done private duty at some previous time. The second line shows that 50 per cent of nurses now in private duty, 45 per cent of nurses now in public health, and 37 per cent of nurses now in institutions have at some time nursed a relative free of charge; and so on down. These figures are of more significance than might at first appear, since they show that public health and institutional positions draw workers constantly from private duty, as well as from each other. Anything which affects the standards of private duty must necessarily, therefore, affect public health and institutional work. It is also worth noting that public health and institutional workers have in such large numbers experienced private duty before going into their present fields that they are thoroughly familiar both with its advantages and its disadvantages. Their comments on private duty, as compared with their present activities, have more than academic value.

13. SUMMARY

The tables and diagrams in this chapter seem to show the following outstanding facts about the rank and file of the nursing profession:

a. The profession contains larger numbers than would normally be expected of nurses whose fathers were born outside of the United States. There is reason to believe that many of them were born either in England or Canada.

b. While half of the nurses have fathers who are either farmers or manufacturers, the per cent is smaller than for corresponding groups of men in the country at large. Men who engage in trade or the various professions, on the other hand, are found with unusual frequency to be the fathers of nurses.

c. Probably about one out of every five nurses actively at work is married. The tendency to continue with work after marriage is particularly marked in the first four years after graduation; but continues to be fairly heavy after that.

d. Nurses are rather like college graduates in their tendency to marry. More of them marry within the first few years after graduation than do college graduates, but after the fourth year the college per cent is higher.

e. Probably about 54 per cent of the nurses go into private duty, 19 per cent into public health, 23 per cent into institutional work, and 4 per cent into other branches of nursing.

f. Probably about one-third of the graduate nurses are under twenty-six years old, and about half are under thirty.

g. Over one-tenth of all the nurses have never been beyond the eighth grade in grammar school; and about one-fourth have never been beyond the first year of high school. Of nurses graduated within the past five years, one-sixth have never been beyond the first year of high school.

h. Almost half have had four years of high school, and 15 per cent have had at least one year of college. Of nurses graduated within the past five years 16 per cent have had one year or more of college.

i. Nearly three-fourths of the nurses were trained in hospitals with a daily average of over one hundred patients.

j. Far more nurses live in the cities than in the country.

k. Almost half of the private duty and institutional nurses are living in the same states where they received their training, but less than one-fourth of the public health nurses.

l. About three-fourths of the institutional nurses and about nine-tenths of the public health nurses have done private duty. Nurses shift from field to field.

CHAPTER 13

WHAT PUBLIC HEALTH AND INSTITUTIONAL NURSES SAY

Public health and institutional nurses talk in an almost totally different way from nurses in private duty. Therefore, in presenting the comments from nurses, it has seemed best not to attempt to follow the topics outlined in Chapters 12 and 14, but rather to arrange the material in groups, according to whom it comes from. Public health and institutional nurses will be quoted in this chapter; and private duty nurses in Chapter 15.

1. Comments From Public Health Nurses About Their Work

Public health nurses are almost uniformly interested and happy, as the following testimony shows:

> CALIFORNIA.—The work itself is broad in scope, and there is room to grow in it. In fact, one must keep on growing to keep up with it.
>
> KANSAS.—I believe it offers the widest field of opportunity—opportunity for advancement as well as for service. Then too I like the work. I find it interesting. It forces the nurse to face her patients as human beings, not as cases. The hours are good, and the outdoor exercise healthful.
>
> PENNSYLVANIA.—Public health nursing has been more fascinating to me than any other branch of nursing, due to the fact that one comes in contact with the patients' families. I think that the nurse grows with her work, for each case is singular in its

character. She develops her personality, her personal integrity, her initiative, and all the finer qualities which make one more understanding.

KANSAS.—I am thoroughly "sold" on public health, otherwise I would not have done it for the past eight years. To me it is the step forward in nursing.

KANSAS.—It is very congenial. There is plenty of opportunity for future development and some self-expression. The financial problem is very well taken care of by tax levy, community chest, and earnings.

KANSAS.—I intend to continue public health work as I thoroughly enjoy it, and I have always been able to get positions. I have left each position for a better one.

PENNSYLVANIA.—To my mind public health nursing is the supreme adventure in nursing, but at my age (55 years) I doubt if my strength would be equal to any branch but the government service.

NEW YORK.—Regular hours, Sundays, occasional holidays, vacation with pay, steady salary. There is a great deal of walking done in this work going back and forth to the schools, and lots of stair climbing, but it is not as depressing as private duty nursing.

WYOMING.—In industrial nursing each day calls for a different expression of one's ability in some line. I find this human contact most satisfying, and almost without exception justifying one's efforts. Last, but by no means least, the working hours are an important item.

CALIFORNIA.—I am a school nurse. From 8:30 to 3:30 or about I am busy at school. Saturday and Sunday are free, and the usual school holidays are my own time. We are employed and paid on a ten months' basis, leaving ten weeks in the summer free for vacation, study, travel, or other employment if desired. Last, but not least, the pay is better than I could ever manage doing private duty. Beside the enjoyment of work that brings me in contact with people engaged in educational work and study, there is perhaps a little prestige to the position of school nurse that I rather like.

PENNSYLVANIA.—In public health work I am out-of-doors more than in any other kind of nursing. It is more healthy, varied, and not monotonous. I have contact with other people and all kinds of people; freedom in which I may arrange my own work, also my time off; time to meet other health and social workers, as a rule; time off Sunday, usually the day off; and I like it for the help I can give others, both in social service and nursing, also the help they give me. It would seem a bigger and broader field with great opportunities for service, and intensely interesting.

KANSAS.—I really selfishly prefer public health for the time allowed at home in the evenings and Sundays.

CALIFORNIA.—I love my babies. It's fun to watch my under-weight kiddies gain, and a real satisfaction to see my foreign mothers respond to teaching.

CALIFORNIA.—You can do more for humanity in public health than in anything else in the world. I could write all day about this.

WASHINGTON.—In my position as county tuberculosis nurse, which includes school nursing, I guess I feel the thrill of covering and sort of mothering the whole county, whereas before my efforts were confined usually to one patient at a time. The interest in public health nursing is so far reaching and has so many angles that it surely holds your interest and never lets that interest wane.

CALIFORNIA.—My work takes me into homes of poverty, and sometimes filthy ones, where they need instruction and advice that I can give them. They almost always seem at a loss to know what to do, because of ignorance, and they appreciate the little service I can give them. As a rule, the doctors never stop long enough to give the family much instruction, and many little things come up that they would like to know about, but they do not like to ask the doctor on the case.

WYOMING.—The attitude of physicians toward nurses is unbearable. They expect catering to their personal practice, and in general look at nurses as beneath them socially. This has all come about because of the great numbers of poorly schooled young women who have been accepted in schools of nursing, and is caused particularly by many of them also having had questionable home background. A principal of a high school recently told me that it would be useless to try to persuade any of their graduates to enter a nursing school, because it is one of the "despised callings." Physicians and the leading lay people do not want nurses who have education or even good minds. They seem to wish to keep them in the servant class.

MASSACHUSETTS.—I find that my worst barrier is having to work with all of the doctors. It is so hard to work with them when I know they do not approve of my doing anything different than they have told me to, whether it is a glass of water or an alcohol rub. As one of the local physicians told me, "If you see any one dying, let him die unless I tell you what to do. If you know the medicine I have ordered is going to kill him the next minute, give it!" Needless to say, I stay clear of this doctor's cases.

WASHINGTON.—The salary in public health is not as good, usually, as that in an institution, but the hours are shorter, giving the nurse more time for other activities. I find that I am able to depend on more time in which these activities may be carried on, and that I am not too tired, usually, to do so. The prevention of disease seems to me to be getting at the root of the situation, and to be preferred to the curative phase of the work.

WASHINGTON.—Public health nursing has only one drawback—poor, poor salaries! ($1520—grad. 1913).

KANSAS.—Public health work covers such a wide field of nursing endeavor that it should appeal to every nurse as a challenge to give "her best" to it. As a life work public health nursing seems to hold more advantages than private duty or other nursing activities. However, it should pay better salaries for experienced staff nurses.

NEW YORK.—Public health nursing is intensely interesting and has many opportunities, but the strain is too great to go on unless one has a strong physique.

The above was written on receipt of your questionnaire, after a hard day's work. Now, after ten hours of sleep, I have no intention of giving up, but hope to die in the harness, for there is no work that can begin to touch it.

2. Public Health Versus Private Duty

Of every 100 public health nurses, 88 have tried private duty. Their comments on the differences between the two fields are illuminating.

CALIFORNIA.—The difference between public health nursing and private duty is that one is living, and the latter existing. Private duty means (I had fifteen years of it) going to bed at night too tired to care about study, recreation or anything further than a few hours' respite in sleep. Twelve hours is not as bad as formerly, however, even that leaves no margin of time or energy for the higher things. The work is uncertain and the pay all too frequently much delayed, or possibly fails to come altogether. The only compensation as I look back on it is the wonderful friends made by this type of nursing.

Public health! Oh, there is movement, initiative, getting out into the open, regular salary, eight hours of intensive and intensely interesting work, time for one's friends, to keep up one's clothes, to take extension courses; time to manicure one's nails, to vote and to know why; two weeks or a month's vacation on pay each year. The wonder is that there are any private duty nurses left, and there wouldn't be if the poor girls were not too used up to get out of that rut.

CALIFORNIA.—The shorter hours during which a public health nurse is on duty, make it possible for her to maintain her own good health, to eat and sleep regularly, and have some time for study and recreation. A private duty nurse may take time off duty, but she always feels that she is losing money by doing so. I have found that not until I began to teach health habits to other people, did I observe them myself. As a consequence I have ever so much better health, and enjoy my work so much more.

WASHINGTON.—The reasons that come to me for continuing in public health nursing are, that at my age (49), after twenty years in private or bedside nursing, and alternating occasionally, for a change only, with institutional nursing, I find a wider scope for my personal tastes, a more independent life, a life more free from restraint, a life that doesn't keep you guessing whether you are going to be called on a case today, tomorrow, or next week, and its consequent worries.

WASHINGTON.—After graduation in 1907, and until the war, I did only private duty nursing. I used to get very tired physically, and also tired of the monotony of it. The uncertainty and the confinement were getting on my nerves. After seventeen months in service on regular hours, caring for many patients instead of one, I realized that I could never go back to bedside nursing.

KANSAS.—I intend to continue public health nursing indefinitely because I like it best, public school nursing especially. I like the freedom and unrestraint of being "on my own"; the regular hours; regular pay; the variation; no monotony as found when on private duty; the contact with different kinds of homes and parents, and the associations with the public schools and teachers; the limitless possibilities for promotion and advancement; the term of nine months (paid twelve months) and five-day weeks; the varied duties, no monotonous, eternal routine and grind; the outdoor life; the substantial salary.

CALIFORNIA.—My choice of public health nursing was due first to my physical condition. I had done night duty a great deal in private nursing, also several years of 24-hour nursing, and I felt the need for shorter hours and day work. Now I find it very interesting and would not like to change. I really feel that I'm worth something to my community in health education and disease prevention. Formerly I felt sometimes that I was a mere machine, and often a worn-out one at that.

CALIFORNIA.—I am doing school nursing and am very happy in it. It exceeds by far any other kind of nursing I have done. There is time enough outside of my work so that I can have other interests, and in that way life doesn't become monotonous and I can have friends, which I found rather impossible to do when doing private nursing. My health is very much better as my hours are regular. I get the proper amount of sleep uninterrupted, and I am out of doors part of the time, since I make home calls. My daily associates are very agreeable, since I come in contact with teachers who serve as a mental stimulus. In general, I would say that life seems very much worth living.

CALIFORNIA.—There is a great deal more freedom and opportunity to express one's self in public health work than there is in private duty or hospital nursing. I have never borrowed money since I gave up private duty nursing.

CALIFORNIA.—The public health nurse's income is more certain than the private duty nurse's. Her position is more secure, and her salary regular. The school nurse has a contract for the school year exactly as a teacher has. During the summer she may work or not as she chooses, for the Health Department gives employment to nurses who are doing satisfactory work. There is never that unsettled feeling of not knowing where she is going to lay her head the next night, or whether she is going to be able to "lay it" at all or not. No summons in the middle of the night to get up out of bed, cross town, and become a member of a strange household. There is a chance for home life and some social life.

CALIFORNIA.—I like school nursing immensely, and after 25 years of hard work, mostly private duty, it is impossible for me to take any longer the responsibility for life and death. Hours are very attractive, and contact with the sick is negligible.

CALIFORNIA.—I like school nursing work, and yet it lacks the satisfaction of the actual nursing of sick people back to health.

CALIFORNIA.—I am happier in this work than I was in private duty. My contact is with an entirely different class of people. They learn to lean on me and bring their problems, whether those of illness or otherwise, to me. There is greater satisfaction in doing for these poor unfortunates than in catering to patients that have lived lives of pampered luxury. Also there is no monotony in this work, as there was bound to be in some private cases. I felt that there was no future to private duty. In the eight years of that work I had come to work for the best doctors in the community, and had choice patients, but there was nothing greater to strive for. I believe the regularity of income also is conducive to happiness. When one has dependents it is a great worry not to be sure what the next month's income will be.

KANSAS.—Public health is most interesting because you meet a class of people who need your care and advice in planning a way out of their difficulties as well as with sickness. One is more appreciated. For one thing, the pay does not come, as a rule, from the one who received the attention of a nurse. The nurse is also allowed to use her own judgment. No matter how disagreeable the patient or the task, it lasts only an hour at a time. No time is spent in "entertaining" a patient, or that period of a nurse with a convalescent "just sitting." There is more time for the nurse to live her own life, and to improve her mind and physical condition. I did private duty ten years and thought my working days were over, but I have been so well and happy the five years I have done public health work.

3. What Institutional Nurses Like About Their Work

All through the comments from institutional nurses can be sensed their keen interest in nursing technique, in medical progress, and in the education of students. Comparisons with private duty are frequent.

CALIFORNIA.—I'm receiving an education every day. A good hospital is a most inspiring place to work.

PENNSYLVANIA.—It is my intention to continue in institutional work until I am fifty years old. I like hospital work because it enables me to know about all that is new in the treatment of patients, and because of the varied interests it presents. From a more practical point of view, I like it because it is physically possible for me to do this work, while I should be unable to do certain other kinds of nursing, such as district work or private duty.

WASHINGTON.—One keeps in touch with the newer methods and treatments, and can also compare the different diseases and operative and post operative progress under the different doctors' care.

PENNSYLVANIA.—Institutional life appeals to me the most because my personality at twenty-one years, when I graduated, rebelled at the manner in which nurses were treated in the home, though strange to say, I never noticed it in the hospital because I was always so intensely absorbed in the thing I was doing. I think institutional work offers great opportunities to the nurse for professional advancement, while the social life is of necessity limited due to the long hours, etc. However, I have always been very happy in my work. If I were beginning all over at the present time, I should still choose nursing with the exception of planning a better educational foundation.

PENNSYLVANIA.—I think that institutional life is fine and broad if you have the energy to take advantage of all it may offer, for you are more easily in touch with all of the nursing organizations and progress than in any other lines of work.

CALIFORNIA.—It is to my mind the best way to "keep up" with modern methods of nursing, and being both an instructor and an assistant superintendent of nurses, I enjoy the contact with the student nurses to the utmost, and am also learning administration of a school of nursing. These things, I think, more than offset the hard work which seems to be the big objection to institutional work.

California.—I am in my eighth year as operating room nurse. I have had plenty of knocks; I have worked like a horse; been fatigued almost to the point of unconsciousness; but I will be blessed if I ever stopped liking it. I have been kicked out one door for distemper only to politely walk in another and start in again.

California.—I could not think of anything more desirable than surgical supervisor or first assistant in a large hospital.

California.—Personally I find more satisfaction and enjoyment in operating room work than in any other branch of the nursing service I have been in. I like the detail, accuracy, and routine of the operating room, and find a much better outlet for my capacities in that field than any other I have tried. I have felt the need of a change several times and have tried office work, private duty, and a small amount of public health, but after a very short time I have always returned to surgery. I enjoy private duty for only a short time for I never seem to be using but a small part of my ability. My chief aim is to become a doctor's surgical assistant for I feel that I am not enough of an executive to handle a great many students. I haven't enough patience to allow for their errors, and the constant changing of persons would be difficult for me to cope with. Operating room work with a permanent staff is what I am supervising now, and I like it very much.

California.—Because of the variety of associations, the daily contacts with younger nurses, their interest and enthusiasm, I am able to enjoy my work and to keep young in heart, if not in body.

California.—The regular hours and stated salary

are more desirable. Due to regular hours I have time, peace of mind, and energy left to take an interest in nursing and other activities, also to carry some classes in order to complete high school education, and possibly do some university work. Institutional life offers innumerable opportunities for association with people interested in the progressive and vital things of life. It keeps one up to date in medicine and nursing.

CALIFORNIA.—I find my associates and my superintendent of nurses more of an inspiration than I received from any source while doing private nursing.

CALIFORNIA.—I prefer institutional work to other types of nursing that I have done, because one can usually save more as the income is steady, full maintenance is usually furnished, the work is full of interest, and most of all, I enjoy the contact of the student so full of enthusiasm.

KANSAS.—From a financial standpoint there isn't any doubt but that the nurse doing institutional work saves a great deal more money at a regular salary than the private duty nurse, who is only employed about half the time, does.

KANSAS.—Uniform duty hours, excellent living conditions, medical, surgical and hospital care, including X-ray and laboratory when ill, if necessary one month sick leave on pay, one month leave each year on pay, increase of pay with service, opportunity to travel, both in the United States and abroad, and retirement at age of fifty after twenty years of service.

PENNSYLVANIA.—I did private duty for about a year, and under best conditions I detested it. It is a dog's life. Institutional work in a small hospital is lonesome, because there is no one who understands or appreciates your work. Institutional work in a larger hospital is less lonely. Its problems are not less or more than those of a small hospital, merely different. I have been an executive in both small and large hospitals.

Institutional work is of advantage financially. It gives steady employment, and even a small salary is better in the end than private duty. Institutional work is trying but it is always interesting and usually exciting. There are many compensations in the love of your students and the joy of their success, which follow you all of your life. I was superintendent of the hospital for a time, but I am less interested in the business part of an institution than in the human side, and the development of the nurses. I have taught nurses a great deal and just love it.

California.—The hours in this hospital are good: eight hours with one day off per week. Regular monthly salary with maintenance, good food, and a chance for advancement. This is a large general hospital, so there is always something new to learn.

New York.—While I have never tried other forms of nursing than institutional work, I feel that as a life work I couldn't wish for any position in the nursing field that offers as much satisfaction as my operating room work. Steady hours, supervisory and executive work, and opportunities for better positions, leave nothing to be wished for in this work.

California.—I prefer institutional work on account of the regular hours and income.

Kansas.—I especially like the regular hours and work, but responsibility with only limited authority becomes irksome at times.

Pennsylvania.—My personal experience is that there is less strain, and more chance for a normal life, than in living in a room somewhere alone doing private duty. My experience for five years has been in taking care of nice people in lovely homes, long hours, most of them, but I found later that my institutional work was more pleasant. I also enjoyed educational work with the student nurses. One feels that such work justifies one's existence.

New York.—Institutional nursing—hours shorter, work easier, learn more every hour. If you are living in an up-to-date institution, it is like living in a home. You save more money also as your salary is a stated sum.

Pennsylvania.—I much prefer institutional nursing as I have regular hours on and off duty, regular pay, and an opportunity to attend college at evening. It also gives me a home where I can entertain my friends under conditions more nearly normal than in any other type of nursing.

Pennsylvania.—Being able to keep up with the newest methods of nursing, having a stated salary each month, the companionship of other nurses, and the homelike conditions which you can have when off duty, are some of my reasons for preferring institutional work.

California.—It is the most strenuous of any work I have done, but the satisfaction is greater, and I believe the future is very big.

California.—My reasons for determining to continue institutional nursing are—(1) A keener interest in my profession, engendered by contact with professional people. I would stress the very interesting and valuable contact with student nurses. (2) The educational opportunity offered by fixed hours of duty, allowing study courses, etc., as against the uncertain hours and conditions of private duty. (3) For economic reasons, I may reasonably expect to increase in value to the institutions where I work as my experience and knowledge grow. Can this be said of private duty?

4. What Institutional Nurses Do Not Like

Institutional nurses speak repeatedly of the strain of too heavy responsibility; and the friction in hospital groups. Some quotations throw light on why good nurses hesitate to try general floor duty.

CALIFORNIA.—My objections to institutional work and operating room work in particular would be: Lack of opportunity for recreation, and lack of opportunity to meet and mingle with the public in a normal way. We live in a world of our own and most times a rather narrow one.

CALIFORNIA.—I believe that most women engaged in institutional work become selfish after a while, because of the fact that maintenance and many other services usually go with the position, thus sparing her the necessity of thinking of the expense of her living. Most of us live under conditions which are better than we could afford to provide for ourselves, but we soon learn to take it as a matter of course. Also, we are very liable to "get into a rut" unless we make a definite effort to keep up to date.

CALIFORNIA.—Doctors expect perfection from nurses, though nurses may know and see many, many mistakes, and bad ones, that doctors make, these are covered up by the profession. A nurse's mistakes are never overlooked and "call downs" and insults are showered by the doctors in many cases, whereas perhaps on the very same patient the doctor has made a worse mistake than the nurse! It is too hard to see a student so treated by a doctor, and have to stand by as a supervisor and hear it, the blame not being with the student so much as the fact that she had more patients to think of than she could handle.

PENNSYLVANIA.—I dislike the restrictions of an institution. There is rarely an opportunity to entertain one's friends as much as one would like to do. One must always be an example to a student nurse when off duty as well as when on duty. I dislike the atmosphere among the head nurses in most institutions. They are always "gabbing." I feel the need of recreation, of meeting people in other lines of work, but do not have the energy and time to take advantage of opportunities. The atmosphere in a hospital is so depressing any way.

I want to say that there are some things in a hospital which I love and enjoy—the contact with the student nurses in the classroom and on the wards, and the contact with the patient when teaching the nursing.

I believe we need more social life among the officers and staff in an institution. If we all "played together" once a month or so we might work in a better spirit.

CALIFORNIA.—As long as it is possible for me to live at home I find that I can escape the narrowing influence that hospital life tends to have on institutional workers. My associates who live in a nurses' home never get away from their work, but live with it day and night. If I should have to do that again, and I have done it in years gone by, I would exchange for the field of public health where the worker is expected to have a home away from his work.

WASHINGTON.—A 55-hour week spent in charge of a busy obstetrical department was more than I felt able to stand. I worked at it only one year, and had the great satisfaction of making some progress in the administration of that department. I secured active cooperation of the medical staff in improving O.B. technique and practice in the hospital. I am writing this to let you know that I did not leave obstetrical work as a failure. I simply felt that what ability I had would soon be lost by an over-strenuous professional life. I felt myself beginning to view things in a lopsided way and decided to look further.

In my present position I plan an eight-hour work day for myself. Some days I spend seven hours in actual classroom work, other days only four. I do the regular "school teacher" thing and try to spend Saturday and Sunday in rest and recreation. Such a position gives one the opportunity to live a well-rounded life and to enjoy one's work.

California.—At present I have a very good position which I find intensely interesting because I really like to teach. But the greater part of the time in the past has been very unhappy because I was nearly always expected to do more than it was possible for me to do, and nearly all of my off-duty time found me in a state of exhaustion, so that I was unable to act or feel like a normal individual. I feel that there are very few positions for nurses where it is possible to stay for more than one or two years. We have just had a young graduate return from her first position, saying that she was expected to care for nine patients on general duty, and one of them delirious.

Washington.—I believe that if we could have regular eight-hour duty, day and night, with changes every two weeks instead of every five or six, institutional work would be much more pleasant. The hours should be arranged straight through as 7–3, 3–11, 11–7.

California.—Duties in this institution (54 beds) require day and night work. Sleep in the hospital and always called at night.

California.—As soon as possible I expect to take up some other work outside of nursing. The long hours and constant association with the sick, and the status the nurse has at present with the majority of lay people and some doctors, are the reasons I no longer have the love for the work I did. Instead of a profession it is ranked with unskilled labor in many cases, although demanding high education and ideals in training for it.

CALIFORNIA.—For the great responsibility of supervisor and nervous strain one is under, the salary is too small.

PENNSYLVANIA.—I like institutional work as a life work, as it has many advantages to offer. Most of these have been offset for me by the following disadvantages: Low status as instructor as compared to other institutional positions which require less preparation and less financial expenditure. Low salary as compared to that of assistant superintendent and superintendent who have no special preparation and who have not expended a cent for preparation. My salary has remained the same for five years ($1500) in spite of the fact that I have in the meantime secured my B. S. and have given body and soul to my work.

PENNSYLVANIA.—I work very long hours but it is largely my own fault that I do not have more recreation.

CALIFORNIA.—The responsibilities of the supervising nurse are so manifold that it keeps one in a state of tension. The vacation of two weeks is hardly a sufficient length of time for one to feel ready to resume duties for the ensuing year.

CALIFORNIA.—The institution with which I am connected allows only two weeks of vacation. I feel I must get into some kind of work which allows more than that in order to do good work.

CALIFORNIA.—The pettiness that is practised in hospitals among the members of the staff towards the private duty nurse is unbearable to one that tries to live and let live.

New York.—A great detriment to the graduate nurse in any institution is the employment of so many slightly trained girls and women, who cover the wards and rooms at a starvation wage. A visitor is unable to determine who is the trained nurse or who is not. Needless to say, the patient also pays for this in many ways.

The private duty nurse is very much to be pitied. A large percentage depends upon a registry. The registries play favorites, in fact, patients and doctor ask for a young attractive nurse, etc. Efficiency is an outside factor. (I ran a registry for four years.) Here again steps in the undergraduate who works for less money and longer hours, destroying the morale of the graduate nurse, and we must work if we want to exist. In a few words, a graduate nurse between the age of twenty-two and thirty years can and will find employment enough to provide a good living, and after that she will earn only enough to get along.

New York.—Why should nurses go in training for three years and endure the hardships, when maids are hired here on the same salary as a graduate nurse? Absolutely never have given a bath, made a bed, or taken temperatures, cannot comprehend, do not know what the word responsibility means, and personally feel they are on a par with the graduate nurses. After they are here a while they go out as practical nurses and get practical nurses' salary.

State Unknown.—There probably will be a time when I will be asked to go over to the General Hospital to help out students on the floor. I'll resign. I am not going to return to my student days.

State Unknown.—Furthermore, ladies of refinement refuse to work in training schools with ex-chambermaids as head nurses. Scullions, cooks, and pot washers fill the hospital training schools. Refined women refuse to affiliate.

California.—I am leaving temporarily because I need a change from the strain of the multiple duties which always seem to accumulate for me. I am too prone to do other people's work to last well in a small hospital. Also, I am tired of friction which seems to abound in hospitals. I'm always finding myself in a "mess," though in no way responsible for it.

Washington.—Institutional nursing could be made far more attractive were it run on a more standardized scale. By this I mean that the whims and ideas of a single person as head are different in each institution. If she or he happens to be the ultraconservative type, the whole school is affected. There is no higher authority to which one can appeal for aid and be sure to get it. It is not always the request of additional funds that is turned down but most often a suggested change in the system of some routine ward work. School systems other than those for nurses vary little throughout the country. We are still governed by autocrats and we don't like it.

California.—I am leaving institutional work for a while because there is a strain about the executive and educational work which I have had to do that is wearing, and I feel that I need a change. Also, everywhere I've been there seem to be friction and frequent upheavals and I do not like that. I always seem to get into hospitals during their crises. Also, I am too easily imposed upon to work where there is so much chance for overdoing and taking on extra work as there is in a hospital, particularly a small one. It's not the atmosphere of sickness, but the burden of too varied responsibilities that has worn me out.

California.—Students of this school resented the fact that we appointed as preliminary instructor a nurse who had been on general duty. They said this appointment lowered the standard of the school. However, they admitted the appointee in question was an excellent woman, a good nurse, and that she gave promise of being a good teacher.

CALIFORNIA.—While the nursing organizations and the public in general have done so much in recent years to abolish the exploitation of the student, there are still institutions which are being run on a purely commercial basis. I was recently told by the superintendent of such a hospital, "I don't care a damn about the students, it's my reputation I'm looking after."

5. Institutional Versus Private Duty

Institutional and private duty nurses have in common a genuine love for bedside nursing.

CALIFORNIA.—I had no desire for institutional work of any kind. Really I looked down upon general duty nursing as I felt only transient nurses and worn-out nurses would do it. After so many years of private duty, which I really enjoyed, I became too tired and nervous to be confined with one patient. Since I have been doing mostly night duty on surgical ward I like night duty, as I sleep well and one gets away from the noise and confusion of day work. So for an "old worn-out nurse" I suggest institutional work, regularity with fairly good pay and shorter hours.

CALIFORNIA.—I prefer a large family to one patient.

PENNSYLVANIA.—In institutional nursing there are no worries, as the board, room, laundry, telephone bills, etc. In case of illness one is usually taken care of free of charge with full salary, that is, if illness doesn't continue to last. One knows just where she stands as to time to work, off duty, etc. And the annual vacation of a month with pay, usually. There is no time to be lonesome in an institution.

CALIFORNIA.—From 1910 to 1917 I did private duty exclusively. I loved my work and being happy in it I gave more of my strength than I should have. Of course, at that time we did not have the twelve-hour duty. I was supporting a mother and helping to educate two younger brothers, father having died. Naturally with these responsibilities I could not save and realized if I was to keep up with the situation I must rest at least 48 hours between cases. The first 24 hours were always spent in bed, then a jolly show or stimulating recreation, then back to work, as I was out $3.56 every 24 hours that I did not work. Then the hospitals paid no attention to the collection of the special nurse fee. During these seven years I lost $500.00 or salary for 20 weeks' duty and practically all of this time was spent with difficult cases. Lucky to get four hours sleep out of the 24. Using a mattress on the floor for my bed on two occasions, insufficient bed clothing, and usually dirty quilts. Poorly cooked food and an hour or two off in the afternoon if there was some one to train to relieve me. The hospitals relieved three hours out of each 24. My expenses during the twenty weeks were $375.00.

During the above period I was on the watch for institutional work for the sake of regulated hours, but the salary was too small as the hospitals provided room and board. My own situation demanded that I pay rent for my family, so I was obliged to remain in private duty.

Then 1 year, 2 months Red Cross Home Nursing Classes, salary $100 a month. Nip and tuck to make ends meet. Six months Army. Had a taste of regular hours. Nine months private duty and decided to do institutional work as a position finally opened that paid enough so I could afford to take it.

I appreciate my clean bed, my somewhat regulated life—plain but well-cooked food. Have gained 25 pounds. Don't look as old as I did nine years ago. Have been able to accumulate some property. Have been ill only three days in ten years.

I am grateful for my private duty experience. It taught me to see the other person's side. It taught me poise and ability to judge and to always be on the alert and pay attention to detail. I recommend four or five years of it to every graduate nurse.

Self-preservation is the law of nature, and I really believe that the nurse will have better health, more working years, and be able to save a little for later years if she does some form of industrial, school, public health, or institutional nursing.

Pennsylvania.—In private duty I have found myself in a family where there was no one to manage the household but me. This was on two occasions, and beside the patient I had the housekeeping and much of the actual work for the family. It was distasteful to have to work for well people. In a hospital one can do any menial work and feel it is for the sick. Beside, the patient was left alone while I washed dishes and removed ashes from the range.

California.—To me private duty had more the aspect of a high priced servant or maid. People usually want their money's worth. In an institution a nurse's position to her patient is on a more superior status.

Kansas.—I prefer institutional work to private duty because you have your regular hours on and off duty. Your patients are being cared for and treatments carried out while you are off duty, which so often is not the case when doing private duty, especially out of the hospital. A doctor is always available in case of emergency. Always plenty of supplies (sterile goods, linen, drugs, etc.) and materials to work with and to make your patient comfortable.

Pennsylvania.—I prefer institutional work to private duty because you have your regular hours, regular week-ends, and when you go to bed at night you know that you can usually stay there until morning. Because in the locality where I come from the nurses are still doing mostly 24-hour duty, and one cannot work all day and be up at night too. In the first place, you cannot do justice to your patient, and why make a martyr of yourself? When you are doing private duty nursing you cannot plan from time to time, as your work is too uncertain. While in institutional work your pay is also regular whether the institution is full or not so busy. And with the price of rooms and apartments these days, it is a big thing to have your room and board. I did private duty for eight years and find that I can save more by doing institutional work.

New York.—I have better food. I do not wish to grow old doing private duty. I did private duty in New York City for five years. I was in a "rut" that took a six months' post-graduate course to get me out of.

California.—I much prefer surgery to public health nursing or private nursing, because of better hours than private duty and not so confining a life. Public health nursing I did not like because of the quantities of red tape involved and necessary conversational qualities.

California.—Time spent with patients is actual care and not satisfying whims or acting as maid.

California.—At the present time I am doing night duty, having charge of one floor of the hospital, which contains about 30–35 beds. I like general night duty, because it is steady work and fairly good pay. I find I make more money this way than I did while doing private nursing.

I dislike private nursing thoroughly, because you never know when you are going to be called or where you may have to go. The uncertainty is maddening to me.

California.—When I was younger I was extremely partial to private duty. I still am of the opinion that the private duty nurse and the general duty nurse are the only real bedside nurses that we have. A thorough course of the theory of nursing could amply fit one for the position of an institutional nurse; but to become a capable bedside nurse, one must have the bedside instruction and practice.

The institutional nurse holds an important position. Her importance is not in bedmaking, nor in bedside nursing, but it is in the management of herself and of other people. If a nurse has not poise, education, and diplomacy, she is doing the institution for which she works an injustice to accept any sort of a position therein.

California.—The hours are too long and the work too heavy to suit me, but the uncertainty of private duty makes institutional work more suitable to me.

Washington.—Until I happened by accident to fill my present position six years ago as superintendent of this sanitorium (the former superintendent left suddenly and they had no one in view and picked me from the hospital nursing staff), I had done nothing but private duty nursing in hospitals and homes. I was unable to earn a decent living besides finding the work nerve-racking, exhausting, and confining. I have gone seventy-two hours without removing my clothing many times (I'm not keen on these endurance contests) and when fortunate enough (?) to get a strenuous twelve-hour case (the patient's condition was usually grave or they would not consent to a twelve-hour system), I was too tired for any social life—even a picture show, just had enough ambition left to cross the city in a street car to my room (usually took an hour or more from leaving patient's bedside before getting home, waiting for street cars, transferring, and dressing in street clothes before leaving home or hospital, all taking time). Getting home at eight o'clock is not too soon for hot bath and bed as it must be remembered that you must be up by five-thirty to be back in the morning by seven.

I will never return to private duty for the above reasons, plus the antagonistic attitude of the hospitals to a strange nurse. You are treated as though you were not wanted and were very fortunate to have the opportunity of gracing their fair portals. It always meant delay and annoyance in getting lemons, oranges, sufficient linen, etc., for your patient. Graduates of the hospital were more fortunate as they knew how to steal what they could not get otherwise for their patients. If you had to leave the hospital to procure your meals or for your hours off on a twenty-four hour case, no one gave your patient any attention, and rather than find them neglected or have additional work on your return you would go without meals or bring a sandwich. In many homes, especially the homes of the poor, your hours off were limited to a minimum as you were afraid to leave the patient in the hands of the unskilled and often had to sleep on a makeshift bed.

My present work is much happier and far more remunerative, although entailing much responsibility from hiring help and inspecting their work to ordering all the supplies and groceries, but even so is far superior to private duty. My working hours are shorter and easier but, of course, there are drawbacks, the principal ones being that I must remain in charge of the institution half of the evenings of the week, and every other Sunday in absence of house physician. However, when I am off duty I hop in my car (a necessity as I am six miles from town—although within walking distance of an interurban), which an assured monthly salary of $150 has made possible.

NEW YORK.—Institutional work to me is wonderful.

I like to watch my hospital grow. We are like one big family knowing the weak points and the strong ones. The hospital is my family with patients as children to be watched and studied, worried over and then be proud of. The nursing staff is the other. Who wouldn't enjoy themselves watching young girls adjust their lives and win out or lose as the case might be? The thrill of graduation and then another group of nurses joining the ranks.

Private duty to me is essential—very hard and quite tiresome. It has a sameness of one case after another. I like to feel that I am a part of the big machine and in my small groove help to keep things running smoothly. It is wonderful to know the different departments trying, but not always succeeding, in working together. I enjoy the romance in the hospital, with its thrill of this famous patient or the tragedy of that.

CHAPTER 14

HOW DO NURSES LIKE THEIR JOBS?

Having secured this composite picture of who the graduate nurse is, and what she is like, the next step was to gather certain facts as to her economic status. Does nursing pay, in terms of dollars and cents? Can nurses look forward to a long professional life of economic independence, with enough money saved at the end so that they can retire when their active years are over and live in reasonable comfort? Or must they, if they undertake this profession, plan rather definitely to secure charitable aid from their less altruistic relatives? Of the three main branches of nursing, which offers the most attractive financial returns? The following pages throw light upon some of these questions.

1. How Much Rent Does the Nurse Pay?

Very few institutional nurses have the rent problem to contend with, since it is almost universal for hospitals to supply maintenance to their workers. The plan of making a cash living allowance in addition to the salary and permitting workers receiving it to live outside, seems to be rapidly growing in favor, but apparently the number of institutions which have as yet adopted it is small. Except in the rare cases where a private duty nurse is serving on a long, chronic case, all private duty nurses find it necessary to have a regular room of their own with telephone connections. The typical private duty nurse spends an aggregate of five months in twelve out of work, and during these periods, which may last from one day to several weeks, she must have a place to live. One-fourth of the private duty nurses pay $17.42 or less a month for room rent, half of them pay $24.71 or less, and three-fourths pay $33.56 or less. Similar figures for public health show that one-fourth pay $18.66 or less, one-half $27.32 or less, and three-fourths pay $39.27 or less. Both among private duty and public health nurses there are many who live at home and pay either no rent at all or only a small sum, and there are a few who have hired apartments and pay fairly large apartment rentals.

Rentals increase in amount with the size of the city. For both private duty and public health nurses rentals in cities of under 25,000 are in the $15.00 to $20.00 group. In cities from 25,000 to 500,000 population, rentals for the private duty group are between $20.00 and $25.00, and for the public health group between $25.00 and $30.00. In cities of 500,000 and over, the rentals for private duty nurses are between $25.00 and $30.00, and for public health nurses between $30.00 and $35.00. These figures are for the median or middle nurse in each case. Half of the nurses in the group are paying the amount specified or less, and half are paying the amount specified or more.

As might be expected, the rents paid by public health workers vary according to the position of the worker. Floating nurses pay between $15.00 and $20.00, staff nurses between $25.00 and $30.00, supervisors $30.00 to $35.00, and directors $35.00 to $40.00.

2. What is the Size of Her Laundry Bill?

Institutional nurses ordinarily have their laundry taken care of by the hospital, but private duty and public health nurses must pay their own costs. In private duty the amount of the laundry bill depends directly upon the number of days the nurse works. The March, 1927, study called for a complete work record for the week just ended when the nurse answered the questionnaire. Among nurses who worked one day during that week, the typical nurse paid a laundry bill which was more than fifty cents, but less than $1.00, while among the private duty nurses who worked all seven days of the week studied, the typical laundry bill was between $2.00 and $2.50. For all private duty nurses together, regardless of how many days they worked, the typical bill was $1.89. In public health the typical bill was $1.13, and the number of days the nurse worked made no difference in the size of the bill.

3. Does She Help Support Some One Else?

Most of the private duty studies were made in March, 1927. Comments on the backs of the questionnaires indicated so frequently that the nurse was responsible for the support of some one other than herself that it was deemed worth while to send a follow-up questionnaire in the month of August, 1927, to study, among other problems, the extent of this liability.

Figures are not available for public health or institutional nurses, but among the private duty nurses who were reached by the second questionnaire, it was found that 47 per cent were not responsible for helping support any one else, but 53 per cent were. Of the 53, 41 reported that they were responsible for the partial support of one or more people, and 12 that they had one or more people entirely dependent on them. The total number of dependents is so large that if it were possible to distribute the dependent group evenly among all the private duty nurses, we should then be able to say, "Every private duty nurse helps support some one else." It is almost a one to one relationship.

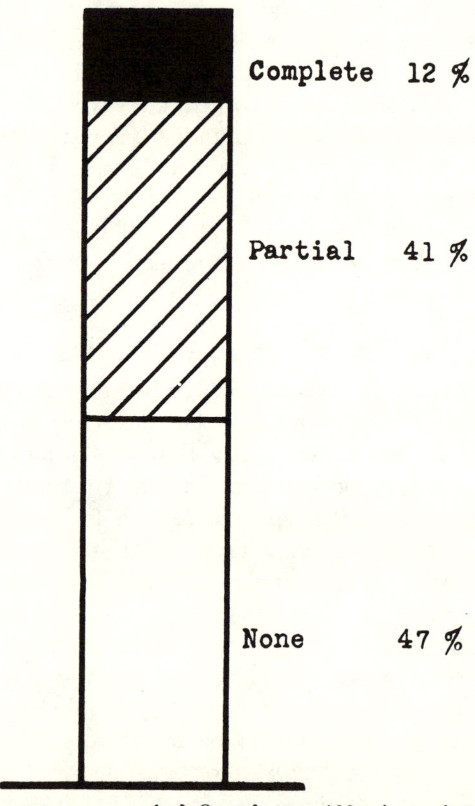

Diagram 34.—Support some one else? Out of every 100 private duty nurses, 47 have no one dependent upon them; while 53 contribute to the financial support of some one else. Twelve of the 53 have one or more people completely dependent upon them for support

4. How Much Has She Saved?

The nurses were asked, "Have you as much as $200 set aside which you could use in case you became ill?" "Have you as much as $500?" "$1,000?" The returns were as follows:

TABLE 56. PER CENT OF NURSES WHO REPORTED EACH AMOUNT OF SAVINGS

Savings	Private duty	Public health	Institutional	All
$200—No	27%	24%	18%	24%
$200—Yes	28	28	23	27
$500—Yes	16	16	17	16
$1,000—Yes	29	32	42	33
Total	100%	100%	100%	100%

It will be seen that private duty nurses are consistently least fortunate in their amounts of savings, and institutional nurses are most fortunate. In all three groups, however, a fair proportion belongs in the $1,000 or more class. The popular impression that nurses do not know how to save does not appear to be justified by these figures. The savings are particularly impressive when one realizes what a large proportion of all the nurses have been out of training school less than ten years.

The savings figures were tabulated for different population groups and for years out of school. In private duty and in public health the size of the city apparently makes no difference in the amounts of savings. In institutional work nurses working in the larger cities have larger sums of money saved. In all three branches savings increase regularly with the number of years out of training school.

Comparisons have been made of the amounts saved according to the positions held within the general field.

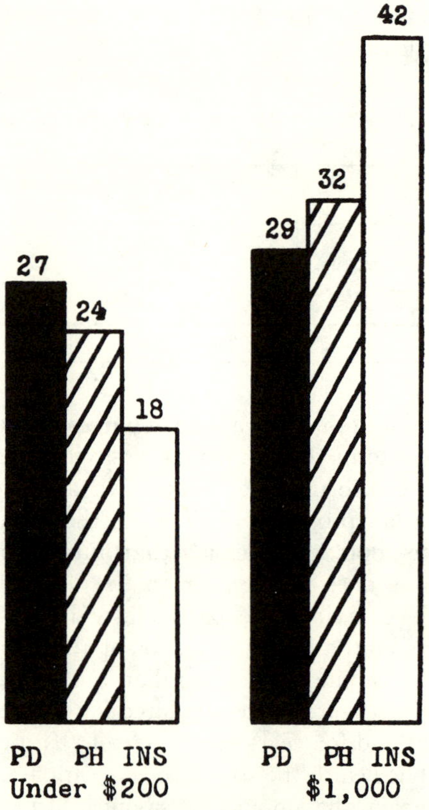

Diagram 35.—Per cent of nurses in each branch who have saved less than $200, or as much as $1,000

The following figures give the information for public health.

Public health—Savings

Staff nurses...........	31% haven't $200;	but 23% have $1,000
Floating nurses........	40% haven't $200;	but 30% have $1,000
Supervisors...........	19% haven't $200;	but 38% have $1,000
Directors.............	6% haven't $200;	but 59% have $1,000

Similar tabulations for nurses in institutional work give the following results.

Institutional—Savings

Superintendents of hospitals..................	9% haven't $200;	but 62% have $1,000
Superintendents of nurses..	9% haven't $200;	but 59% have $1,000
Assistant superintendents..	23% haven't $200;	but 46% have $1,000
Instructors and supervisors.	19% haven't $200;	but 33% have $1,000
Staff nurses..............	32% haven't $200;	but 29% have $1,000
Head nurses..............	22% haven't $200;	but 33% have $1,000
Nurses in special service....	18% haven't $200;	but 26% have $1,000
Administrative and clerical.	19% haven't $200;	but 63% have $1,000

5. Does She Have to Borrow?

Nurses were asked, "Did you have to borrow any money last year to live on?" Fourteen per cent of the private duty, 8 per cent of the public health, and 3 per

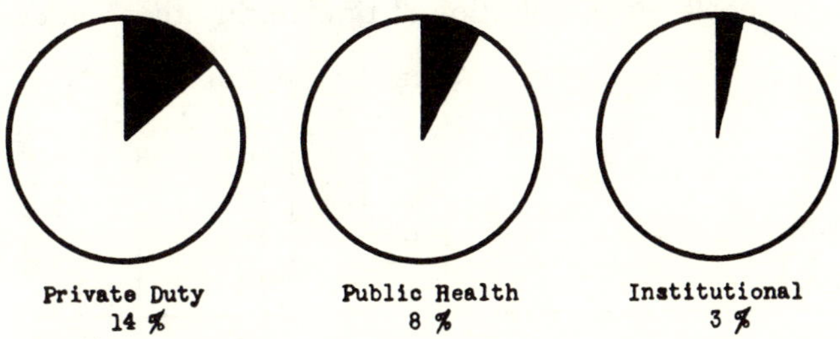

Diagram 36.—"Did you have to borrow any money last year to live on?" 14% of the private duty nurses answered, "Yes"; 8% of the public health nurses; and 3% of the institutional nurses. Public health and institutional nurses belong to regularly organized staffs, and therefore receive regular pay checks. They know each week what they can count upon

cent of the institutional nurses answered "Yes." For nurses in general 9 per cent were obliged to borrow. As might be expected, borrowing decreases with the number of years in service.

For public health nurses the returns show:

Staff nurses	10% borrowed
Floating nurses	11% borrowed
Supervisors	6% borrowed
Directors	2% borrowed

Institutional nurses answered the same question as follows:

Superintendents of hospitals	1% borrowed
Superintendents of nurses	2% borrowed
Assistant superintendents	2% borrowed
Instructors and supervisors	4% borrowed
Staff nurses	6% borrowed
Head nurses	3% borrowed

6. What is Her Working Week?

The first studies of private duty were made to cover the last week in March, 1927, which was taken as a period when sickness was near its height. The following table shows the distribution of time during that week.

TABLE 57. DAYS NURSES WORKED DURING ONE MARCH WEEK

	Private duty	Public health	Institutional
Worked	5.1 days	5.7 days	6.1 days
Waited	1.0	0	0
Sick	.4	.1+	.1−
Rested	.5	1.2	.8
Total	7 days	7 days	7 days

It will be seen that the typical private duty nurse worked less, worried more, was sick more, and rested less than the nurses in the other two fields.

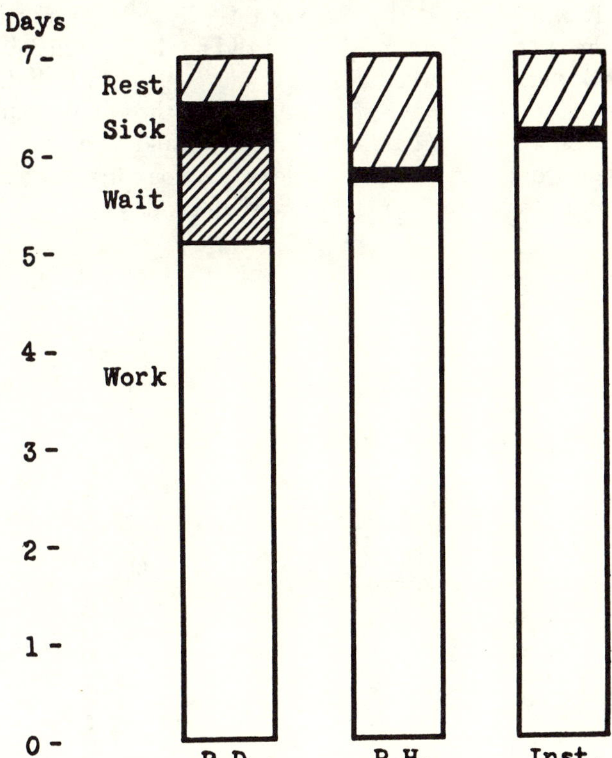

Diagram 37.—The typical March week. Private duty nurses worked less, worried more, were sick more, and rested less than the nurses in the other two groups. Figures for last week in March, 1927

The table which has just been given shows the week for a typical nurse in each group. That is, half the nurses worked more than is shown and half less. The actual days worked for all nurses are shown in the following table.

It will be noted that among the private duty nurses there is a fairly large group which did not have a full day's work during the week and a very large group which did not have a full day's rest. Almost all of the public health nurses worked for at least five days, and very few of them worked more than six days. Among institutional nurses almost half worked more than six days.

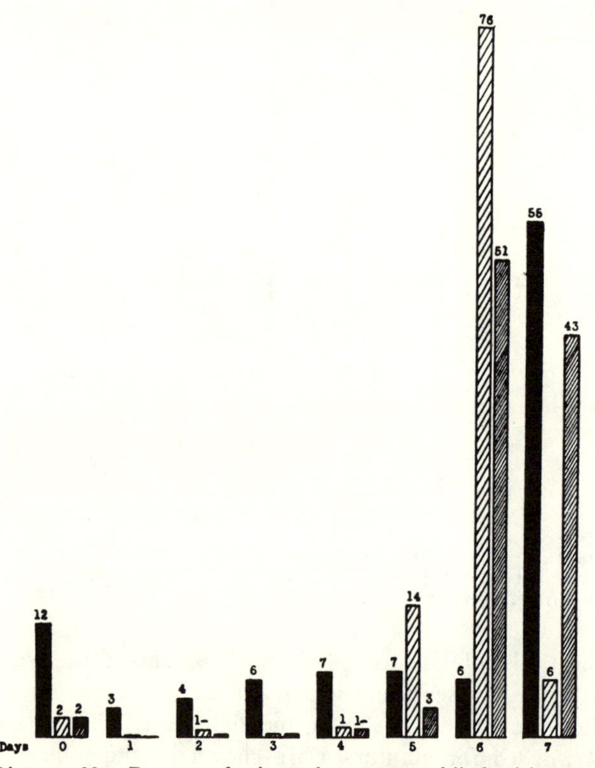

Diagram 38.—Per cent of private duty ▬, public health ▨, and institutional nurses ▨. who work each number of days

TABLE 58. PER CENT OF NURSES WORKING EACH NUMBER OF DAYS DURING THE MARCH WEEK STUDIED

Days	Private duty	Public health	Institutional
0	12.3%	2.1%	1.6%
1	2.5	.2	0
2	4.1	.6	.5
3	5.6	.5	.4
4	7.0	1.0	.8
5	7.1	13.9	2.5
6	6.2	75.6	51.2
7	55.2	6.1	43.0
Total	100%	100%	100%

Notes from institutional nurses suggest that while in theory they have a complete day off each week, in practice, when work is heavy, they are frequently obliged to forego all or part of the weekly holiday.

Because there was evidence that private duty is seasonal and irregular, a second questionnaire was sent out in August. The returns show that while there was more unemployment in August than in March, the general type of distribution remained the same.

TABLE 59. PER CENT OF PRIVATE DUTY NURSES WHO WORKED EACH NUMBER OF DAYS IN THE MARCH AND AUGUST WEEKS

Month	Days worked								Total
	0	1	2	3	4	5	6	7	
March	12	3	4	6	7	7	6	55	100%
August	30	2	3	4	5	5	6	45	100

The "typical" private duty week for the two months is also shown in the following table.

TABLE 60. DAYS WORKED BY TYPICAL PRIVATE DUTY NURSE IN ONE WEEK IN MARCH AND ONE WEEK IN AUGUST

	March	August
Worked	5.1 days	4.1 days
Waited	1.0	.7
Sick	.4	.4
Rested	.5	1.8
Total	7 days	7 days

It will be noted in these studies that data were gathered for the amount of time lost during the week because of illness. Lost days because of illness are much higher among private duty nurses than in either of the other groups, and the time of year seemed to make no difference in the amount of illness. In one March week the typical private duty nurse lost .36 of a day, the typical public health nurse .13, and the typical institutional nurse .09. Apparently age makes no difference among private duty nurses so far as sickness is concerned until the nurse has been out of training twenty-five years or more. From that point on, sickness definitely increases.

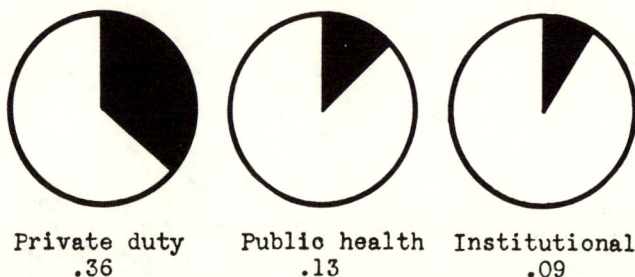

Diagram 39.—Days too sick to work. Each circle represents one day during the March week studied. The black portion shows what per cent of a day was lost by the typical private duty, public health, and institutional nurse because of illness

7. What are Her Hours of Work?

Special data were gathered for the private duty nurses concerning the number of cases handled in a week and the number of hours worked. Of 2,657 private duty nurses who reported on this question, 2,287, or 86 per cent worked on only one case during the week, 307, or 12 per cent worked on two cases, 53, or 2 per cent on three cases, 9 or .3 per cent on four cases, and one on five cases.

Apparently most cases are either in the hospital or in the home, and there are comparatively few which start in one location and transfer to the other. Fifty-three per cent of the nurses reported that their cases were in the hospital, 42 per cent in the home, and only 5 per cent in both hospital and home.

The question of whether a nurse works "12" or "24" hours a day seems to depend rather closely on whether the case is in the hospital or in the home. For hospital cases 52 per cent of the "days" were 12 hour day duty, 36 per cent were 12 hour night duty, and only 12 per

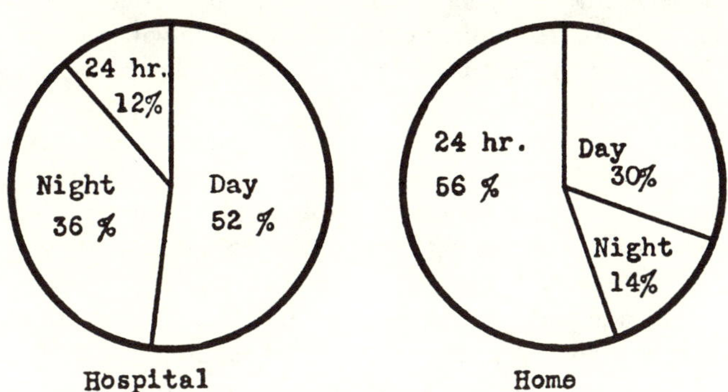

Diagram 40.—Per cent of hospital nursing days, and of home nursing days, which were on 12 hour day, 12 hour night, and 24 hour service

cent were 24 hour duty. For cases in the home, however, 30 per cent of the "days" were for 12 hour day duty, 14 per cent for 12 hour night duty, and 56 per cent for 24 hour duty.

It should be noted in thinking about these figures that 12 hour day duty is usually thought of as including two hours of rest, although nurses testify that in practice they are frequently unable to secure any such free period. Twenty-four hour duty in theory includes four hours of rest and at least a few hours of sleep at night. Here, again, however, nurses report that in many cases they are unable to get either free time in the day or an adequate amount of sleeping time at night. The actual rest periods in private duty apparently vary so greatly that no adequate statement can be made concerning them. It seems safe to say, however, that the more difficult and nerve-wracking the case, the less likely it is that the nurse will be able to take her allotment of free time. Neither in hospitals nor homes is provision usually made for relieving the special nurse, and if the patient is seriously ill, and the nurse conscientious, she will not leave him unless she knows that some other thoroughly competent person is in charge.

The question arises at this point whether it should not be a recognized practice in all hospitals to provide for regular relief periods for special duty nurses. The charge which the hospital makes is based on the assumption that the hospital will provide an amount of nursing service adequate for the average patient. If the patient secures a special nurse, it is on the assumption that he is in need of more service than can be given by the regular staff, but in theory this supplements the regular nursing service and does not supplant it. Otherwise, if it were understood that by engaging a special the patient relieved the regular nursing staff from its regular responsibility for caring for him, the hospital would, of course, be in honor bound to charge him less than it charges patients with similar accommodations who do not supply their own special duty nurses. That hospitals do not always recognize the obligation of supplying a reasonable amount of nursing service to all patients, regardless of whether or not they have specials, has been repeatedly brought to the attention of the Committee by patients, physicians, and nurses. It would seem that a legitimate method for meeting this obligation, at least in part, would be to provide regular relief periods for special nurses and so cut the special nurses' day to 8 or 10 hours instead of 12 without leaving the patient uncared for.

Among institutional nurses the hours worked are often more than the theoretical working week. During the March week studied the typical nurse in each of the nine institutional positions reported hours as follows:

TABLE 61. AVERAGE HOURS WORKED IN MARCH WEEK BY TYPICAL INSTITUTIONAL NURSE ACCORDING TO POSITION HELD

Position	Average hours worked
Superintendent of hospitals	62
Superintendent of nurses	59
Assistant superintendent	56
Instructor or supervisor	56
Staff nurse	60
Head nurse	59
Nurse in social service	54
Nurse in administrative or clerical work	52
Others	51
All	58

In public health the typical working week (according to the census recently taken by the National Organization for Public Health Nursing) is 42 hours.

8. How Much Does She Earn?

Each nurse was asked how much money she earned in 1926. Of the private duty nurses, 43 per cent were unable to answer the question, because they had not kept track of their actual earnings. Most of the public health and institutional nurses, who are on regular stated salaries, were, of course, able to answer, since all that was needed was to multiply the amount of the monthly pay check by twelve. The diagram shows the average salaries received by private duty, public health, and institutional nurses for each number of years out of training school. It should be noted that throughout this discussion institutional salaries are computed on a cash-received basis and then are increased by an allowance of $500 to cover maintenance. This is because, with a few exceptions, practically all institutional salaries include maintenance. The allowance of $500 is extremely conservative, since it means less than ten dollars a week for board, lodging, and laundry. In many cases nurses are receiving maintenance which is probably worth two or three times this figure.

The diagram shows that while there are individual variations, the typical private duty nurse continues from year to year at almost an even level of pay. The average throughout her professional life is $1,311. Public health nurses begin at about $1,450 and rise steadily, though not rapidly, according to their years of service. In institutional work the average salary begins at about $1,750 and rises rapidly for the first fifteen years, remains on a level for the next fifteen, and then drops. The average salaries for public health and institutional nurses are $1,720 and $2,079 respectively.

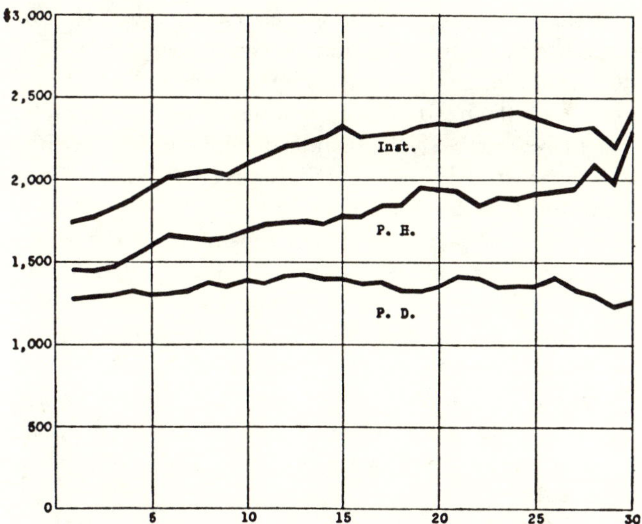

Diagram 41.—Years out and Year's Pay. Average salaries received by private duty, public health, and institutional nurses who have been out from training school each number of years. Institutional salaries include a flat allowance of $500 a year for maintenance. Averages for whole group: Private duty $1,311, public health $1,720, institutional $2,079

The diagram represents "average" salaries. The average is a figure which seeks to tell what the condition would be if all nurses were alike. A somewhat different figure is the median, which shows the half-way point, where the middle nurse stands. In most of the salary data the median is below the average, because the median is not affected by the few very high salaries, which must be included when averages are being computed. The median salaries for private duty, public health, and institutional nurses are $1,297, $1,685, and $2,000 respectively. This means in each case that half the nurses received that or more, and the other half received that or less. In private duty one-fourth the nurses had $1,010 or less in 1926, and another fourth received $1,612 or more. In public health one-fourth received $1,503 or less, and the top fourth $1,892 or more; while among institutional nurses the lowest fourth received $1,724 or less, and the top fourth $2,338 or more.

The size of the city in which the nurse works has a direct bearing upon private duty earnings, but seems to have relatively little bearing in the fields of public health and institutional nursing. In private duty the typical nurse living in towns under 10,000 earned $1,177 in 1926. The amount increases until the typical private duty nurse in a city of 500,000 or more earned $1,413. In public health and institutional work, however, no such increase is apparent.

The size of the school in which the nurse was trained has apparently very little influence upon salaries in private duty or in institutional nursing, but there is a definite influence in public health. The typical public health nurse who was trained in a school with a daily average of less than 50 patients, earned between $1,500 and $1,600 in 1926. The typical public health nurse who was trained in a school of more than 50 but less than 300 patients, earned between $1,600 and $1,700; while those coming from larger schools earned between $1,700 and $1,800.

In private duty the amount of education a nurse has had seems to make little difference as to the amount of money she is able to earn. In public health and institutional work, however, there is a definite increase with increased years in school. The following table shows the pay of the median, or half-way, nurse for each educational group in private duty, public health, and institutional work.

TABLE 62. SALARY RECEIVED IN 1926 BY THE MEDIAN OR MIDDLE NURSE IN EACH EDUCATIONAL GROUP

Schooling	P. D.	P. H.	Inst. (Incl. $500)
Under 8th grade	$1,275	$1,567	$1,850
8th grade	1,350	1,608	1,922
1 year high school	1,261	1,647	1,852
2 years high school	1,268	1,671	1,829
3 years high school	1,347	1,664	1,989
4 years high school	1,289	1,669	1,981
1 year college	1,290	1,740	2,053
2 years college	1,275	1,846	2,045
3 years college	1,150	1,875	2,399
4 years college	1,467	1,860	2,114
1+ post-graduate	..	1,850	3,550

As was stated at the beginning of this discussion of salaries, 43 per cent of the private duty nurses do not know how much they earned in 1926. It is interesting to note that the amount of education the nurse has had seems to have no bearing upon whether or not she has kept track of her yearly earnings. The groups which had the highest per cent of definite answers on this point were the private duty nurses who had had less than 8th grade education at one end and those who had had four years or more of college education, at the other.

The range of salaries for private duty nurses was from no salary at all to one nurse who earned $3,600 in 1926. The range for public health nurses was from $0 to over $6,000. The range for institutional nurses was from $0 to $9,200 (including $500 for maintenance).

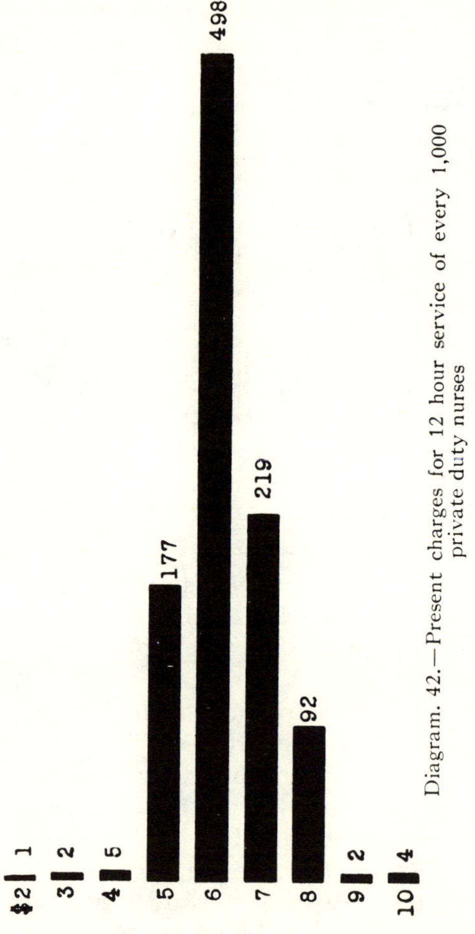

Diagram. 42.—Present charges for 12 hour service of every 1,000 private duty nurses

For 24 hour service in private duty, charges have increased from $3.00 a day ten years ago to $7.00 a day now. For 12 hour service charges have increased from $3.00 a day to $6.00 a day. For all services combined, the median is $6.00.

Typical earnings for the median, or middle, nurse in public health and institutional positions are as follows:

Among public health nurses

The median staff nurse receives between $1,500 and $1,600 a year
The median supervisor receives between $1,800 and $1,900 a year
The median director receives between $2,200 and $2,300 a year

Among institutional nurses ($500 has been included for maintenance) the median

Superintendent of hospital......	receives between $2,600 and $2,700
Superintendent of nurses........	receives between $2,500 and $2,600
Superintendent of hospital and nurses......................	receives between $2,400 and $2,500
Assistant superintendent........	receives between $2,000 and $2,100
Instructor or supervisor.........	receives between $1,800 and $1,900
Staff nurse....................	receives between $1,600 and $1,700
Head nurse..................	receives between $1,700 and $1,800
Nurse on special service.........	receives between $2,000 and $2,100
Administrative or clerical.......	receives between $1,800 and $1,900
Others......................	receive between $2,000 and $2,100

9. How Much Charity Service Does the Private Duty Nurse Give?

Since the typical, or median, private duty nurse charges $6.00 a day; and since she earned $1,297 in 1926, we are able to find how many days she was employed. The computation gives us a total of 216 days—or approximately seven months. This does not allow for any regular rest periods, because in private duty there is no regular arrangement for rest days, and every holiday the nurse takes means that she loses a day's pay.

She also, however, loses pay for certain days when she is hard at work. A study was made of the number of free days of nursing care given by private duty nurses during the six months ending in August. Of all private duty nurses who reported, 38 per cent had given no days of nursing care during that time, but 62 per cent had given one or more days. The range was from those who gave no time at all to 2 per cent who gave four months or more out of the six months studied, without pay. For the group as a whole the average was 14.6 days for six months, which would be the equivalent of 29.2 days, or practically one full month of free nursing service a year. If we

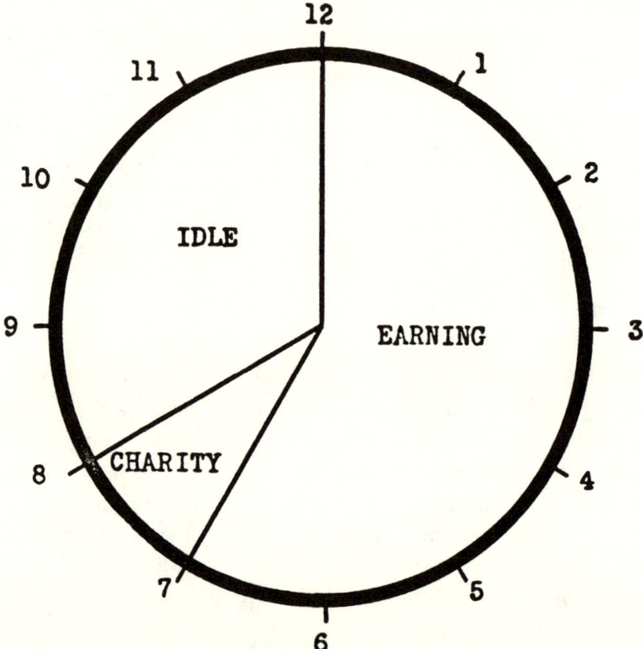

Diagram 43.—Months in each year which the typical private duty nurse spends in earning money, giving charity, and living on her savings. The typical private duty nurse must live for five months on what she earns in seven

assume that this work was worth \$6.00 a day, it means that these nurses are giving the equivalent of \$175 worth of free service each year, or one-seventh of their total year's earnings.

It is worth remembering in this connection that the private duty nurse works on only one case at a time, and since her working day is twelve hours long, or more, she cannot make up for her charity cases by taking on a few extra paying cases at the same time. Nor, if she is to maintain her professional standing, can she balance the free service she gives to a needy patient by taking on a wealthy patient and charging him double! Her charity comes out of her own pocketbook.

10. How Does She Like Her Job?

At the bottom of each questionnaire the nurse was asked, "Do you intend to keep on indefinitely in private duty?" or, "In public health?" or, "In institutional nursing?" The replies were as follows:

	Private duty	Public health	Institutional
Stay	55%	86%	82%
Hesitate	9	6	7
Go	36	8	11
	100%	100%	100%

The figures indicate that public health and institutional nurses are in general fairly content in the fields in which they are working and are not particularly anxious to change, but almost half of the private duty nurses are either definitely intending to leave private duty or are seriously considering doing so.

Other returns give further evidence as to the dissatisfaction among private duty nurses. Apparently popula-

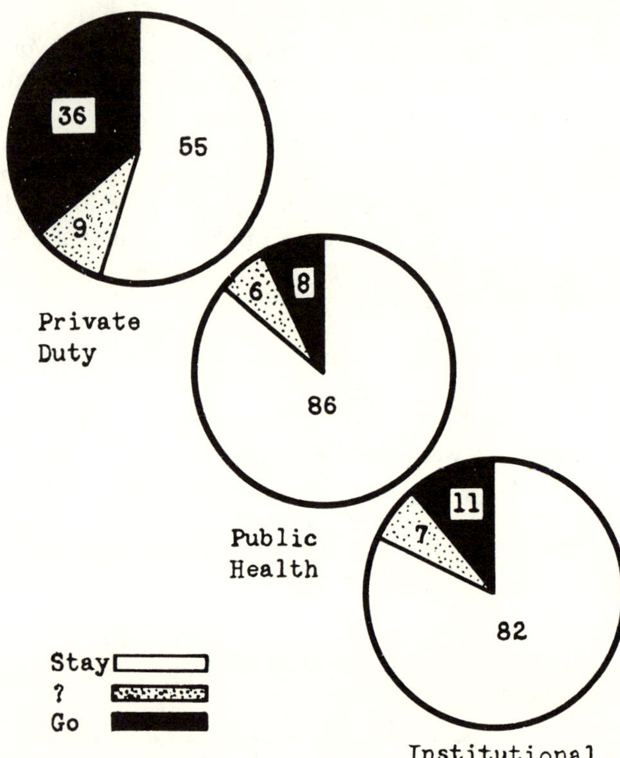

Diagram 44.—"Do you intend to continue indefinitely in this type of work?" Of the private duty nurses, 55% plan to stay and 45% are either hesitating or definitely planning to leave the field. Among public health nurses the corresponding figures are 86% and 14%; and among institutional nurses, 82% and 18%

tion makes no difference, but there is a definite connection between the age of the nurse and the amount of her education, and her desire to stay or to leave the private duty field.

Among private duty nurses:

0– 5 years out	43% want to stay
6–10 years out	54% want to stay
11–15 years out	63% want to stay
16–20 years out	69% want to stay
21–25 years out	71% want to stay
26–30 years out	79% want to stay
31+ years out	77% want to stay

The implication of the table is that the more recently the nurse has been graduated from training school, the less satisfied she is with private duty, and the more anxious she is to get into either public health or institutional work. Many nurses who do not like private duty leave early. Those who stay like it, or become accustomed to it, or stay because, as many have written to the Grading Committee, they are "too old to learn anything else."

In private duty there is also a fairly definite connection between the amount of education the nurse has had and her desire to stay or leave.

8th grade or less	67% want to stay
1 year high school	58% want to stay
4 years high school	52% want to stay
4 years college	38% want to stay

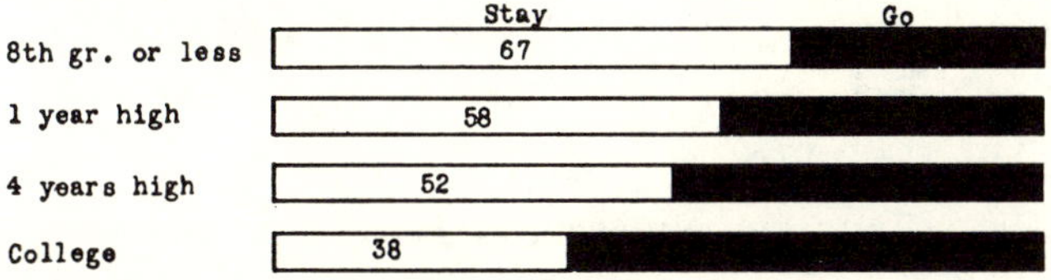

Diagram 45.—"Do you intend to continue indefinitely in private duty?" The returns classified according to the amount of schooling each nurse has had, show that the better the nurse's education, the less likely she is to be contented in the private duty field

In public health and institutional nursing, on the other hand, there seems to be no relation between population, age, or educational background. In these branches nurses are happy, and about equally satisfied throughout the groups.

Several people who have seen Diagram 45 have suggested that perhaps the Grading Committee ought to hesitate about making this particular series of figures public. One said, for example: "The educational requirement in this state is very low. We have tried and tried to raise it. The objectors—physician owners of small hospitals—refuse to accede because, 'if a nurse is educated she doesn't want to work,' and to them the private duty field is the only one in which a nurse has to work. The nurse, if educated, and therefore lazy, doesn't want to work and consequently she leaves private duty. That is the argument in favor of eighth grade education for nurses. It seems to me that this diagram strengthens this argument."

The Committee might agree that these figures are dangerous if it had never made a study of what physicians really want. No thoughtful person, however, could look at the figures and diagrams in Chapters 8 and 9 or read the many hundreds of frank comments on the backs of returned medical report forms now in the Committee's files without being impressed with one outstanding fact.

Physicians Want Intelligent, Well-Bred, Well-Educated Nurses for Their Patients

They are concerned about problems of cost, and supervision, and distribution, and they make many suggestions for solving them, but when physicians are thinking in terms of their own patients they do not want practicals; they do want R.N.'s. They do not want servant girls; they do want well-bred, intelligent young women.

And thoughtful physicians everywhere realize that intelligent daughters of families above the servant class are no longer contented with an eighth grade or one year high school education. It is probably perfectly true that poorly educated, low grade nurses are more apt to want to stay in private duty (where there is great independence, and no one to check up on the quality of their work) than to go into public health or institutional nursing. But very few physicians will welcome nurses of that type. The private duty nurses about whom the physicians grow really enthusiastic are (if they are young) rather apt to be high school or college graduates.

11. SUMMARY

The outstanding facts in this chapter may be summarized as follows:

a. Practically all private duty nurses, as well as public health nurses, either live at home or pay rent. Most institutional nurses live rent free.
b. Laundry bills are higher for busy private duty nurses than for public health nurses. Institutional nurses pay no laundry bills.
c. More than half of the private duty nurses help support some one else.
d. Institutional nurses save most, and private duty nurses least.
e. Private duty nurses are more apt to borrow money to live on than nurses in public health or institutional nursing.
f. During the busy season private duty nurses work less, worry more, are sick more, and rest less than nurses in the other two fields.

g. In private duty, most hospital duty is on 12 hour and most home duty on a 24 hour basis. The weekly hours are 84 or 168, with undetermined and irregular rest periods. In public health the typical working week is 42 hours. In institutional it is 58. The suggestion is made that hospitals might properly provide relief service to reduce the hours for specials on hospital duty.

h. Half the private duty nurses earn $1,297 or less per year; half the public health nurses $1,685 or less; and half the institutional nurses (if $500 is included for maintenance) $2,000 or less.

i. In public health and institutional nursing the beginner may look forward to increased pay. In private duty she may not.

j. The typical private duty nurse works for pay seven months a year, gives charity service for one month, and is resting or waiting for work for the remaining four months. What she earns in the first seven months must support her in the remaining five.

k. Well over four-fifths of the public health and institutional nurses want to stay on in their branches of the profession. Almost one-half of the private duty nurses want to leave.

l. The younger and better educated the nurse, the more apt she is to want to get out of private duty.

CHAPTER 15

WHAT PRIVATE DUTY NURSES SAY

It has not been necessary to look at the face of a questionnaire in order to know whether it came from a private duty, a public health, or an institutional nurse. The sorts of comments made on the backs of the questionnaires have been of such markedly opposite types that it has been possible to tell which was which at first glance. The tone of most public health and institutional replies has been happy. The tone of most private duty replies has been rather evidently unhappy.

1. Like Private Duty—Enjoy Bedside Nursing

In spite of the prevalent discontent among private duty nurses, one fact has stood out clearly, so clearly, in fact, that it has been genuinely impressive. NURSES LIKE BEDSIDE NURSING. They do not like their hours, or pay, or conditions of work, but most nurses honestly enjoy taking care of really sick patients. It is this fact which throws a ray of hope through all the pages which follow. It should never be lost sight of. In spite of the constant criticisms and the prevalent bitterness in the private duty field, many of the women who are in that field are at heart real nurses who care deeply about their work and have never lost the essential spirit of nursing.

MASSACHUSETTS.—It is a grand feeling after hours of strenuous nursing to see that steady climb to health which only a private duty nurse can glory in.

NEW YORK.—I like the responsibility which a private nurse in a home must assume in absence of the doctor.

MASSACHUSETTS.—Personally, I like private duty even though it is harder; you come in closer touch with your patient and see better the results of your work.

NEW YORK.—I love it but feel we could do more and last longer for the public were things adjusted a little.

MASSACHUSETTS.—I really do love the care of a patient and I don't think one can give the same real care in a hospital that one can give in a home. Also, it has more responsibility, and when a nurse has been a graduate for a lot of years, she likes to feel that she has had enough experience to be able to nurse in a house and again, one is not so much a piece of machinery. This is the way I truly do feel and I do love my nursing.

WASHINGTON.—One does meet many interesting patients and when one hears "Oh! I feel so comfortable now," or "I just don't know what I would have done without you when I felt so badly," one feels almost as well repaid as when the "check" eventually rolls one's way. And what is more satisfying than to see a patient after a hard night—a night when one did not know if the patient would live to see the morning dawn—see the patient relax and drop into an hour of restful sleep?

LOUISIANA.—I will keep on private duty nursing because I love the work. It brings me the opportunity to perform many acts of charity and it is such an interesting study. I learn something new on every case.

NEW YORK.—There is a great deal to be said for private nursing, especially in the home of the middle class. There I think a real nurse can prove herself what people have so often called us—Angels of mercy. One becomes very near and dear to patient and the family. My specialty is children: I love them.

MASSACHUSETTS.—I feel a great satisfaction in entering a home where all is confusion, due to sickness, then, by being as tactful as possible, get things straightened out. I feel that we can help the entire family as well as the individual. Then, too, I feel more independent as I can have a complete rest when I am off a case. (Am sick a good deal with a kidney condition so have to be very careful and not get run down.) While on general duty or industrial work or hospital staff, it is almost compulsory to be on duty, even though you don't feel equal to it.

MASSACHUSETTS.—I think we older nurses like the home and get a closer and more sympathetic relation and feeling toward the patient and family.

NEW YORK.—I do not proclaim it a life of ease but I do consider it worthwhile labor.

WASHINGTON.—Gynecology is my work and has been for the past 12 years, also care and feeding of infants. I have given much time and study to the latter and like it very much. I like private duty nursing because I have no trouble obtaining cases. I very seldom go on call, perhaps twice in a year, and some years not at all. I get the greater part of my work through ex-patients, and in eight years' nursing in Washington I have not had one single complaint about the nursing fee. I do not nurse constantly. I find it too hard. I arrange to take plenty of rest between cases.

NEW YORK.—It is interesting to me to meet all classes of people and hear their opinions on different topics and get their views in general on everything.

I would not give my private duty experience for a million dollars.

NEW YORK.—I love my work. I don't regret that I have taken up nursing as a profession, but I do ask for a square deal.

2. Like Freedom

Perhaps the most attractive aspect of private duty is its freedom. Nurses who have had three years of necessarily close supervision in the nursing school revel in the complete absence of such supervision after they are graduated. They like to be free to move from city to city, to choose cases as they wish, to take a day off whenever they feel like it, to try one unexpected adventure after another. It is the very fact that nursing is a free lance occupation which attracts many nurses to it. They would rather, many of them, have freedom than have the advantages which regularly organized work would bring.

CALIFORNIA.—I like private duty nursing because it leaves me more free to go about. But I don't see sense to these questions.

NEW YORK.—I like private duty nursing because I have time between cases; also I am my own boss.

NEW YORK.—My home is in California so I prefer private duty work because I can take longer vacations than I could get in any institutional or industrial position.

CALIFORNIA.—I do night work mostly because I help support a home and a five year old boy, and in that way am at home with him during the day.

KANSAS.—I much prefer hospital work, but I have an aged mother to care for. We own our home and my mother refuses to leave it for any other.

I am her only child left and she has depended upon me for her support for about thirty years.

New York.—I suppose it is a selfish reason, but I like to feel that when I finish a case I can take one or more days off duty without having to ask permission. The hours are, of course, long—what other class of people work twelve hours?—and when on call every time the phone rings my heart jumps into my throat, and if it happens, as it does in my case, that there is no one but myself to answer the phone, why I have to stay in the house after I once register. Taking all things into account, isn't it true that some one has to do private duty nursing? We cannot all do charge duty, public health work, or such like. Isn't it perhaps well that there are some of us who prefer "Private Duty Nursing"?

California.—I do it because it gives me the chance to make a small home for myself and indulge my domestic complex when off duty. Also it gives me opportunities of rest not possible in a home with other nurses.

California.—I like private duty. Have always enjoyed my cases. And if my little girl is ill, it is much easier to get relief than if I am doing any other branch of nursing.

California.—Being a mother of three children and having a home to keep and a mortgage to pay, necessity made private duty more attractive to me because it may be regular or irregular and affords me time at home if I desire it.

State Unknown.—Yes, I enjoy private duty and it leaves me freer to take care of friends and relatives than institutional nursing would.

California.—I intend to do private duty indefinitely because I have two children and desire to be with them as much as possible. Private duty gives me a few days between cases to be with them.

MASSACHUSETTS.—I have had a sick husband and we are just beginning to get to the top of the hill. He will need a complete re-education and that means four years of work evenings for him and I shall continue where I am unless I can find executive work which leaves me as free as this does.

MASSACHUSETTS.—My main reason for continuing private nursing is to be able to partly satisfy my wanderlust nature. My permanent residence is with my parents near Boston, but I enjoy traveling and can while doing private duty as in no other way. In other words, I can come and go as I wish. Have spent one winter in Washington, D. C., and have crossed the country three times in the past seven years.

MASSACHUSETTS.—I especially enjoy private duty nursing from the time I get my check until I have to register again.

NEW YORK.—I am still my own boss.

3. Hours

The protests against the long hours of private duty nursing were almost unanimous. Hardly a return was received which did not somewhere voice the universal conviction that even the 12 hour day is inhumanly long. It is believed that, if the one matter of hours could be arranged so that nurses would either work on a regular 8 hour shift, or if working in longer "takes" could have equally long rest periods regularly provided for every seven days, the major part of the present unhappiness in private duty would disappear.

NEW YORK.—I think private duty nursing is darned hard work, on account of the hideous hours. The nursing is all right, but I am a wreck after every hard case and bored after every easy one.

The easy ones are as "hard as the hard" ones on account of the hours. Can't something be done to give a little relief in a 12-hour day?

California.—I am on a 24-hour case now where it is absolutely necessary for some one to be with the patient all the time, but no provision has been made for the nurse's hours, and, it being very rude to walk off at the time, I am obliged to stay.

Kansas.—Of course, you are allowed four hours off but when your patient is bad, who will give him the care that you would if you were with him during that time? No one! Usually the relative or friend disturbs the patient to such a degree that the nurse (if she is conscientious) hesitates about leaving the patient for such a length of time.

Then again she must be up all hours of the night getting little, if any, sleep, and then keep it up the next day. People as a rule (especially the working or laboring class) cannot afford two nurses on a case and when they want a nurse you may rest assured the patient is very ill. I think a nurse certainly earns her $6 a day when she usually works or is on 24 hour duty. Of course, an "easy" case may be had once in a while but they are few and far between.

New York.—If I had a sister I should not want her to endure the hardships and trials of nursing. For the past few months I have been nursing at a hospital on the east side. I get up at 5:45 a. m., take a cross-town bus and then the subway and am on duty at 7:00 a. m., 12 hours of duty and then home at 7:45 p. m. I may have a uniform to get ready or a few stockings to darn or mending to do and then to bed. If I go out for the evening, I am too tired for my next day's work. I am not crowded on the buses or subways in the mornings, as maids, clerks, and most others go to work at 9:00 a. m.

WASHINGTON.—All shop girls enjoy shorter hours than we do; they are protected by legislation. Why not the nursing profession?

NEW YORK.—The hours of private duty are perfectly ghastly—14 hours from the time one leaves home until one returns at night, but industrial and hospital positions do not pay a living wage.

MASSACHUSETTS.—While any kind of nursing is fine work in itself, to think of spending a life as a private duty nurse would be for me a terrible thought. The life is too abnormal, too dreadfully one-sided. It is not the work but the time one gives to it. After a day which begins by my taking the car at 6:15 a. m. and ends with my return home at 8:00 p. m. I am literally exhausted body and mind. No, I hope that it will not be necessary for me to keep on indefinitely in private duty nursing. No one but a sister of charity, perhaps, who has deliberately renounced the world should be expected to do so.

NEW YORK.—Our first impulse is to say that we hate private duty nursing when in reality it is the long hours we hate. If we could only have an eight hour duty, I think in the majority of cases private nursing would be ideal but I see no hope for it now although there is no reason why hospital patients could not be cared for by institutional nurses for at least two hours each day. When one thinks of having to work 12 hours a day and under such trying circumstances sometimes, it really seems to be nothing short of criminal. But who cares? The laboring man or factory girl is protected by law from having to work over eight hours, unless they get paid accordingly. (I can hear some sweet, dignified nurse with the Florence Nightingale spirit saying, "Oh, but we would not think of comparing ourselves with this class of people!")

Nowadays few nurses work for the love they have

of it. Most of them have been disillusioned, especially when they look around and see women who have been out for 20 and 30 years still plodding along trying to meet expenses—women who have 24 hour duty most of the time and who have worn themselves out unnecessarily so that they have had to take long vacations in order to rest. This makes me think that it would not hurt us to pocket our pride until we wake up our principal citizens and make them feel that we are only human too.

NEW YORK.—Am 54 years old and am a private duty nurse and shall continue to do special nursing in homes and hospitals. I realize now (too late) that I should have taken a hospital position several years ago when I was in better health.

I consider the long hours of duty cruel and inhuman and would take less money for nine or ten hours. I think the problem could be worked out by the Training School's cooperation. The student nurse could look after the patient (in hospital cases) after 6:00 p. m. and until 8:00 a. m. Private patients do not like to be awakened until 8:00 a. m., and my work is finished at 5:30 or 6:00 p. m.

NEW YORK.—On account of long hours I can work only about 16 or 17 days a month as I have to rest between cases.

CALIFORNIA.—I sometimes have to start out at 5:45 a. m. and not get home before 8:15 or 8:30 and that leaves very little time for any recreation, mental or physical, and if work is slack, one has to go on call immediately on finishing a case, and that means you have to sit in the house, ready, night and day, sometimes weeks. There is very little time for any social life. You cannot plan anything ahead, and so naturally one is apt to get into a rut, and grow narrow and that is tragic both for one's self and the patient. It is so essential for a nurse to be fresh and bright and optimistic and to put her best and noblest effort into her work, and how can she with such long tiring hours?

New York.—Even 12 hours is too long to work and keep up a sunny disposition and good health. Getting up at 5:30 a. m. and returning at 8:15 p. m. leaves little time for recreation and even an opportunity to enjoy sunshine. I graduated ten years ago and feel that I've been fairly successful and happy in doing my work. I cannot see any reason why most of the hospitals cannot provide a relief for a graduate for 2 hours every day so that the 12 hours will be cut to ten hours a day when the patient's condition permits.

New York.—As I am an out-of-town graduate, I get only calls for night duty and I can't do much of it at a time for I can't get more than three hours' sleep during the day-time.

New York.—At my first opportunity I intend to give up private duty nursing. My health has failed me and I weigh only 103 pounds due to long hours and the worry and indefiniteness of being on call. My work is as interesting to me as it was at first but long hours and lack of funds are the two most important drawbacks about it.

Washington.—The loss of friends. People are too busy to bother to keep up friendship with a person who is never able to say her time is her own. If I could start over again, I wouldn't even consider nursing as a life work. There are more pleasant and profitable professions open to women at the present time.

California.—I have been enthusiastic about nursing until I took up private duty. I like private duty nursing in itself much better than the general floor duty because the patient gets all the care he needs and the nurse has an opportunity to study the case thoroughly. But after only one year's experience as a private duty nurse, I have had my enthusiasm cooled. A private duty nurse lives a slave's life; she cannot engage in social activities since she never knows whether she will be off or on a case, and while on a case she is too worn out to do anything except work, sleep, and get ready for work. The hours are inhuman and the pay is ridiculous. Any washwoman earns fifty cents an hour and doesn't have to take a four-year high school course nor a three-year training school course nor does she have to leave her home at all hours of the night and in addition she gets her Sundays off, etc. As private duty nursing is today, it is not a fitting life work for any nurse.

State Unknown.—Twelve hour duty with no relief. I got up at 5:45, went to breakfast at hospital at 6:35, on duty at 7:00. Reached home at 7:45 p. m., making my day 14 hours long with no intermission.

California.—I like nursing but I think 12 hours are too long for any person to work. When I get off duty after working 12 hours on a hard case I am too tired to go anywhere but to bed. If I had shorter working hours I could plan ahead and go to hear some good lectures, or see a good show, or go to night school and improve my education, besides participating in community activities and enjoying life. As it is, I just exist.

New York.—The state makes laws for other women to work only 8 hours a day. A nurse on 12 hour duty, if the case be any length at all, is overtaxing her strength and is away from fresh air and sunshine, to say nothing of recreation, too long at a time. A nurse cannot with certainty ever make a date for some future time unless she goes to the expense of paying another nurse to take her place. While she is resting from a hard case her income stops and if she takes a case too soon she is undermining her health.

KANSAS.—Can't plan on anything. Have had to give up almost all social connections. My friends outside of the nursing profession have about quit inviting me to their social affairs.

NEW YORK.—I am leaving private duty nursing, for the 12 hour duty is absolute slavery. No negro or man would ever work 12 hours. The mental strain is too much for any woman, especially in private homes, where you have to listen to all the sorrows and sympathize and give your body and soul to others. I have nursed in mining camps and in Fifth Avenue mansions; it's all the same, fatigue poisoning finally gets the private duty nurse.

MASSACHUSETTS.—A woman doing private nursing is practically cut off from all social contacts of the world. She cannot attend church regularly, or even think of going to club meetings! I am very much interested in music and am sure if I could possibly find time would enjoy studying music at least half or an hour a day. It is entirely out of the question at the present. I am only a high school graduate and there are languages and sciences I should love to know and would be willing to go to night school to study, but doing private nursing I shall have to be content with my knowledge from books which I am able to read once in a while.

STATE UNKNOWN.—Twelve hour duty, seven days a week, I find too fatiguing for any human being. I have tried 24 hour duty; generally it is worse. I have stayed for 12 years at private duty nursing because I really love my work, but I will soon have to change because of long hours. I could be busy every day in the year, as I work only for one busy surgeon, but my income rarely exceeds $1500. I am too tired to work more steadily. I do not think this sufficient income after 12 years' experience.

NEW YORK.—The hours are so long that one never

gets direct sunshine. When I am off a case I must stay in to listen for a call. I have no porch, as I share an apartment. If I only go out to buy food I may miss a call. If I buy food I may not have time to cook it, as when a registry calls they always say you must get there inside one hour. It often takes longer to get there by trolley, elevated or subway or all combined. It is almost impossible to get one's bag into the subway trains. If you ever travel in the early morning when all the laborers are going to work, you will find it almost impossible to squeeze yourself in and stand in all the fumes of smoke and smell of garlic. But there is no fear of having their company when we nurses are returning at nine and if the night nurse is 10 minutes late it is more often nearly 10 o'clock when I get home.

California.—Of course, the long hours, leaving no time for the development of outside interests, getting up so early, having no regular hours off duty and no regular days off duty are our chief complaints. When we have a few days off our friends are working; we haven't much opportunity to make friends outside the profession. No wonder private duty nurses are such a narrow-minded bunch—it is forced on them. They are not allowed to develop individuality.

State Unknown.—I have been doing private duty nursing for 14 years but feel that I cannot stand the long hours indefinitely. I do love my work and that is why I have not made a change and hate even now to think of doing so. One must work steadily to make a decent living and these long hours, seven days a week, are drudgery.

Washington.—So little time for recreation, reading, sleeping, or anything a human being ought to have in this world. All other women's work is eight hours, while ours is 24.

4. Pay

An extraordinary thing is noticeable in the comments on the nurses' earnings. Almost half—43% to be exact—of the private duty nurses have kept no records of their pay, and have only the vaguest idea of how much they actually earn in a year. Because their weekly wage is often large—$42 or $56 or sometimes considerably more—some nurses feel that they are earning large amounts of money, and will even state that the chief reason they stay in private duty is because they can earn so much more than in any other field. A careful scrutiny of individual records shows that this statement was in almost all cases made by a nurse who acknowledged that she had no idea of how much she earned in 1926. Most of the nurses, however, know that their incomes are inadequate.

> STATE UNKNOWN.—To be kept busy is the most profitable way of meeting expenses. Also I like the work very much, although I do find the hours long when my patient is convalescing.

> STATE UNKNOWN.—I prefer private nursing because I can take time when I feel that I need it. Also, I find that I can save more even though I do not work steadily, and I do not care for the institutional atmosphere which one has to contend with in hospitals.

> NEW YORK.—I can earn as much working two weeks as institutions pay in a month. My home expenses are the same whether I work or not, or whether I live at the hospital.

> STATE UNKNOWN.—I prefer private nursing because when I leave a case my time is my own, and I can earn more money in private nursing.

> NEW YORK.—I am contemplating giving up private duty because of the uncertain income, the long hours, and mostly because of the almost constant discussion

about the private duty nurse's salary, and the general attitude of the public that she is overpaid.

CALIFORNIA.—Private duty nursing as it stands at present is too much a game of chance. The nurse has nothing behind her. She is the buffer between the institutions, medical profession, and the public. She is an absolute necessity to all of these, yet in no way is there protection or assistance rendered her for the many problems that confront her in her daily work. These are my reasons for not only discontinuing private duty but the profession also—very shortly.

NEW YORK.—Nurses just graduating get the same salary as those who have long experience. This is altogether different in the business world.

CALIFORNIA.—A private duty nurse receives only what an ordinary scrub woman gets, fifty cents an hour, and she is supposed to have had an education and special training besides. Work and definite income are too uncertain. You do not know whether you are going to work for two weeks or for the whole month. You cannot count definitely on $150 every month, as you may make only $100 that month. You cannot be positive about either item.

CALIFORNIA.—Another great disadvantage in our profession is the uncertainty of collecting our money. In hospitals the institution will not guarantee our salaries from the patients, although they, at least out here, make the patient pay a week in advance. Often I have been called on cases in a hospital where the patient did not have a cent, and the hospital did not even care to investigate. In this way I have lost in the past three years close to $300.

STATE UNKNOWN.—I am willing to work from ten to twelve hours daily, but I think our salary should be increased, for there are weeks when we do not have any work at all, and our expenses, with meals, go on just the same.

STATE UNKNOWN.—My only reasons for giving up private nursing, or nursing at all, are the long hours and poor pay for what we give. All things considered,—and I think I have been in the profession long enough to judge (thirteen years), private duty, hospital, country nursing, and did not register against anything,—we are the poorest paid and the hardest worked of any class who earns a living—scrub women included. They usually have steady employment, always get $4.00 per day and carfare, and work only eight hours. I like my profession but it needs adjusting.

WASHINGTON.—We do not average as much money as women whose preparation takes six months.

KANSAS.—I have never made $1,000 in any one year nursing.

CALIFORNIA.—I have never been sorry that nursing has been my life's work. It has given me much, but financially I am far behind other women of my age who started life in other fields of endeavor, teachers, stenographers, bookkeepers, saleswomen, etc. I graduated 27 years ago.

PENNSYLVANIA.—I enjoy private duty when I am nursing, but when I am off duty it costs so much to live that I am unable to save for a rainy day. After vacation time has passed I will strive to secure an institutional position.

CALIFORNIA.—I am leaving private duty because my average case lasts three days or nights in the hospital, and five in the home. I find the cases increasingly hard to collect fees from, especially hospital calls, as the management assumes no responsibility of payment when they issue the call to the registry, and some hospitals here refuse to allow the nurse to leave her bill in the hospital office, or to allow the patient to leave the money in the office for the nurse. The patient, when entering a hospital in this state, pays a certain sum for a room by the week and general nursing care, but when he goes on "special" some of the hospitals ignore this "general nursing care" paid for, and resent a student's answering the patient's light if special is busy outside the room, and giving assistance in lifting, etc., when necessary. A two-hour relief of this general nursing care each day would be only fair of hospitals, and a boon to the twelve hour nurse.

MASSACHUSETTS.—To me nursing should be considered as a vocation rather than as a profession. I cannot blame the young girl of today for not getting into such a hard life. Unless she can consider that she will get some consideration in another life for all her sacrifices, she will be very unhappy. For the nurse there is no protection, no bonus, no compensation, no pensions, nothing whatever done for her, no vacation with pay, and the average pay, $7.00 per day for twelve hour duty, with ten per cent to the registry, carfare, laundry, etc., leaves very little for her rent, living expenses, etc.

STATE UNKNOWN.—I sincerely hope that you and the members of your Committee can soon do something to improve conditions for the nurses, especially the private duty nurses, because I am at the point now where even clerking in a store would give me more of a living than what I get out of nursing.

MASSACHUSETTS.—I have very seldom had a patient that I did not enjoy taking care of. It is very hard to be compelled to wait for money when through with a case, if one has room and board to pay for.

MASSACHUSETTS.—I would never advise any young girl to go into training. After three years of strict discipline and hard work she is given a diploma. There are two things she may do, general floor duty or private duty. (Provided she does not put in another year or so preparing for a special study.) In this district she gets $70 a month at general, works from 7:00 in the morning until 7:00 at night, and is indeed fortunate if she can get off at that time, works holidays and Sundays, and for all that receives an average of $18 a week. Private duty is the most lonesome work any one can do. Always a stranger coming into a saddened and worried home, and between cases wondering what is next, unable to make plans or engagements. To an older woman who can find her joy in life in the work of nursing itself, it may be an ideal vocation. For the ordinary young girl who wants to live her own life, the commercial world can offer a far better inducement.

New York.—Is there anything that can be done regarding more prompt payments of fees on compensation cases?

California.—In spite of my 21 years of private duty nurse's experience I am condemned to keep on working for from twenty to twenty-two hours each day. One year, my first out here, I earned $204.

California.—I will land in the poorhouse at my present mode of living. I hope to go back to secretarial work, the work I did before becoming a nurse.

5. Dependents

No records have been gathered for the amount of dependency among relatives of public health and institutional nurses. References in the early studies to people who needed support were so frequent in the private duty replies that a special study was made of this point. The comments which follow are typical of many which were received.

WASHINGTON.—I have to support two besides myself (my mother and cousin) so I must stay with the line of nursing that brings in the greatest returns.

STATE NOT KNOWN.—Must do private nursing to cover living expenses and obligations at home.

WASHINGTON.—More money than in general duty. (I have a son of whom I am the whole support.)

STATE NOT KNOWN.—Having a mother and invalid sister to support, it is necessary for me to work steadily. Therefore I am continuing at the work I am used to and brings me the best financial returns.

KANSAS.—I have now regained my health, but making a living for myself and adopted girl is hard work here. I am well enough that I feel able to do a moderate amount of private nursing. (I like the profession when I am able to do it.) I have had a few cases in the last six months, but there is very little nursing in this small town. I am planning to sell and move to a larger place, where I may be able to get nursing, sewing, and other work until my girl is through school. (She is just ready for high school.)

NEW YORK.—I have a mother, father, sisters, and brothers who depend on me for some financial support, and it is my aim to render efficient service and to obtain as steady an income as I can while I am still young and my earning power is at its height.

MASSACHUSETTS.—As I am the sole support of my mother and have been for fifteen years, I find that I can make more money doing private nursing, so have to continue doing that branch for the present and indefinite future.

6. Unemployment

Many nurses frankly enjoy the long idle months when they can go home and live with their families, or if they

have saved money enough, take interesting vacation trips. As the nurse grows older, however, and begins to realize the importance of putting aside some money in the form of savings, she begins to be definitely worried about the many days of unemployment which she must face. It seems to be true that nurses belong more or less to separate groups. This is probably controlled by the chief activities of the hospitals through which they get most of their cases. Some nurses seem almost to specialize on one, two, and three day cases, whereas other nurses seem to have cases which ordinarily run for two or three weeks at a time. If the short cases and the long could be equitably distributed so that each nurse had her share, there would probably be less suffering among certain groups.

NEW YORK.—I like private duty nursing when I am working, but it is that "on call" that kills—work one week or two and stay home on call for sixteen days. One has to live during that time. Expenses are going on; one is afraid to buy an extra pair of stockings or to go to some place of amusement for fear one has not enough money to buy food until one does get a case.

CALIFORNIA.—There were many, many hours, not possible to count, when I was not free, when I was on call, when I had expected to go back on a case and was notified at the last minute, too late for another case. If a large corporation were selling our services, they would figure our wasted time as overhead, and the public would pay. As it is now, our prices are considered exorbitant. The public considers sickness as a misfortune. The other disasters—auto breakdowns, plumbing breakage, fires—are all paid for, but our work should be done for love. I have given five of my best years. I am twenty-eight, and now at the end of them I have less nervous stability, fewer friends (no time to give to them, we soon drift apart). I have only a few pieces of household furniture.

New York.—When on call the telephone is a torment to me at times. I dread the outcome of it. Perhaps because I am thoroughly tired out and far from well. Folks think nurses make wonderful pay. Maybe we do, but when off a case money has to be spent, and it can be reckoned as the sum spent plus the money one should make. I am going home on a forced rest. I have had to borrow $200 from an aunt of mine and also get a loan on my adjusted compensation with which to do it. Private nursing this winter was very slow. I would far rather work overseas, and that was hard, than do private nursing.

New York.—Last fall I was on call at the Official Registry for six weeks. The day I was called I had just gone to the grocery store, and fifteen minutes later I called the Registry to accept, but they had me wait four more weeks before receiving a call.

State not Known.—It is utterly impossible for me to fill out the questionnaire, as I haven't had a whole week's work since June. I had such a hard case then that I did not work during July. In August I had two days one week, one night another week, four nights another week. Although a graduate of ...... I have had to depend on my own doctors or a commercial registry for work. I try to fit in wherever I am, housework, cooking, serving my patient's tray. There is no shortage of nurses. There are many nurses like myself who don't get work because the registrar is partial to her own friends. My work for the last year has not been enough to even pay my rent.

California.—Cannot stand the many short cases of two and three days.

WASHINGTON.—Since I went back on call three weeks ago I have had just three days' work special and five days' day floor duty.

NEW YORK.—The strain on the nerves when sitting at home and listening for the telephone to ring when off duty is enough to drive one to distraction.

CALIFORNIA.—This part of California seems to be overcrowded with nurses or too healthy a climate to get sick in.

NEW YORK.—I have nursed only three months during the last fifteen months, so I could not be of any assistance to you.

PENNSYLVANIA.—I came to this town two years ago to establish a home for my parents in town. A few months afterward my father died and I am carrying on for an aged mother and semi-invalid sister and myself. Have no complaint against private duty in this town, except when work is slack my chances are very poor, as their own nurses get the preference and I may not be called unless by special request from doctors, which I am thankful to say occurs occasionally. The only registries are the two hospitals, and one refused to let me register because I wouldn't go out of town. I much prefer institutional nursing, but private work is more lucrative, and with my responsibilities I must consider that; but even so, I am barely able to carry on.

NEW YORK.—The nurses who register at their own hospital get all the best work, and girls from other cities have to take what comes along.

MASSACHUSETTS.—The out-of-town graduate gets work when the graduates from the local hospitals are busy, very seldom at any other time.

NEW YORK.—I have almost been severely depressed of late over the great number of very short cases, although I have had many excellent patients and some difficult ones too. A three weeks' case at some future date would seem like a most exquisite boon!

Not the true spirit, you say? Why not be frank with facts when they are there. Be assured, however, that I love actual, honest to goodness nursing too well to allow my complaints to travel outside the profession.

CALIFORNIA.—I have been on call at the official registry for five weeks and have not had a call.

NEW YORK.—What are we going to do? For nearly three months I lived on one meal a day.

7. Work Often Exhausting

The good nurse wants to be kept busy. She expects to work hard, but there are limits to her capacity. Especially as the nurse grows older, or as her health begins to be damaged by long hours and irregular methods of living, does she find private duty difficult to stand.

CALIFORNIA.—I have found that bedside nursing so utterly tires me out that I am compelled to give up all outside life while on a case and also to take long periods of rest between cases. I have been quite astonished at this physical phase of special duty nursing.

PENNSYLVANIA.—My experience has been that real nursing is honest to goodness hard work, especially in the home where only one nurse can be afforded. I have been off duty now for four weeks, with excruciating pains in the right shoulder and hand, and although the pains are now comparatively few and far between, I seem to have lost all lifting power on that side. A case of paresis is certainly soul crushing, nerve and back breaking, and I think that it should be up to the doctor and the registry to explain to the people that such cases are more than one nurse can handle.

New York.—I cannot shake the responsibility of patients when off duty, especially if they are very ill. I worry about them off duty and really subject my mind to 24 hour duty instead of 12 hours. The result is that I am more easily tired than those who are not so affected.

California.—I left a good office position to enter a training school, happy in the thought that at last I would be doing something which would benefit humanity. The three years of training were hard and took every bit of energy I had, but I finished the course. I am happy still when I am relieving real suffering, but I know I made a big mistake in entering the profession. As far as my work is concerned, I have made good, but I have not the vitality that the long, strenuous hours require. I cannot work steadily enough to get ahead financially. I am in debt, so at the age of thirty-five years and with no capital I dare not make another change. Therefore, I intend to remain in private duty nursing because I have no alternative.

California.—Since I have had three nervous breaks I am not physically fit for constant work, but do what I can. I usually have to rest between cases if they are critical cases, consequently cannot earn as much as I might otherwise do.

New York.—For every three weeks of nursing duty I must rest one week. I have never been able to pay an income tax. But I wish to continue private duty because I honestly love my chosen profession and I like bedside care more than any other branch of it.

MASSACHUSETTS.—For three and a half years I have not been nursing on account of illness. I am still an invalid. That is what private duty nursing has done for me! I worked too hard. One has to work to pay expenses.

MASSACHUSETTS.—Last year I was sick from April 10 to the middle of November, so only worked 110 days last year. It is impossible for me to work all the time, on account of having to work Sundays and holidays and work twelve hours a day. I am absolutely exhausted after I have worked on a four or five weeks' case.

CALIFORNIA.—I have lifted so many heavy patients that I have been on my back for months at a time. As I cannot lift as I used to, I have little work. No, I would never do private nursing again if I could do aught else, and I know not what I can do.

NEW YORK.—I usually average two weeks in one month, because after that length of time of twelve hour duty I am too tired to go on call immediately for another case.

MASSACHUSETTS.—The amount earned last year, $500, was far below the average, owing to ill health.

MASSACHUSETTS.—This week was a very lazy week, but it follows a ten weeks' obstetrical case. The last four weeks were 24-hour duty in the home, a small one, in which the help was impossible to get, and owing to the mother's age her comeback was poor, so it was necessary for the nurse to be housekeeper, also. The other son, 18 years, was sick in bed a week of this time. This, of course, was not an average case, but I believe it typical of what many of us do occasionally, and such things take a heap of pep out of us.

8. Some Work Not Real Nursing

Even worse than being too busy to the good nurse is the experience of not being busy enough. Nurses like bedside nursing but they do not like to go on cases where they feel they are wasting time.

PENNSYLVANIA.—Too often patients do not really need the services of a professional nurse. So often I find that all they want is some one for company. I am sure I did not take up training for that reason. Quite often patients need the services of a nurse for only a few hours, perhaps to give a bath, or treatment, and the rest of the day the nurse just sits and does nothing really worth while. Give me a really sick patient every time so that I can work. I don't care if there is something to do almost every minute of the day.

CALIFORNIA.—There is too much "lady's-maid" work in private duty nursing, and not enough of that for which we were trained.

STATE UNKNOWN.—I have learned to dislike it very much because I realize that the public at large regards us as servants. However, I think I could rise above this if we could concentrate all of the work and then "clear out." But the hanging around for twelve hours is more than I can stand.

MASSACHUSETTS.—The thing I dislike most in private duty nursing is the tendency the patient has to keep the nurse after she is really better. I like bedside nursing when the patient is really ill; but when it comes to the time when they just need you for a companion, I for one am anxious to get away.

MASSACHUSETTS.—A conscientious nurse cannot leave a really sick patient for three hours in the hands of some utterly inexperienced person and go out and enjoy herself, or even take some well-earned rest. This has been my experience and I have heard many other nurses speak in the same way. Then again we come to the convalescing patient who requires very little real nursing care by day or night, and one sort of feels lost.

California.—I prefer night duty. I always have done so. I don't have to talk. I prefer middle class patients, because they are usually sick when they employ you and I prefer sick patients. Wealthy patients give one the feeling of a lady's maid.

California.—I like the bedside nursing and treatments, but we have very little of it when caring for one patient. Except in cases when the patient is very ill, and in newly operated cases, the trained nurse is very little more than a companion. Our services are of no special value—any intelligent woman could do what we do three-fourths of the time, without any special training. We put in the long twelve hour days, sometimes for months, with persons we do not like, with whom we would have nothing to do if we could choose; persons who bore us to death with their tales of illness and their family troubles; persons with disagreeable personalities; and worse yet, the pampered wealthy people who have always been able to buy everything they want, and find they cannot buy health.

California.—Many times the case is one that doesn't need a graduate, but because of having money, employs a graduate nurse. On cases of the type mentioned I feel my time is wasted. I just spent six weeks on a case of this type.

9. Attitude of Doctors and Patients

It is a pathetic thing to have nurses feeling, as so many of them apparently do, that physicians and patients do not like them. The physician is the only professional person who has any interest in the work of the private

duty nurse. If she cannot feel that he is with her in spirit, she becomes a forlorn and lonely worker. Cases where the nurse has been fortunate enough to work with a physician who is honestly interested not only in his own technique but in hers, show the wonderfully stimulating influence which even the few minutes of his daily visit may give.

CALIFORNIA.—The doctor for whom I nurse is doing wonderfully interesting work (surgery) and he makes us feel that the nursing is most important.

MASSACHUSETTS.—My greatest objection to private duty nursing is the attitude of the public toward the private duty nurse. Most people seem to class nursing as a menial occupation instead of a profession.

NEW YORK.—How little the general public or even the patients who have had the finest skill you possess think of you after it is all over. How few appreciate all you do for them. They are grateful at the time but that is soon forgotten. It is a noble profession and I am happy to be a member of it but when your youth and health are gone then comes the hour of regret.

WASHINGTON.—The general run of people in the western states seem as though they would much rather pay the piper than the nurse. Very little cooperation with nurse and doctor. Doctors rarely standing by nurse.

NEW YORK.—I have noticed that doctors have been far less loyal to the nurses than the nurses have been to them.

WASHINGTON.—Doctors are fighting us tooth and nail because we do not work 24 hours a day and charge $25 per week, and relent only when they have gone too far with an expensive operation and in order to save the patient they have to put on a couple of the hated species and, believe me, from the time she goes on until she comes off she is busy. Unless something is done, our profession is doomed.

New York.—Lack of cooperation from many doctors who resent the nurse's presence while knowing she is a necessity. Lying to the family about the patient's condition and leaving the nurse to try to explain why things go wrong. To illustrate this—one of my last cases, where the patient was in a dying condition when I went on duty. The attending physician, a well-known baby specialist, went out to the mother of the child and told her her baby was in good condition. It died one hour and forty-five minutes after I went on duty and I could not locate the doctor who had left the house to drive the day nurse home!

California.—If the doctors would stand by the nurses, it would make nursing easier.

California.—I think that if there were more cooperation among the nurses and doctors it would be much easier on all concerned. For example, the nurses are taught that it is very unethical to talk to a patient about a doctor, regardless of how good or bad he may be, but, on the other hand, if the patient talks to the doctor about the nurse, he is immediately ready to discharge the nurse and get another one, regardless of her good or bad qualities. We none of us are perfect, but by trying to work together, the road that seems never to have a turning is much easier.

California.—No independence. There is much that is rather servile in the attitude many doctors and hospitals expect of nurses.

Massachusetts.—People think for the money they pay a nurse that she is some kind of a machine.

New York.—The work of a private duty nurse is hard, lonely, and one that does it is just a drudge for others and her work and sacrifices are seldom appreciated by doctors, patients, or families.

NEW YORK.—Have nursed strangers where I have never received one penny, not even a "thank you."

MASSACHUSETTS.—In my years of experience I have found that the medical profession is much less interested now than formerly in helping a woman in her efforts to earn a living at nursing.

CALIFORNIA.—We as private duty nurses do not receive sufficient sympathy and cooperation from hospital superintendents and staff nurses, also the medical profession. We have to defend doctors against criticism of the public, and in turn I fear we do not receive the same support from the medical profession.

10. Practical Nurses

Private duty nurses occasionally come into appallingly close contact with the inferior type of so-called "practical." Reports which follow were frequently prefaced by a note from the nurse explaining that she was not sending in the story in order to be "catty." Apparently there was real fear lest her professional criticisms should be taken as being merely outpourings of jealousy.

KANSAS.—There are too many doctors here putting practical nurses on their cases in the homes instead of graduates, and practical nurses here are charging from $35 to $40 per week.

NEW YORK.—Not so long ago I was "specialing" in a certain hospital in New York, and I had occasion to notice a student nurse who was taking her training at the hospital. She had been there about three months. A few weeks ago I was passing by a registry downtown when this same young lady walked out. I recognized her and spoke and asked her how she was getting along with her training. She told me she was now out on private duty and on call at registry in front of which we were standing, that she was getting plenty of work at $7–$8 per day, the same as the R. N. She also said she had left the training school because she did not receive special time off one day from the supervisor. She also remarked that she thought it absurd to work so hard for two or three years when she was getting just as much consideration, and making just as much money out of the nursing profession after only three months' training as though she had finished her training and received her diploma.

State Unknown.—Girls will not spend 2½ and 3 years at the hardest work a woman can do, only to come out of the school to find the "domestic" or "certified" nurse on the same footing as herself, and receiving the same salary. There are registries in New York and elsewhere that send out "domestic" nurses and tell them to get all they can, although the registries deny this. One large registry on the west side seldom says a nurse is an *undergraduate*. In fact they usually send them out as *graduate nurses*. They are known to keep the undergraduates busier than the graduates. All over New York undergraduates are getting $7 and $8 a day. And many get $10 and even $15 for an alcoholic case. I have met many "domestic" and certified nurses and some have said to me, "Why should we spend so much time in a hospital when we can command as much salary as you?"

An undergraduate went on a serious case with three other nurses who were graduates, receiving the same salary, etc. Neither the doctor, patient, nor other nurses knew she was only a "domestic" nurse. I can tell you of many, many unfair cases like the above. No matter how pleasant the training school life may be, it is how the nurse gets along after graduation that counts with her.

STATE UNKNOWN.—Never has a patient asked me whether or not I was registered.

STATE UNKNOWN.—May I ask how you plan to get data about the very, very vast army of fine nurses who are not registered in this state? They outnumber the local product, I believe, in domiciliary nursing.

MASSACHUSETTS.—I have been followed on several cases by a "domestic" and prices seemed to be higher. To me it is one reason why private nursing is so at a standstill.

MASSACHUSETTS.—I find that private work is the poorest branch of the work. The attendant and undergraduate have spoiled private work in this city, where they get nearly as much pay as the graduates do.

NEW YORK.—In country nursing especially, a trained nurse has a lot to contend with, for instance, practical nurses, undergraduates, and certified. It hardly seems fair to have to work for the same money that one who has little or no training does.

NEW YORK.—The unpleasant feature of private duty nursing in New York City is that the field is overcrowded with foreigners who demean the profession by being servile and standing up for no principles, because they feel that they must have the work. American girls who prefer private duty to other branches of nursing find it difficult to compete with these people and leave private duty for other branches of nursing or go into business.

MASSACHUSETTS.—Because I am not a graduate but registered, I cannot do school or industrial work, which I prefer.

MASSACHUSETTS.—I am an R.N. but not a graduate.

GEORGIA.—Diploma? Yes, from correspondence school.

11. Group and Hourly Nursing

Many private duty nurses are looking eagerly towards group and hourly nursing as being possible solutions for the problem of impossibly long hours. Just what hourly and group nursing involves is evidently not yet clear to many of them, but they are eager to learn.

CALIFORNIA.—I might suggest group nursing as a possible change in private nursing and the only way to give more skilled service to larger groups of needy people; a chance for the establishment of an 8-hour working day; lessened expense for the individual patient to keep private service; and increased payment for the private duty nurse on the whole. In addition there is the grand satisfaction of making one's self useful to a larger number of sick people by giving more actual service. If group nursing could be established, I think I could make private duty nursing my life work.

NEW YORK.—The plan of nursing that really would appeal to me is group nursing. That is where the nurse would have just enough to do to be able to care for the patients properly without causing them the expense of special nursing and still be able to care for her own health.

CALIFORNIA.—I hope to see the group nursing plan now being advocated in our state carried out, thus enabling us to be a truly professional group of women. I think an 8-hour day more desirable, no matter how hard one had to work during those hours. I can thus (by private duty) have a home, and if I am to make it a life-time profession, I want my home and family when working hours are over, just as the doctor has his.

NEW YORK.—If the hours of a private duty nurse were 8 or 10 hours long, with maybe two or three patients, the work would be more attractive, and I am sure many more nurses would be interested.

PENNSYLVANIA.—I really have nothing against private duty except the hours—84 a week. I have been nine weeks on this case, which is very depressing, and I can only work and sleep. Yes, truly it is a terrible life and I would not advise private nursing to my friends as it stands today. Why not try 8-hour group nursing among the poorer patients in the hospital? It would help, I think.

CALIFORNIA.—If the time ever comes when a private duty nurse can work 8 hours a day and earn at least $8 per day and work 6 days a week, board furnished, then she can be a normal human being and live a normal life in the community. This can be brought about by organization and by having patients grouped. The nurse could work hard for that time and then be free to *live* the rest of the time.

I think the nurses themselves are largely responsible for long hours. They won't stand together and seem to think they should be martyrs in the matter of losing sleep and generally overworking. They will have to be educated while in training to see that there is no more reason why a nurse should kill herself working at her profession and not be able to have any time for social life than a school teacher or stenographer should. The idea that nursing is a special sort of profession that demands all sorts of sacrifices more than any other profession is all "bunk." It does demand that under present conditions, but present conditions are "rotten" and should be improved.

CALIFORNIA.—Would be glad to care for two patients, 8-hour duty, *if* given the same remuneration as I now receive for one on 12 hour. Cannot afford to work for less and save anything for later years even if I work 9 and 10 months a year, as I nearly always do.

California.—To my mind the ideal private duty nursing is hourly nursing in a large percentage of cases, even among the well-to-do. The patient would rather have her daily bath and "fixing up" and get the nurse out from under foot, leaving the ordinary care to the family when there is no need of constant skilled attention. And for the average wage-earning family, they could have the luxury of a trained nurse for an hour or so each day, instead of mortgaging the homestead.

California.—I am going to make a six months' trial of hourly nursing in this city, and if the public demands merit it, will continue this line of work. I did a year of this work in another state with success, but there does not seem to be much demand for it here as yet. I intend going before the Parent-Teachers' Associations and Housewives' Leagues with an explanation of the work as well as getting in touch with the local doctors before starting. If the demand does not merit continuing the work after six months' trial, I plan going into a school for chiropody in order to obtain a training that will insure an assured financial return.

State Unknown.—I have heard lots of talk from time to time of group nursing, etc. To begin with, neither patients nor nurses in Buffalo want it, however you speak of the shortage of nurses. If there is a shortage it is not in Buffalo or New York City. I am considered a good nurse, by which I mean that I am conscientious and untiring in my desire to be kind, helpful to my patients, and at the same time give them good nursing care. Never in my nursing experience have I waited so long for cases as I have done this winter. This experience of mine is only one of hundreds of other nurses in the city, so why under those conditions try to figure out a way to fix it so we have still less work?

State Unknown.—There will be fewer nurses in

Detroit if the doctors insist on group nursing. Some doctors wish nurses to have four patients with only $1 extra a day. They make it cheaper for patient, more work for nurses, and complain of nurses' high prices. They get rich; there is never a word about their prices for operations.

California.—I have not been able to plan on attending a good concert, a lecture, or a good play, because I had to cancel my engagements so often, changing from day to night duty, as I take what I can get. We have been talking about 8-hour nursing in our district, and group nursing at the hospital, but we have not been able to work this problem out yet, though most of the nurses would prefer shorter hours, even though more work.

New York.—The hours are too long for the amount of nursing care really necessary for the average patient. I would rather work fewer hours in the day and be busy all the hours on duty. I liked visiting nursing because when the necessary care was given to one patient, one could go on to the next. My hours were 8:30 a. m. to 5 p. m., but I had work for every minute. On private duty the morning care is given at 9:30 a. m., and then I just waste time until the evening care is given. Twelve hours is too long to be confined in the hospital each day when the real working hours are about five.

California.—I do not care for patients who are not sick and would rather feel that I am really doing some good. I like general duty except that one does not have time to do all one would like for patients. I really enjoy caring for sick people and am always sorry to have to present a statement for salary because it does seem hard for people when sick to have such expense, but I certainly do not feel that private duty nurses are overpaid considering that they work long hours and have practically no other life but their nursing. One can not have the outside interests that nurses in other fields have. It seems that if group nursing could be worked out it would be a good thing for both patients and nurses.

NEW YORK.—Private duty is chiefly selling personality, which becomes difficult if you have to do it 12 hours every day during the week. Unless a private nurse does a great deal of variety work and reads medical journals, she finds herself far behind the advances made. Isn't it possible to get the consent and cooperation of a hospital, group of doctors and nurses, and try out the plan of group nursing?

12. Hospital Floor Duty

Apparently most private duty nurses believe that hospital floor duty is less well paid than private duty. This is because they know so little about what the payment in private duty really is. Others would hesitate to take up hospital floor duty under any conditions of pay. It is interesting to follow the implications in many of these reports that if it were possible to do genuinely high grade bedside nursing in hospitals, more private duty nurses would be glad to consider general floor duty.

CALIFORNIA.—I think any nurse is happier with more than one patient.

CALIFORNIA.—Floor duty in hospitals is too hard and often with not enough help, and one has no time to do the little things for patients that often mean much to add to their comfort and health. In short I do not like nursing if it must be done in such haste that the patient feels that it's a matter of carrying out orders and no more. I enjoy private duty but feel that 12 hour duty is too long in many cases. When hospitals arrange to give nurses 8-hour duty with from five to six patients to care for, I shall prefer floor duty.

California.—After nursing 18 years I took floor duty in a new 100-bed hospital to brush up and keep fit.

New York.—I like floor duty best but hours are so long and we have to work so hard that I can stand it only six months at a time.

New York.—I think I prefer private duty to any other form of nursing but find my health is better if I change off every two or three years. When I get tired of private duty, I take a hospital position for a year or so and find it is a wonderful rest.

California.—A nurse, after putting in three years of training, is not strong enough to work day in and day out continuously for the amount that hospitals pay their graduate nurses on floor duty. The average amount that nurses are getting on floor work is \$80–\$85 a month with room and board.

California.—Compared with floor duty, private duty is to be preferred. As a rule, a nurse on floor duty is rushed in the larger hospitals. In country places usually one has not so many patients and country patients are less demanding. The salary is too small for the average floor duty and housing conditions unsatisfactory—two and more in a room.

New York.—A nurse who can stand 20 years of private duty nursing must have had a good healthy body to begin with. I find that private duty is easier than hospital floor duty because there is a little time to relax. Hospital floor duty is usually a mad chase of work from morning to night.

New York.—I will never do institutional work of any kind. Three years of training proved that to me, that I would never care to take a hospital position after graduation.

Washington.—I like general hospital duty but find that the average hospital does not allow enough help on the floor to give every patient all the care required. I despise rushed or half done work and I have found that is the kind of work a great many nurses have to do if they attend to the number of patients assigned.

New York.—The charge positions in general hospitals today are mostly held by first year graduates with little or no experience in nursing, except what they have gained in their 2 or 3 years' course, or by graduates of schools of other states or countries who use this means to get a footing in the city in which they expect to do private duty later. In other words institutional work is so poorly paid that no good nurse who can be busy otherwise will do it.

California.—I intend to keep up my private nursing indefinitely, for I find it is not as hard as floor duty, and I get better compensation for my time put in. On floor duty I am on my feet eight to ten hours and receive from $80 to $100 a month and feel that most hospitals have too few nurses for number of patients and nurse can not do justice to patient, while on private nursing one gets from $6 to $8 per day and at the least one can make as much as $80 to $100 a month and take better care of patients. It seems to me from what I can see of so many hospitals, everything is too commercialized. That's why it's so hard on nurses. "Worked to death." I have done lots of it but no more for me! From now on private duty!

California.—After I registered here for the first private duty I've ever done, I had three short cases—a week (for which I was never paid), three nights, and one night respectively—and then went on with a mental case in a home and have been there for 19 months and 3 weeks at $7 a day, 12 hour duty. All the nurses envy me but I've earned my money although I'm a cross between a valet and a professional entertainer, rather than a nurse. I'm leaving next week before I become deranged myself and am going back to general duty more for variety than because my private duty experiences have been unpleasant. The thing which attracts me at present is 8 hour duty and a day off occasionally. Also I really like caring for a number of different persons in a day. It gives more "scope for the imagination" than a single individual, especially for 12 hours. I have been investigating public health nursing but so far have not decided to take it up. It seems to me to offer better opportunities for advancement and expansion than private nursing does, with better hours and sure money.

California.—I prefer private duty because of the fuller opportunity to do good work. In the institution in which I worked there was always a dearth of workers, consequently the work was hurried and poorly done. Neither the nurse nor the patient was satisfied and the atmosphere was one of constant irritation on both sides.

California.—If general duty was eight hours, six days in the week, $5.00 per day without maintenance, then I would consider general duty. The hospitals do not pay their general duty nurses enough money.

California.—For my part I can see no reason why nurses should work 12 hours or 10 hours on general duty. We are human as other girls and the law seems to protect girls in other vocations from working more than eight hours. We also would like to have the opportunity for recreation (with more time to spend in the outdoors and sunshine). An eight hour day would only mean three dollars more to the patient without meals. I think most of the girls would prefer eight hours instead of board at the hospitals.

CALIFORNIA.—Private duty has this one advantage —you have not so many to please and very few complaints. In general duty, in most hospitals, you are rushed.

13. Male Nurses

The studies of the Committee have dealt almost entirely with female nurses. The numbers of male nurses are so few that no particular discussion has been devoted to their problem. That they have a real problem, however, is indicated by the few comments which follow.

CALIFORNIA.—I am a "male" nurse and consequently the situation presents a little different angle in my case. First, there shouldn't be any male nurses because his services are not in sufficient demand and he is ostracized by the women of the profession. He's a freak of nature in the hospital and eventually will be eliminated. Secondly, it isn't fair for hospitals to ask young men to give up two to three years (the most important) of their lives to the institution and then treat them as social outcasts afterward. Thirdly, the women take every kind of case they can lay hands on (to get the money)—vulgar alcoholics, violently insane, desperate chronic cases, or many bad accident cases—many times to the injury or injustice of both themselves and the patient. But they're like a lot of hungry vultures and will take a chance on their lives rather than let some poor struggling "mere man" trying to support a wife and children earn a few dollars.

MASSACHUSETTS.—I like my profession. I am a married man with five children. I combine massage with nursing and can just live on my wages although I can't save anything.

NEW YORK.—The nursing profession has been disappointing to me from an economic standpoint. I am a married man and have several children to support and I find great difficulty as a male nurse to be kept busy at all times. For the past several years I have come in contact with so-called male nurses, who are not registered in New York State, doing all kinds of nursing service, giving treatments which they are not authorized to do, making it more difficult for me and other R.N.'s to get employment.

ILLINOIS.—I am a male nurse. After graduation from my hospital here I took the State Board and passed with a high average. I am very much interested in my work, well liked by my patients, and as a rule I am busy. But were it not for my own hospital I would be idle most of the time. The registries will not call a male nurse unless so stated that the patient must have one. For a simple appendectomy, gall-bladder, or like cases, they call female nurses. My own hospital calls me for all cases. I would very much like to stay at my work but I do not think it fair the way a male nurse is treated. They give us training, require us to be R.N.'s, but still we are not recognized by the Red Cross nor are we treated fairly by the registry. Don't you think that as long as we are required to go through all these hardships that after graduation we should be placed on an equal status with the female nurse?

14. Keep on?

Every nurse was asked, "Do you intend to keep on indefinitely in this line of work?" The replies from the private duty nurses are pathetic.

NEW YORK.—I intend to keep on doing private nursing because I don't know anything else; wish I never had to see another patient again.

MASSACHUSETTS.—My health does not permit me to do real hard nursing any more, but I can get along very nicely on chronic cases such as I have now and, therefore, I expect to continue as I am doing. I prefer hospital work, but had to give it up some years ago. I enjoy this work, like my patients and am interested in them, but the monotony gets on my nerves sometimes.

NEW YORK.—Yes, I shall keep on as long as I am able—too old and worn out for other work. I would like to add for the benefit of our profession that private nursing is torture!

MASSACHUSETTS.—Nothing else for me to do at my age. Graduated 29 years ago.

NEW YORK.—Have not been able to save enough money to do otherwise and am untrained for any other kind of work and now too old to train.

NEW YORK.—I expect to keep on private duty indefinitely, because I have not been fitted for anything else.

NEW YORK.—I am very tired of private duty nursing, but it is all I know how to do. I have been graduated for 33 years.

CALIFORNIA.—Expect to do private duty when able, as I'm getting along in years and am not fitted for anything else.

NEW YORK.—I intend doing private nursing not because I like it better than other nursing, but because I cannot get a vacancy any place else.

KANSAS.—I want to do something in which I can advance. Let the girls just out of training and the older nurses who have always done private duty do it. I think every nurse should have some experience in private duty, but you never get any further than you were when you started. I intend to look further than this, as I have been out of training only about five months.

CALIFORNIA.—Private nursing is the only thing that I feel competent to do. I break down and have to give it up every once in a while, but go back to it again. I spent six months of last year caring for a half-brother who has diabetes. For this I received no pay.

NEW YORK.—Private nursing is too exhausting. There is no future to it. One cannot save on present salary. It is job work with no advancement for proficiency and skill. Hours too long for proper living conditions. Some of the work is distasteful to me—"lady's maid" cases in particular.

NEW YORK.—Not if I can do better in something else.

NEW YORK.—I do not feel that I can afford to keep on with private duty nursing as I cannot earn sufficient to prepare for the time when my professional life must end because of age and inability to carry on with work which means constant physical exertion. To my mind private nursing cannot be a means to preparing for self-support and independence in later life.

CALIFORNIA.—I do not intend to keep on doing private duty because:

1. Wages are inadequate.
2. Hours are too long.
3. Every day off duty is actual money spent.
4. There is no advancement.

No matter how hard you work or how well you do it, you make exactly as much money as the nurse who "slides by" with as little effort as possible.

NEW YORK.—I hope not.

NEW YORK.—I have to.

CALIFORNIA.—I do not intend to keep on doing private duty nursing, because when I see older nurses who do private duty and have fallen into such a rut the only things they can find to talk about at meals is their patients, treatments, etc., well, I feel ashamed of them and vow I'll not talk shop; and the best way not to talk shop is to keep a broader outlook than is possible doing private duty.

15. What of the Future?

It is often stated that "every nurse ought to do some private duty, but no good nurse ought to stay in that field more than a few years." The question for the profession is whether private duty should be considered only as a temporary occupation, and if so, how can the profession provide adequate employment for ex-private duty nurses in public health or institutional work? Should it be true that there is no future in bedside nursing, or is there some way in which the nurses who love to take care of sick patients may find either in private duty or in hospital floor duty a life-long opportunity for them to practise not administrative work, nor teaching, nor prevention, but the definite nursing art of taking care of sick patients?

NEW YORK.—I love nursing. It was my desire for years to study it, and I enjoyed every bit of my training, but I would discourage any young woman I knew going into the profession, for there is no future in it for any woman.

CALIFORNIA.—People prefer young special nurses. Private duty nursing is no work to grow old in. If I keep in the nursing profession, I shall specialize in laboratory work.

CALIFORNIA.—While there are times when I am oppressed by moans and groans and think to myself, "Oh, Lord, how long—how long must I do this sort of work?" yet I know in my heart there is no work in which I so delight as private duty nursing. It is my chosen field, and from the beginning of my training I planned for it.

Yet I know now something that I did not understand before, *i. e.*, a nurse must not be old or young, just in between, and alas! I am about to grow older.

CALIFORNIA.—I am middle aged and many doctors and hospital superintendents make a practice of calling the registry for *young* nurses, which leaves the older nurses to take what they can get.

CALIFORNIA.—The first ten years I worked most of the time, 24-hour duty. Then my health broke and in the next seven years had four major operations. In between these operations I worked quite steadily. Income varied. Now, however, conditions have changed. All calls must come through Central Registry. The superintendents of hospitals are calling the alumnæ, and a few favored ones of the older girls. The superintendents of hospitals discourage the doctors calling the nurses they want for private cases and are calling the recent graduates of their training schools. Naturally we older women, who have carried the brunt for years, are left out of the picture. I am not nursing a grouch, as that is inevitable in all lines of work. Youth must be served. Other lines of nursing are open, so will look elsewhere for work.

CALIFORNIA.—I must earn a living and so continue doing the only work I am fitted for. The outlook is not good, and work grows scarce, with short cases. I suppose more or less the young graduate must take our place. What is to become of the older nurses? Many of us have had responsibilities and could not save; others have not saved. I wonder what is to be done!

CALIFORNIA.—The question in my mind is—will I still be desirable in the nursing field in another five years, when I shall be forty years old?

CALIFORNIA.—The doctors as well as the people demand young, energetic nurses. One could continue to hold a position after 45 or 50, whereas at this age the private duty nurse is passé.

MASSACHUSETTS.—Private duty nursing is the hardest work in the profession. The hours are long and tedious. The salary so uncertain, and the biggest objection to it is it has absolutely no future. A nurse can do private duty for twenty years and in the end that is all she is. Institutional or public health work is better.

WASHINGTON.—I am forty-eight years of age and have the best of health. I never lost a day because of illness all through my three years' training and have been sick only a day or two once in a while since then. I feel quite peppy, but I can see this is the age of youth, and I want to give up nursing before I get to be a tired old nurse that people pity.

I have some other work in mind which will necessitate my going to school for two years. I have been saving up for this for some time and hope to be able to take it up this autumn.

I love nursing—especially private duty—and if I had my life to live over again I would be a nurse, but the day I graduated I would take out an endowment policy for $5,000 and see that I saved enough money to keep it paid up.

CHAPTER 16

WHO PRODUCE THE NURSES?

The character of nursing education is, in the last analysis, determined by the women who control it. This chapter attempts to give a picture of 1,400 such women. The tables cover

274 R.N. Superintendents of Hospitals
608 R.N. Superintendents of Nurses
518 R.N. Superintendents of both Hospitals and Nurses

Including 31 incomplete returns, the total replies equal 1,431, or 47% of the 3,034 requested. These returns cover the entire country in representative proportions.

1. How Big Are Their Hospitals?

Superintendents of Nurses work in larger hospitals than either the R.N. Hospital Superintendent or the R.N. Superintendent of both services. Less than one-fifth of the Superintendents of Nurses are in hospitals with under 50 patients as compared with almost half of the R.N. Superintendents of Hospitals, and almost three-fourths of the R.N. Superintendents of both Hospital and Nursing service. Forty-eight per cent of the Superintendents of Nurses, 77% of the R.N. Superintendents of Hospitals, and 94% of the R.N. Superintendents of both services are in hospitals with less than 100 patients daily average.

2. How Long Have They Been Out of School?

Nearly 13% of the Superintendents of Nurses (who are practically all principals of nursing schools) and over 15% of the Superintendents of both services (three-fourths of whom are principals of nursing schools) were student nurses themselves not more than five years ago.

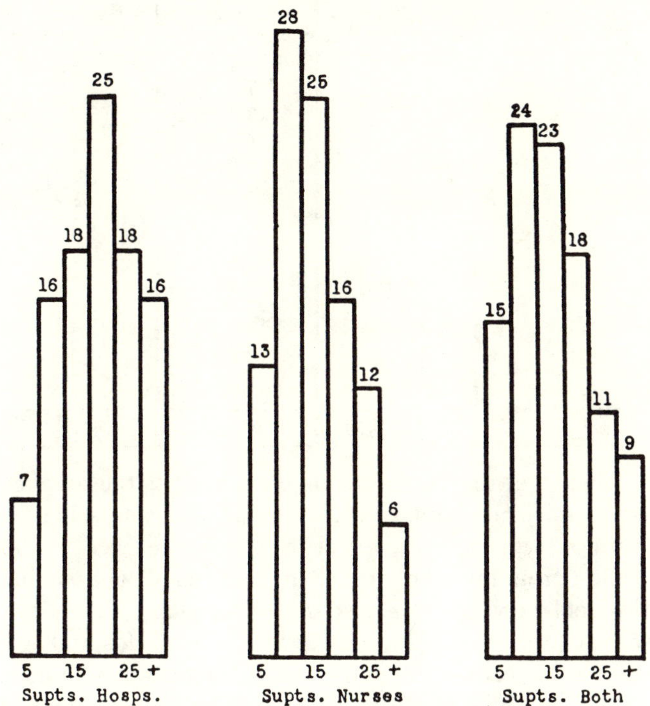

Diagram 46.—Per cent of each group of superintendents who have been out of training school 5 years or less, 6–10, 11–15, 16–20, 21–25, and over 25 years

While we do not know the exact ages of these women, the figures suggest that they are probably less than 26 years old. One wonders whether young women so relatively immature are capable of conducting really high grade educational institutions!

TABLE 63. PER CENT OF R.N. SUPERINTENDENTS OF EACH TYPE WHO HAVE BEEN EACH NUMBER OF YEARS OUT OF NURSING SCHOOL

Years out of school	Hospital Superintendent	Nurse Superintendent	Superintendent of both services
Under 1	.3%	.3%	.7%
1	.8	1.0	.6
2	..	2.3	3.3
3	1.1	2.2	2.8
4	1.9	3.7	2.7
5	3.0	3.0	5.1
6	2.6	5.5	4.8
7	3.0	6.5	6.1
8	3.0	3.6	3.3
9	3.0	6.4	5.8
10	4.6	6.3	3.7
11–15	18.4	24.8	22.6
16–20	24.8	15.7	18.4
21–25	17.7	12.2	11.3
26–30	10.5	5.0	6.2
31+	5.3	1.5	2.6
Total	100%	100%	100%

The age of the Superintendent—or rather the number of years which she has been out from training school—does not seem greatly to affect the size of her school. The median or middle Superintendent of Nurses has been out of school 12 years, the median Hospital Superintendent 17 years, the median Superintendent of both Hospital and Nurses, 13 years. Apparently Superintendents of Nurses or Superintendents of both services tend to be definitely younger than R.N. Superintendents of Hospitals.

3. How Many Different Hospitals Have They Worked In?

While the "average" R.N. Superintendent has worked in only three or four hospitals, there is wide variation on this point, which is more marked among Superintendents of Nurses than among members of the other two groups. With the R.N. Hospital Superintendent, the typical woman five years or less out of training has worked in only two hospitals, including the one in which she is trained, while the woman who has been out six years or over has typically worked in only three.

For the Superintendent of both services, the typical woman out five years or less has worked in two hospitals. One out from 6 to 20 years has worked in 3 hospitals and one out more than 20 years has worked in 4. Figures for the typical Superintendent of Nurses, however, go from 2 to 5 in the same period of time.

So many of these Superintendents stay for long years in one position that the average number of hospitals worked in is usually 3. Some interesting exceptions, however, have been noted. Among R.N. Hospital Superintendents, 1 Superintendent who has been graduated within the past 5 years has already worked in 8 hospitals, 2 graduated 8 and 9 years ago respectively have worked in 9 each, while 1 who was graduated 27 years ago has worked in 40.

Among the Superintendents of Nurses, 1 Superintendent who has been graduated 3 years has already worked in 5 hospitals, 1 who has been out 8 years has worked in 12, and 1 who has been out 13 years has worked in 18 hospitals.

For the Superintendents of both Hospital and Nursing service, 1 nurse who has been graduated 10 years has worked in 12 hospitals, and 1 who has been out 18 years has worked in 15 hospitals.

4. How Well Is She Educated?

There are older women among the R.N. Superintendents who have never gone very far in high school and yet who are among the most valuable women in the nursing profession. Many of them would be counted as educated even though they do not happen to have academic credits.

Since their day, however, conditions in this country have changed so markedly that, with rare exceptions, it is no longer possible for a woman to be socially respected unless she has gone beyond the first year of high school. Professional women of any pretense to culture and breeding must, *if they are less than 30 years old*, have at least a high school education; and it is rapidly becoming true that if they wish to have the respect of their colleagues, they must have had a year or two of college as well.

It should therefore be a matter of real concern to those who are interested in the progress of the nursing profession to note that among the R.N. Superintendents of Hospitals who have been graduated from training school 10 years or less 23%, or nearly one-fourth, have never been beyond the first year of high school. One wonders how many of these women can be skilful and intelligent hospital administrators. That some of them are of this type may, of course, be true; but it would seem highly improbable that most of this young executive group could be handling these positions of extreme difficulty and responsibility successfully. The girl of today who has neither the intelligence nor the ambition to go beyond the first year of high school, would seem a sorry choice for the superintendency of a hospital!

The records of the R.N. Hospital Superintendents are far worse in this regard than those of the R.N. Superintendents of Nurses, or of both Hospital and Nursing service combined. Throughout all of these studies it will be noted that the Superintendent of Nurses is apt to be better educated than the Superintendent of either of the other groups. The Superintendent of both Hospital and Nursing service ranks slightly below her; and the R.N. Hospital Superintendent markedly below.

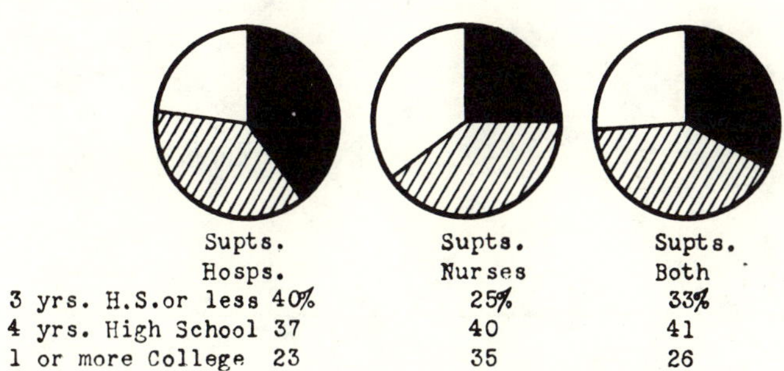

	Supts. Hosps.	Supts. Nurses	Supts. Both
3 yrs. H.S. or less	40%	25%	33%
4 yrs. High School	37	40	41
1 or more College	23	35	26

Diagram 47.—Per cent of all R.N. superintendents who have had 3 years of high school or less; who have had 4 years of high school; or who have had 1 or more years of college

Although records for the two other types of Superintendents are far better than those for the R.N. Hospital Superintendents, it is nevertheless a serious thing that, of those who have been graduated 10 years or less, 6% of the Superintendents of Nurses and 9% of the Superintendents of both Hospital and Nursing service have never gone beyond the first year of high school!

The following table shows the number of years of education of the Superintendents of each of the three groups. It should be noted in connection with this table that while the totals include some Superintendents who are connected with hospitals without training schools, the number is very small and the per cents having each amount of education are not materially changed when the tables are made for those having training schools only.

TABLE 64. PER CENT OF R.N. SUPERINTENDENTS OF EACH TYPE WHO HAVE HAD EACH SPECIFIED AMOUNT OF SCHOOLING

Education	Hospital Superintendent	Nurse Superintendent	Superintendent of both services
Under 8th grade	.3%	—%	.9%
8th grade	8.2	3.4	5.9
High school, 1	11.6	4.0	6.3
" " 2	10.1	9.4	10.3
" " 3	9.7	8.3	9.8
" " 4	36.9	40.1	40.8
College, 1	6.7	9.8	8.2
" 2	9.4	11.2	9.9
" 3	1.1	2.2	2.7
" 4	5.6	10.9	5.0
Post-graduate, 1+	.4	.7	.2
	100%	100%	100%

Diagram 48 shows for all three types of Superintendents graduated within the past 10 years the per cent who have never been beyond the first year of high school and, in contrast, the per cent who have had at least one year of college.

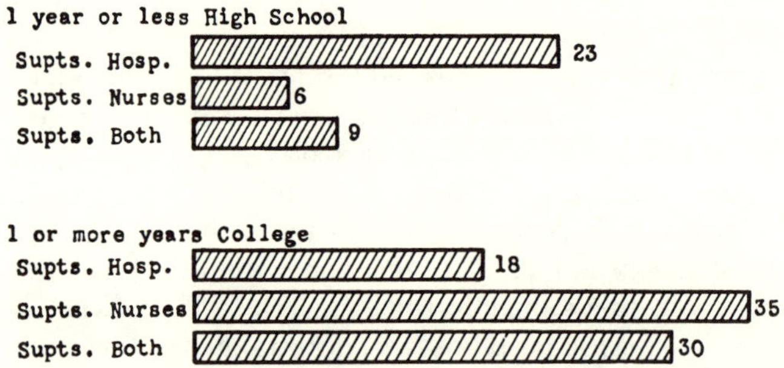

Diagram 48.—Per cent of R.N. superintendents who have been graduated from training school *within the past ten years*, and who have had 1 year of high school or less (upper bars) or 1 year of college or more (lower bars)

There is one feature of the educational situation in regard to Superintendents of Hospitals which should cause grave concern, at least until some adequate explanation is found. Among Superintendents of Nurses and Superintendents of both services the per cent who have had one year of high school or less is definitely lower among recent graduates than among those who have been a greater number of years in the profession. This is what would normally be expected, since educational standards throughout the profession are steadily rising. For nurse Superintendents of Hospitals, however, it is found that among those who have been graduated from training school *within the past 10 years*, 23 per cent have never gone beyond the first year of high school, as compared with 19 per cent of the older women in the same field. It would seem that in this group educational standards are falling. The numbers upon which these per cents are based are, of course, relatively small, but their trend is so definite and their contrast to the results secured with the other two groups of R.N. Superintendents so complete, that they would seem to have something more than accidental significance. The problem is one which should be pursued further.

5. Have They Taken Special Courses?

Half of the Superintendents of Nurses, and more than half of the other Superintendents, have never taken any course in institutional management or in educational methods.

27% of the Superintendents of Hospitals
30% of the Superintendents of Nurses, and
20% of the Superintendents of both services

have taken courses in institutional management.

31% of the Superintendents of Hospitals
42% of the Superintendents of Nurses, and
28% of the Superintendents of both services

have taken courses in educational methods.

59% of the Superintendents of Hospitals
51% of the Superintendents of Nurses, and
64% of the Superintendents of both services

have taken no courses in any branch.

In these particular figures the records of the Superin-

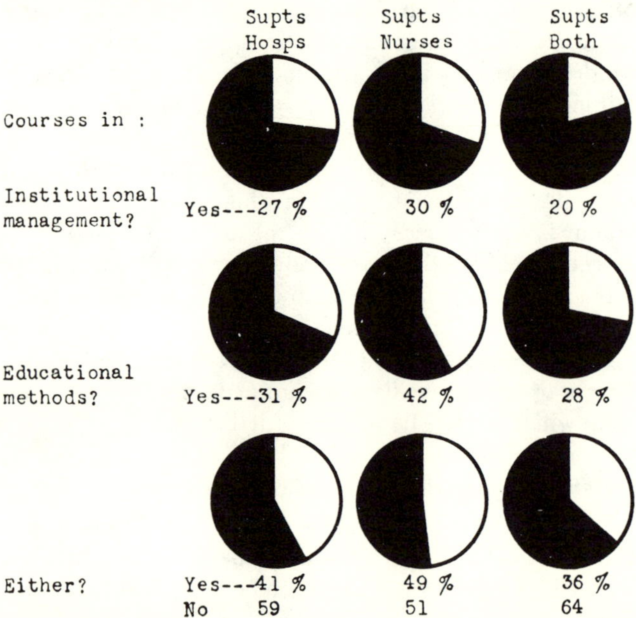

Diagram 49.—Per cent of all R.N. superintendents who have taken courses in institutional management or educational methods

tendents of both services are somewhat poorer than those of the Superintendents of Hospitals, which may be accounted for by the fact that when one woman occupies both positions, she finds it extremely difficult to secure leave of absence for post-graduate study of this type.

6. How Much Do They Earn?

The highest salaries reported in this study were for R.N. Hospital Superintendents, $6,000; for Superintendents of Nurses, $6,000; and for Superintendents of both services, $8,700. All three give maintenance in addition to the cash.

In general, it may be said that the R.N. Hospital Superintendent is slightly better paid than the Superintendent of Nurses and the R.N. Superintendent of both services. The typical R.N. Hospital Superintendent receives $2,100 plus maintenance. One-fourth of the women in her field receive $1,800 plus maintenance or less and one-fourth $3,000 plus maintenance or more. For Superintendents of Nurses the typical salary is $2,000 plus maintenance. One-fourth of the Superintendents receive $1,800 plus maintenance or less, and one-fourth $2,400 plus maintenance or more. For the Superintendents who combine the two positions, the typical Superintendent receives $1,920 plus maintenance. One-fourth receive $1,800 plus maintenance or less, and one-fourth $2,400 plus maintenance or more.

It should be noted in connection with salaries that maintenance is so regularly provided that it may almost be taken for granted in all three fields. Hospitals assume, in other words, that the Superintendents will reside in the hospital buildings, where, presumably, they will be continuously on call.

The size of the hospital makes a difference in the amount of money which the Superintendent receives.

The hospital with a daily average of less than 50 patients is apt to pay from $1,500 to $2,000 plus maintenance, regardless of whether it has one Superintendent to handle both the Hospital and the Nursing administration, or whether it has two people to divide the work between them.

The hospital with from 50 to 99 patients is apt to pay its R.N. Hospital Superintendent from $2,500 to $3,000, its R.N. Superintendent of Nurses from $1,500 to $2,000, and if it has one Superintendent for both positions, she is apt to receive from $2,000 to $2,500.

For Superintendents of Hospitals or Superintendents of both services in hospitals with over 100 patients, the typical payments are from $3,000 to $3,500 plus maintenance, while for the Superintendent of Nurses the typical payment is from $2,000 to $2,500 plus maintenance.

In general the salaries in the Middle Atlantic, the East North Central, and the Pacific states tend to be somewhat higher, and salaries in New England and the Southern states are slightly lower than in other parts of the country.

Similarly, the amount of the R.N. Hospital Superintendent's schooling, or the special courses she may have had, seem to have no effect on the salary she is able to secure; while for Superintendents in the other two types of work there is a distinct increase for college women as compared with those who have never gone beyond high school; and for those who have taken special courses as compared with those who have not.

7. How Fast Does Their Pay Increase?

The typical Hospital Superintendent has held her present position for 5 years and has received a $500 cash increase in her salary. The typical Superintendent of both Hospital and Nursing Service has held her present position for 3 years and has had an increase of $300 in her salary, while the typical Superintendent of Nurses has held her present position for two years and has had an increase of $220 in her salary. These figures do not include data from members of religious sisterhoods.

8. How Many Years Have They Held Their Present Positions?

Almost two-fifths of all Superintendents of Nurses have held their present positions one year or less and over half have held them two years or less! In the table which follows the data for Superintendents who are members of religious sisterhoods are omitted. If they were included, the average tenure of office would be slightly, but not markedly, increased.

TABLE 65. PER CENT OF SUPERINTENDENTS IN EACH GROUP WHO HAVE HELD THEIR PRESENT POSITIONS EACH NUMBER OF YEARS. (Data for Sisters in Religious Orders Omitted)

Years	Supt. of Hospital		Supt. of Nurses		Supt. of Both Services	
	%	Cum.	%	Cum.	%	Cum.
Less than 1	7.2	7.2	20.6	20.6	11.3	11.3
1..........	7.2	14.4	16.9	37.5	12.5	23.8
2..........	11.5	25.9	13.7	51.2	16.0	39.8
3..........	10.6	36.5	10.6	61.8	11.1	50.9
4..........	11.0	47.5	10.0	71.8	9.4	60.3
5..........	8.2	55.7	6.0	77.8	8.0	68.3
6..........	5.3	61.0	5.2	83.0	6.7	75.0
7..........	4.8	65.8	4.1	87.1	4.0	79.0
8..........	7.7	73.5	3.0	90.1	3.5	82.5
9..........	2.4	75.9	1.7	91.8	1.7	84.2
10..........	3.4	79.3	1.1	92.9	3.4	87.6
11–15..........	9.1	88.4	4.0	96.9	7.5	95.1
16–20..........	5.8	94.2	1.8	98.7	3.6	98.7
21 and over....	5.8	100.0	1.3	100.0	1.3	100.0
Total........	100%		100%		100%	

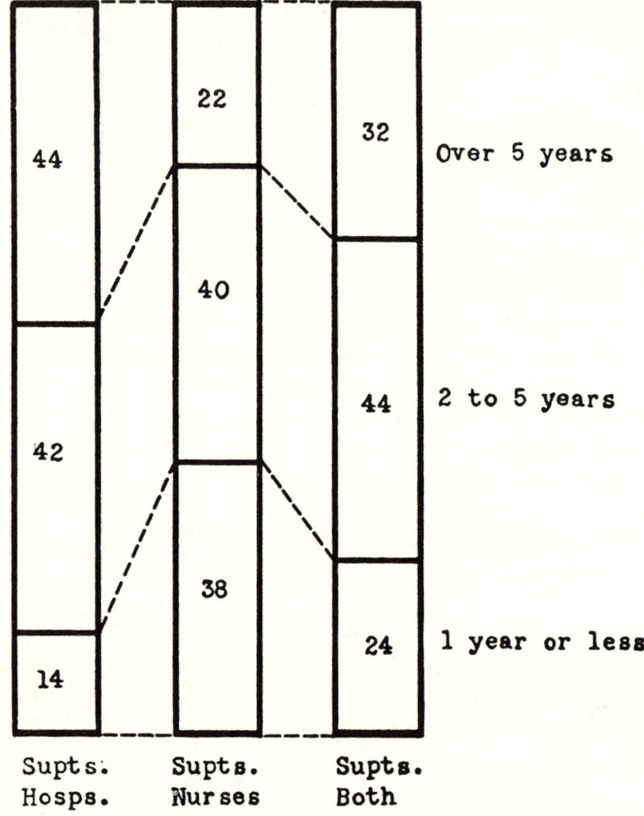

Diagram 50.—Per cent of R.N. Superintendents who have held their present positions each specified number of years

Apparently there is no connection between education and tenure, since the one year high school product and the college woman seem to stay in one position for about the same number of years.

Table 65 indicates that Superintendents of Nurses are

apparently less contented, and find their positions more difficult to hold, than Hospital Superintendents or Superintendents of both services. It would seem that nursing education must suffer seriously when practically three-fourths of the Superintendents of Nurses have stayed with their present schools five years or *less*.

9. What Are Their Relations with Their Boards of Trustees?

Only 18% of all the Superintendents of Nurses report that they have a nursing committee to whom they are directly responsible. Most Superintendents of all types are directly or indirectly responsible to the hospital Board of Trustees.

The typical R.N. Hospital Superintendent attended 8 out of a possible 11 meetings of the Board of Trustees in 1927. The typical Superintendent of both services attended 9 out of a possible 12 meetings; while the typical Superintendent of Nurses attended only 3 out of a possible 12.

Since the nursing service is so intimately connected with almost every phase of hospital administration, it is difficult to conceive of the Board of Trustees holding any regular meeting without discussing nursing in some form. One wonders whether the extremely high turnover in Superintendents of Nurses might not be somewhat cut down if the presence of the Superintendent herself were encouraged at board meetings. Such dissatisfaction as results in 51% of the Superintendents of Nurses quitting their jobs before the end of the second year would seem to indicate that there must be some lack of team play between the members of the Board and the Superintendent of Nurses which might perhaps be remedied if the point of view of each were automatically presented to the other through direct and frequent informal discussion. At least 20% of the Superintendents of Nurses were so included, and did attend all the meetings of their Boards of Trustees during the year.

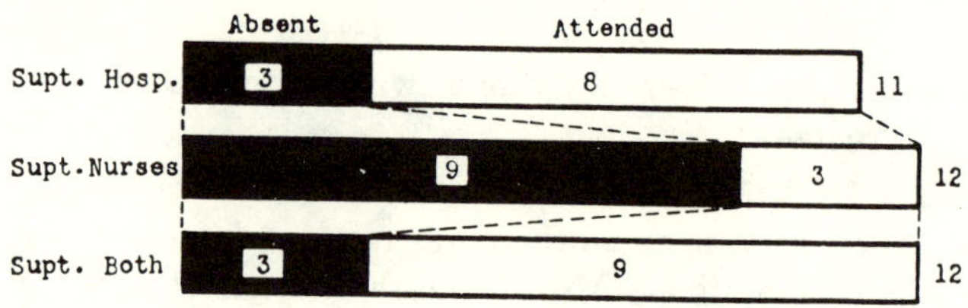

Diagram 51.—Average meetings of Boards of Trustees in 1927, and average attendance at these meetings of three types of all R.N. superintendents

10. Do They Want to Keep On?

R.N. Superintendents of all three types are reasonably happy in their work and inclined to continue in the same field. Ninety-two per cent of the R.N. Hospital Superintendents, 91% of the Superintendents of both services, and 89% of the Superintendents of Nurses answer "Yes" in reply to the question, "Do you intend to continue in your present line of work?" Age seems to make comparatively little difference in these replies except that there seems a distinct tendency for the youngest group of Superintendents of Nurses and Superintendents of both services to be a little more discouraged and the youngest group of R.N. Hospital Superintendents to be a little more optimistic than the older women in the same lines. The amount of education which the nurse has had has even less effect than her age upon her desire to stay or leave. Superintendents in all three groups who have never been beyond the eighth grade seem to be just about as contented as are those who have had one or more years of college.

11. Have They Training Schools?

Two-thirds of the R.N. Hospital Superintendents, practically all of the Superintendents of Nurses, and about three-fourths of the Superintendents of both services have training schools.

The numbers of schools having each size of student body are shown in the table which follows.

TABLE 66. SCHOOLS HAVING EACH NUMBER OF STUDENTS AS REPORTED BY EACH TYPE OF SUPERINTENDENT

Number of Students	Supt. of Hospital	Supt. of Nurses	Supt. of Both	Total	Per Cent	Cumulative Per Cent
1–9	10	22	53	85	7.5	7.5
10–19	30	68	112	210	18.5	26.0
20–29	33	83	88	204	18.1	44.1
30–39	24	86	54	164	14.5	58.6
40–49	25	66	19	110	9.7	68.3
50–59	11	45	13	69	6.1	74.4
60–69	12	48	9	69	6.1	80.5
70–79	10	38	4	52	4.6	85.1
80–89	4	28	3	35	3.1	88.2
90–99	5	15	4	24	2.1	90.3
100–109	4	16	1	21	1.9	92.2
110–119	2	15	..	17	1.5	93.7
120–129	..	17	1	18	1.6	95.3
130+	6	45	2	53	4.7	100
Total....	176	592	363	1,131	100	

The middle or median Superintendent of Nurses is connected with a school of 46 students; the median R.N. Hospital Superintendent with a school of 36 students; and the median Superintendent of both services with a school of 22 students. For all Superintendents combined, the median school has 34.

Superintendents with schools were asked whether they

needed more students. It is clear from the replies that there is no serious shortage of students, since 72% of the Hospital Superintendents, 68% of the Superintendents of both services, and 63% of the Superintendents of Nurses say that they have all they need. The demand for students is slightly greater in large hospitals than in small ones.

12. Do Their Schools Use Affiliation?

Superintendents were asked whether their schools give all the types of training necessary for state registration or whether they are obliged to send their students away. Of the R.N. Hospital Superintendents, 50% reported that their schools give all types of training, 9% secure affiliation in their own cities, and 41% send their students to other cities for affiliation. Among the Superintendents of Nurses, the corresponding figures are 55%, 15%, and 30%. Among the Superintendents of both services, the corresponding figures are 40%, 8%, and 53%. It seems probable that these differences are rather closely connected with the fact that the Superintendent of Nurses is apt to be in the largest hospital and the Superintendent of both services in the smallest. Clinical material in the small hospital is often so scarce that affiliation is necessary.

Most of the Superintendents agree that students sent to other cities for affiliation usually return to their own cities afterwards in order to practise nursing. There is, however, a marked difference on this point between the R.N. Superintendents of Hospitals, only 4% of whom say that affiliating students are apt to remain away indefinitely, as compared with the Superintendents of Nurses and the Superintendents of both services, 12 and 11 per cent of whom say respectively that students are apt to stay away.

13. Have They Raised Their Entrance Requirements?

Ninety-one per cent of the Hospital Superintendents, 89% of the Superintendents of Nurses, and 87% of the Superintendents of both services report that their schools have raised the entrance requirements within the past 10 years. Apparently the tendency for greater strictness is almost universal. The raising of requirements has oc-

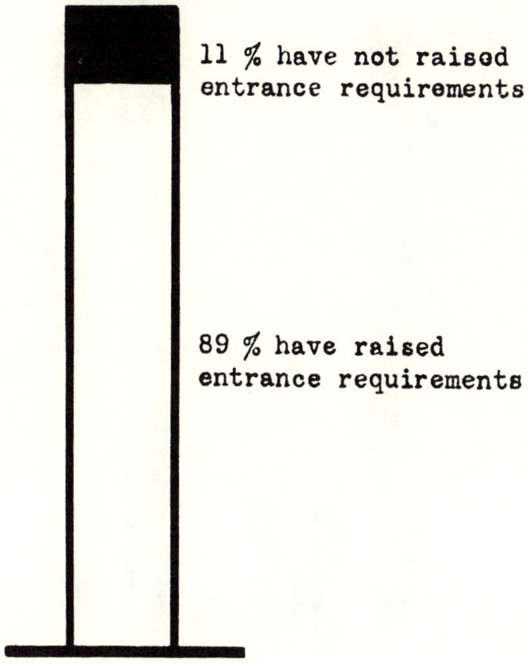

Diagram 52.—Has your school raised its entrance requirements within the past 10 years?

curred in the very small hospitals as well as in the largest.

The Superintendents who have raised their entrance

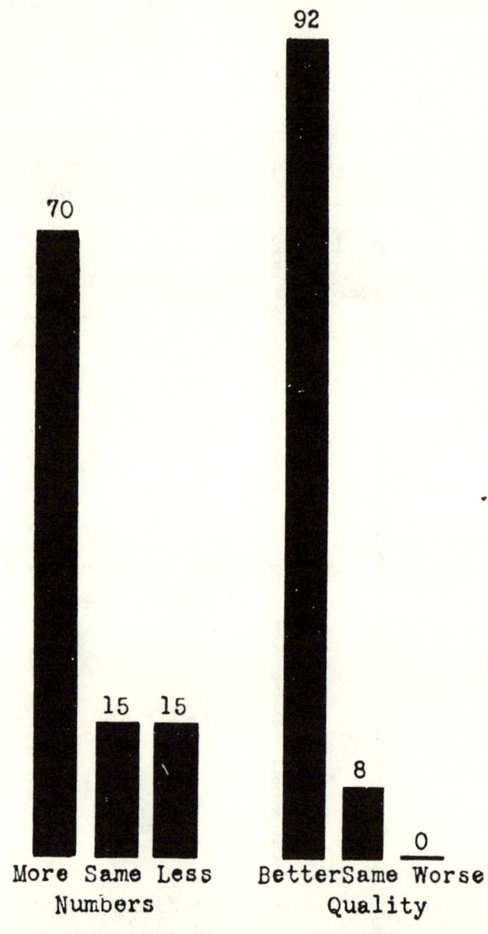

Diagram 53.—Per cent of superintendents of nurses answering the questions, "Did the fact that your school raised its entrance requirements result in more or less applicants for admission? Did it raise or lower the quality of applicants?"

requirements were then asked what effect the higher standards had had on the number and quality of applicants.

	Supt. of hospital	Supt. of nurses	Supt. of both
Number of applicants increased....	67%	70%	65%
Number of applicants decreased....	15	15	18
No change......................	18	15	17

Superintendents seem to agree that, in at least two-thirds of the cases, the effect of raising entrance requirements has been to increase the numbers of applicants for admission to the training school. This seems to have been true even in the very small schools.

Superintendents were also asked whether the raised requirements had actually made any difference in the quality of students who apply for admission—quality, of course, implying not merely better academic preparation but better all-round types of womanhood. On this point the Superintendents of Nurses were most enthusiastic, with a 92% vote for improved quality. The Superintendents of both services reported improved quality in 87% of the cases, and Superintendents of Hospitals in 83%. Practically all of those who did not see a definite improvement in quality stated that there had at least been no reduction in quality caused by the raised standards. Not over 1% in any of the three groups felt that the quality had been lowered.

14. How Many Graduate Nurses Have They?

In certain European countries it is taken for granted that students go to nursing school primarily for the purpose of being taught how to become good nurses, and not primarily for the purpose of staffing the hospital. In those countries it is understood that the student nurse supplements the graduate nurse. It was desired to find out to what extent in the United States student nurses supplement graduate nurses. (In these studies the statements for the R.N. Hospital Superintendents are omitted, since

Table 67.—Schools Reported by Superintendents of Nurses and by Superintendents of Hospital and Nurses, as Being Connected with Hospitals Where Each Number of Graduate Nurses is Employed (Not stated cases are omitted)

Graduate nurses employed	Schools reported by		Total	Per cent	Cum. per cent
	Supts. nurses	Supts. both			
0	20	9	29	3.0	3.0
1	16	27	43	4.5	7.5
2	38	41	79	8.3	15.8
3	36	41	77	8.0	23.8
4	36	55	91	9.7	33.5
5	27	52	79	8.3	41.8
6	37	38	75	7.8	49.6
7	38	21	59	6.2	55.8
8	29	21	50	5.3	61.1
9	22	11	33	3.4	64.5
10	28	10	38	4.0	68.5
11	16	7	23	2.4	70.9
12	32	4	36	3.8	74.7
13	12	3	15	1.6	76.3
14	23	2	25	2.6	78.9
15	16	3	19	2.0	80.9
16	7	3	10	1.0	81.9
17	7	2	9	1.0	82.9
18	5	1	6	0.6	83.5
19	3	..	3	0.3	83.8
20–29	63	10	73	7.6	91.4
30–39	28	4	32	3.3	94.7
40–49	16	1	17	1.8	96.5
50–59	11	..	11	1.2	97.7
60–69	5	..	5	0.5	98.2
70–79	5	..	5	0.5	98.7
80–89	1	..	1	0.1	98.8
90+	10	1	11	1.2	100.0
Total	587	367	954	100%	

many of them have R.N. Superintendents of Nurses in the same hospitals who answered the questionnaires, and it was desired not to duplicate returns for the schools.)

The returns showed that when all types of graduate nurses except the Superintendent herself are considered, nearly one-fourth of the schools have 3 graduate nurses or less, one-half have 6 or less, and three-fourths have 12 or less.

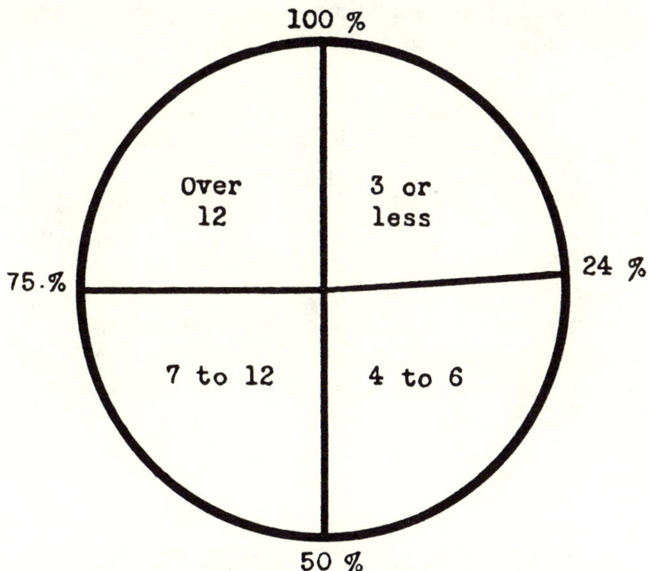

Diagram 54.—Per cent of schools where the total graduate nurses employed by the hospital (exclusive of the R.N. supt.) are 3 or less, 4 to 6, 7 to 12, or over 12

For schools run by Superintendents of Nurses, 94 per cent have more students than graduates in the hospital, 2 per cent have equal numbers, and in 4 per cent of the cases there are more graduates than students. In schools run by Superintendents who handle both services 97 per cent have more students than graduates, 1 per cent an equal number, and 2 per cent more graduates than students. In 3 per cent of the schools run by Superintendents of Nurses and in 2 per cent of the others, with the exception of the Superintendent herself, there is no graduate nurse employed by the hospital.

Some of the extreme instances where student nurses are being educated with apparently very little R.N. guidance are:

1 school of 171 students with 2 graduates in the entire hospital
1 school with 100 students with 3 graduates
1 school with 200 students with 3 graduates
3 schools with 80, 72, and 61 students respectively, and no graduate nurses at all except for the Superintendent herself.

15. Students with Floor Duty Nurses?

Sixty-seven per cent of the schools conducted by Superintendents of Nurses and 83 per cent of those conducted by Superintendents of both services report that there are no graduate nurses whatsoever on general floor duty in their hospitals.

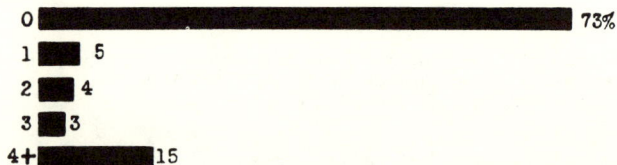

Diagram 55.—Per cent of hospitals reported by superintendents of nurses and superintendents of both services as having no graduate floor duty nurses, and one, two, three, or four or more

The schools were classified in groups according to the numbers of students, with 1–9 students, 10–19, etc., up to schools with over 130 students. In every case it was found that the middle school in each of these groups did not employ a single graduate floor duty nurse. These figures do not mean that graduate floor duty nurses are never employed in hospitals with training schools. One school with 388 students employs 90 general floor duty nurses; another with 230 students employs 80 graduates; and one with 2 students employs 23 graduates on general floor duty. Cases of this sort, however, are so unusual that they do not affect the truth of the statement that most hospitals with training schools expect the students to carry the entire nursing load of the hospital.

16. Students with R.N. Teachers?

Thirteen per cent of the schools conducted by Superintendents of Nurses and 15 per cent of those conducted by Superintendents of both services report that they have no R.N. teacher for their students. (They may, of course, have lectures by doctors or by other teachers who do not happen to be nurses.) Approximately half of the schools conducted by Superintendents of Nurses and two-thirds of those conducted by Superintendents of both services have either no teacher at all or only one. If all the students and all the teachers in these schools were combined into two aggregates, so that the teachers would be evenly distributed throughout the total student body, it would be found that there were 33 students per teacher in schools conducted by Superintendents of Nurses, and 22 students per teacher in those conducted by the Superintendents of both services. The typical school with less than 50 students has one R.N. teacher; schools of between 50 and 110 students have two R.N. teachers; and those above 110 students are apt to have three R.N. teachers for the entire student body.

17. Students with Supervisors and Head Nurses?

Although in theory there is a distinct line of demarcation between the supervisor and the head nurse, it was clear early in the study that the difference between the two is not generally accepted, and it was, therefore, decided to get the number of both combined. As contrasted with general floor duty nurses and with teachers, the number of supervisors or head nurses has a close relation to the number of students. The following table shows the number of supervisors and head nurses in the middle school of each group.

TABLE 68. SUPERVISORS AND HEAD NURSES IN THE MEDIAN SCHOOL OF EACH GROUP WHERE SCHOOLS ARE CLASSIFIED ACCORDING TO THE NUMBERS OF STUDENTS

Number of students	Median supervisors and head nurses	
	Supt. of nurses	Supt.of both
1– 9	2	1
10– 19	2	2
20– 29	2	3
30– 39	5	4
40– 49	5	4
50– 59	6	5
60– 69	7	9
70– 79	8	..
80– 89	8	..
90– 99	11	..
100–109	9	..
110–119	18	..
120–129	13	..
130+	21	..

For all the schools under both types of Superintendents there is an average of nine students for every supervisor or head nurse.

18. How Much Do They Pay Their Graduate Nurses?

The typical, or middle, hospital pays $96, with maintenance, for graduate nurses on general floor duty. The returns are nearly uniform, as the following table shows.

TABLE 69. PER CENT OF SUPERINTENDENTS OF EACH TYPE REPORTING EACH AMOUNT OF SALARY PAID IN ADDITION TO MAINTENANCE, TO GRADUATE GENERAL DUTY NURSES

Pay	Supt. of hospital	Supt. of nurses	Supt. of both	Total
Under $70	1%	1%	1%	1%
70– 79	10	8	7	8
80– 89	28	24	27	26
90– 99	31	24	27	26
100–109	22	30	32	29
110–119	5	4	2	4
120+	3	9	4	6
	100%	100%	100%	100%

The size of the city in which the hospital is located seems to have practically no influence upon the cost of the graduate floor duty nurses, except that in cities of 100,000 and over but less than 500,000, reports from all three types of R.N. Superintendents indicate that the pay for general floor duty nurses is about $10 higher than in the largest cities, or in cities of less than 100,000. The South Atlantic, East South Central, and West South Central states also are apt to pay between $100 and $110, instead of between $90 and $100 which is the rule for the rest of the country.

19. How Much Do They Pay Other Workers?

While there are a few hospitals where practical nurses and orderlies receive as much or almost as much as graduate nurses, these cases are apparently rare.

TABLE 70. PER CENT OF PRACTICAL NURSES, ORDERLIES, WARD HELPERS, AND WARD MAIDS RECEIVING EACH AMOUNT OF MONTHLY SALARY, PLUS MAINTENANCE

Monthly Salaries	Practicals	Orderlies	Ward Helpers	Ward Maids
Under $30	3.4%	1.3%	7.4%	14.1%
30– 40	4.0	4.8	21.7	29.1
40– 50	15.3	21.7	39.8	34.9
50– 60	21.7	22.8	17.0	13.4
60– 70	33.9	27.0	10.3	6.6
70– 80	13.0	9.8	1.9	1.2
80– 90	3.4	5.4	1.1	.5
90–100	1.3	4.2	..	.2
100 +	4.0	3.0	.8	..
Total	100%	100%	100%	100%
Median	$62	$60	$45	$42

20. Which Do They Prefer—Students or Graduates?

Approximately 500 Superintendents of Nurses replied to the question: "If you had your choice, which would you rather have to take care of your patients—student nurses or graduate nurses?" Seventy-six per cent replied emphatically that they would prefer student nurses, and only 24 per cent voted for graduate nurses.

These figures were taken from an earlier study made in March, 1927, and addressed to Superintendents of Nurses in the ten states to which the original nurse studies were confined. The purpose of this particular inquiry was to discover the attitude of Superintendents of Nurses towards the employment of graduate nurses in hospitals. The vote in favor of the student nurse increased directly

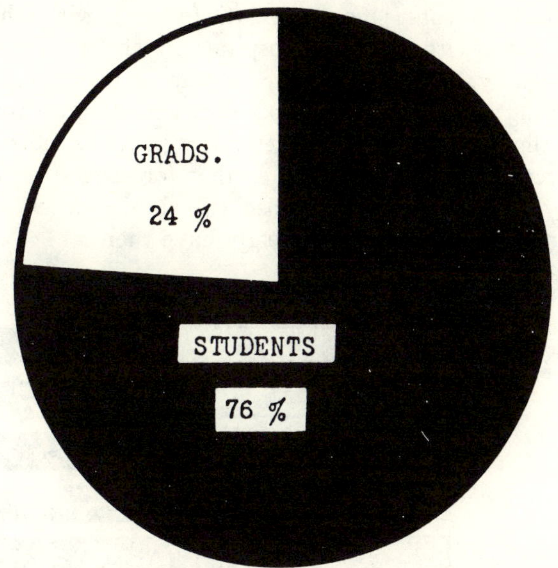

Diagram 56.—Five hundred superintendents of nurses answered the question, "If you had your choice, which would you rather have to take care of your patients, student nurses or graduate nurses?"

with the size of the student body, but even in hospitals where there were no students at all 43 per cent of the superintendents would have preferred students to graduates. Some reasons given for this astonishing and overwhelming vote will be found in the chapter which follows.

21. Separate Dining and Sitting Rooms?

Superintendents were also asked: "Do you have or want a dining-room for the specials separate from that for the regular nurses?" For Superintendents with schools, 19 per cent already have separate dining-rooms, 34 per cent want separate dining-rooms, and 47 per cent do not. The vote is more emphatic for those with schools than those without. For hospitals which have no students, only 22 per cent have or want separate dining-rooms as compared with 78 per cent who do not care for such separation. In the large training schools, however, the vote is almost reversed, so that for schools with as many as 80 students, almost two-thirds either want separate dining-rooms or already have them.

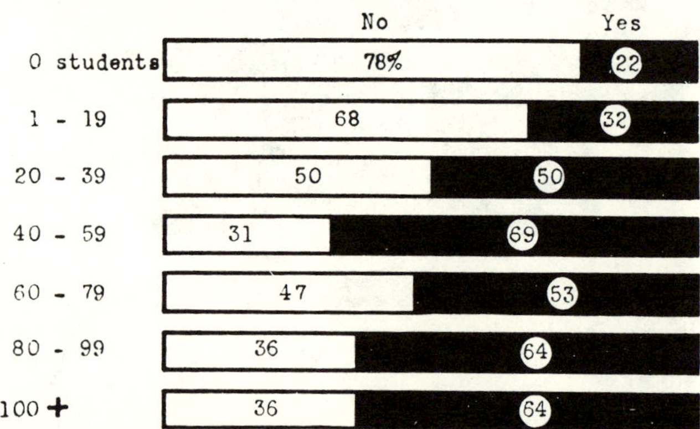

Diagram 57.—Six hundred superintendents of nurses answered the question, "Do you have, or want, a separate dining-room for special nurses?" Schools with few students do not feel the need for separating specials from students, but as the number of students increases the "specials" problem apparently becomes pressing

Superintendents were also asked: "Do you have or want sitting-rooms available for specials?" The difference between the hospital with a school and the hospital without is much less marked here than in the case of votes on dining-rooms. Forty-one per cent of the hospitals without training schools want separate sitting-rooms for their specials, as compared with 72 per cent in hospitals with schools of 80 or more students. For the entire group of hospitals with schools, 23 per cent already have separate sitting rooms for their specials, 46 per cent want them, and 31 per cent do not. Here, again, some of the reasons for these votes are given in the following chapter.

22. Do Their Students Care for Private Room Patients?

Because of the prevalent interest in group nursing and the consequent discussions of the number of private room patients who can adequately be cared for by a single nurse, the question was asked: "How many patients does a student take care of *when the patients are in separate rooms?*" For the entire group of schools the typical school reported that under these conditions students could care satisfactorily for four patients at a time. Reports of what the students were actually doing are as follows:

In % of the schools	patients are cared for by	student	
In 1% of the schools	0 patients are cared for by	1 student	
1	1	1	When the patients are in separate rooms
9	2	1	
43	3	1	
33	4	1	
8	5	1	
4	6	1	
0	7	1	
1	8	1	

In discussions of group nursing, the objection is frequently made that the plan is impracticable because "In order to have one nurse care for more than one private room patient, it would be necessary to rebuild the hospital." The table and diagram here presented would seem to show that not only is it possible, but it is the accepted practice for nurses to care for several private room patients at a time. If student nurses can successfully care for three or four private room patients without having the hospital rebuilt, it would seem reasonable to believe that graduate nurses could do so also.

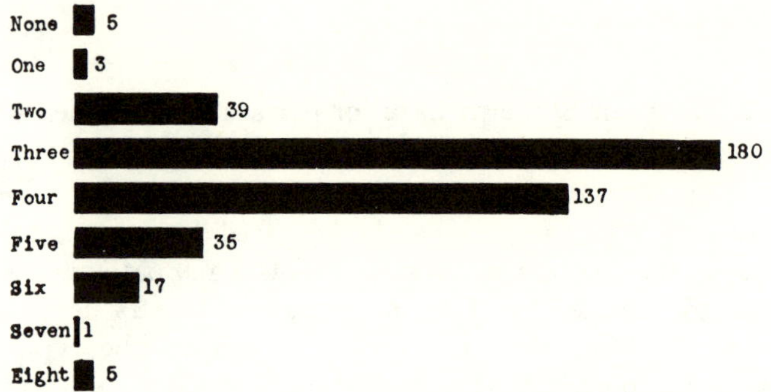

Diagram 58.—Four hundred twenty-two superintendents of nurses answered the question, "In your hospital about how many patients does a student nurse take care of *when the patients are in separate rooms?*"

This report does not attempt to discuss either of two frequently debated questions: the first, whether students learn enough in private room nursing to warrant this use of them, and second whether group nursing by graduate nurses is feasible and desirable. It does not even attempt to define what group nursing is! It does suggest that each problem would seem a fruitful field for further study.

23. Do They Need, and Can They Get, Extra Nurses?

Finally, the Superintendents were asked: "How many extra nurses for general floor duty did you need last week? How many did you get?" (The week referred to was the last week in March, 1927.) Of 512 nurse Superintendents who answered the question, 402 said that they did not need any extra nurses for general floor duty; and 110 needed a total of 677 general floor duty nurses but secured only 347, or 51 per cent of their needs. The size of a training school, or the absence of a school, made no difference in the number of hospitals saying that they needed extra general floor duty nurses. The need was slightly greater in large cities than in small ones.

In this connection it is worth remembering that many Superintendents of Nurses are not given the power to engage extra floor duty nurses in pericds of pressure. They are expected to perform the administrative miracle of having all work handled by the existing staff regardless of how much work there is to do. This fact probably accounts in part for the 49 per cent of extra nurses who were needed but not secured. While definite figures are not available, the testimony seems to indicate that in many instances had the Superintendent of Nurses been given funds from which she could hire extra graduate floor duty nurses as needed, she would probably have been able to secure them.

There is another reason, however, for what occasionally seems to be a real shortage of graduate nurses for general duty. In spite of the fact that general duty pays better than private duty, it is one of the most unpopular branches of the nursing profession. Nurses who honestly prefer bedside nursing to any other occupation will still hesitate to try general duty. Until the hospitals are able to make general duty really respectable in the eyes of the nursing profession, they will always find it difficult to persuade high grade nurses to work for them in that capacity.

24. SUMMARY

The findings of this chapter may be summarized as follows:

a. Superintendents of Nurses are attached to larger hospitals than R.N. Hospital Superintendents or R.N. Superintendents of both Hospital and Nurses. Less than one-fifth of the Superintendents of Nurses serve in hospitals with less than 50 patients, whereas almost half of the R.N. Superintendents and almost three-fourths of the R.N. Superintendents of both services work in the smaller hospitals.

b. Thirteen per cent of the Superintendents of Nurses, and 15 per cent of the Superintendents of both Hospital and Nurses have been out of school only five years. Positions of exacting responsibility are being held by relatively immature and inexperienced young women.

c. Although the "average" R.N. Superintendent has worked in only three or four hospitals, there are wide variations within the general classification, notably among the Superintendents of Nurses.

d. Among R.N. Hospital Superintendents who have been graduated from training school 10 years or less 23 per cent, or nearly one-fourth, have never been beyond the first year of high school. How can they satisfactorily solve the problems of hospital administration with such a limited background? Six per cent of the Superintendents of Nurses and nine per cent of the Superintendents of both services who have been graduated 10 years or less have never had more than one year of high school.

e. Half of the Superintendents of Nurses and more

than half of the other Superintendents have had no special work in institutional management nor in educational methods.

f. The typical R.N. Hospital Superintendent receives $2,100 plus maintenance, the typical Superintendent of Nurses $2,000 plus maintenance, and the typical Superintendent of both services $1,920 plus maintenance. On the whole, salaries in the Middle Atlantic, the East North Central, and the Pacific states tend to be somewhat higher, and those in New England and the Southern states somewhat lower than in other parts of the country.

g. Almost two-fifths of all Superintendents of Nurses have held their present positions one year or less, and 51% two years or less. Superintendents of Nurses change their positions somewhat more frequently than Superintendents of both services, and much more frequently than R.N. Hospital Superintendents.

h. The typical R.N. Hospital Superintendent attended eight out of a possible 11 meetings of the Board of Trustees in 1927; the typical R.N. Superintendent of both Hospital and Nurses attended nine out of 12 meetings; and the typical Superintendent of Nurses attended only three out of a possible 12. May the fact that Superintendents of Nurses meet so rarely with their Boards partially account for the excessive turnover of women in that position?

i. Ninety-two per cent of the R.N. Superintendents of Hospitals, 91% of the Superintendents of Hospital and Nurses, and 89% of the Superintendents of Nurses want to continue in their present line of work.

j. The majority of training schools for nurses seem to have about as many students as they want.
k. The typical school has 34 students.
l. Approximately nine out of 10 schools have raised their entrance requirements within the past 10 years.
m. Two-thirds or more of the Superintendents where entrance requirements have been raised report that the number of applicants for admission has increased.
n. Considering all types of graduate nurses except the Superintendent herself, nearly one-fourth of the schools have three graduate nurses or less, one-half have six or less, and three-fourths have 12 or less.
o. Most hospitals with training schools expect and require the student nurse to carry the entire nursing load of the hospital. Sixty-seven per cent of the schools conducted by Superintendents of Nurses and 83% of those conducted by Superintendents of both services report that not a single general duty graduate nurse is employed in their hospitals.
p. Approximately half of the schools conducted by Superintendents of Nurses and two-thirds of those conducted by Superintendents of Hospitals and Nurses have either no R.N. teacher or only one.
q. The number of supervisors or head nurses is governed in a large measure by the number of students in the school. For schools of both types there is an average of nine students for every supervisor or head nurse.
r. The typical hospital pays the graduate nurse on general floor duty $96 plus maintenance.
s. Of every 100 Superintendents of Nurses, 24 prefer

graduate nurses for the care of patients, and 76 prefer student nurses! They would rather train new students than utilize their own finished product.

t. More than half the Superintendents of Nurses want to segregate their special nurses by means of separate dining rooms.

u. While extra nurses for general floor duty are often needed, Superintendents of Nurses have not the funds to engage them in time of stress. Moreover, although it pays a higher rate than private duty, general floor duty is unpopular among nurses. Until hospitals are able to make general duty really respectable in the eyes of the nursing profession, they will always find it difficult to persuade high grade nurses to work for them in that capacity.

CHAPTER 17

WHAT THE R.N. SUPERINTENDENTS SAY

1. The Problem of Being a Superintendent

The frank recognition of a need for preparation in advance of that to be secured during the regular training for the administrative positions is thoroughly wholesome and shows a fine spirit.

New York.—The position of superintendent should be limited to administration of the institution alone. The school of nursing should have its own administrative head.

Pennsylvania.—The combined position of superintendent and superintendent of nurses is not an altogether satisfactory one, as it also includes many hours of teaching. But you do have the advantage of being able to make plans that no one interferes with.

Massachusetts.—I hope to continue this work with all attention to the training school left off. The two cannot be combined and do justice to both.

New York.—Personally I prefer supervising to administrative work, but I was told by friendly members of the profession so many times that I was side-stepping my responsibilities that I was more or less dragged and pushed into my present position.

Massachusetts.—The nurse superintendent is the only one capable of managing small or medium-sized hospitals at the time they are organized, stretching funds, giving personal contact to the patient, organizing the school, its teachers, and educational standard. There is so much to be done in this field and so few who are capable and willing to do the job well. Men as superintendents of these hospitals are usually failures.

MISSOURI.—Even though many irritations have been removed there is still the matter of the superintendent who feels that the principal is merely one of her assistants, and who (having had nursing experience) knows all there is to know about every phase of nursing. Yet I still say it is a very pleasant life.

VERMONT.—I find the responsibility of a training school extremely wearing after eight years in the service. I am speaking from the point of view of the small hospital superintendent who is housekeeper, teacher, directress of the training school, and also superintendent of the hospital.

MICHIGAN.—I go on duty in the morning feeling certain that an intensely interesting day is before me, and I am never disappointed. The superintendent of the hospital is thoroughly in sympathy with the school of nursing, and gives me absolute support in developing our educational program.

GEORGIA.—I like hospital administration work better than any other line of hospital work when I have the cooperation of the Board of Trustees. My present cooperation is splendid.

NEW YORK.—There is no form of work so full of interest, human and personal, as that of the superintendent of nurses, and none so satisfactory where conditions are right in the hospital, and the connection with Board and Medical Staff. Very few schools, however, offer these ideal conditions. Mine does, I am proud and happy to say.

PENNSYLVANIA.—The Board of Trustees has given me a free hand to develop both the nurses' school and the hospital, and I can count upon their encouragement and support as well as the cooperation of the physicians. I have not found that my duties as hospital superintendent conflict with those of superintendent of nurses, and I have been able to do more to raise the standard of the nurses' school here than I was able to do in two other positions where I was serving as superintendent of nurses.

MAINE.—I find it hard to work here as the superintendent of the hospital, a man, does not appreciate the problems involved in building a training school and I cannot build the school as I choose, for what I consider its betterment.

NEW YORK.—I have learned to enjoy my hospital work as I enjoyed private nursing, although I was practically forced into the position of superintendent in the first place, to help my hospital in time of need. They have been very tolerant and patient with me. As I have been brought up with my staff and Board we know each other's shortcomings which we overlook, and we pull together pretty well. There is no monotony in hospital work, and there is always the opportunity of service to others, which is really the greatest joy of living.

PENNSYLVANIA.—I feel that if one chooses administrative work as a life work one should not attempt it without first taking a course in preparation of hospital administration. I like the work and expect to follow it after I receive my Bachelor of Science degree.

KENTUCKY.—If I were doing it again I would take a course in administration, and have a degree from a college. If we are going to put our schools of nursing on University basis, first those in executive positions must qualify. Working for your degree after several years of hospital experience is like working on a house and putting in the foundation later.

GEORGIA.—I am planning an administration course in the near future so as to check up on myself.

VERMONT.—A man in the hospitals I have had would have been utterly worthless, owing to the conditions which called for nurse qualifications. But she must be qualified in the same sense required of a man, plus her nurse's training, if she plans on entering the specialized work required of a hospital superintendent. The thrill of pioneer work is largely gone, and under the widespread public knowledge of hospital organization and methods only women of excellent mind and proper preparation can successfully carry on. Brilliant minds and little breeding are a poor combination and have hurt our profession. By all means hospitals and training schools should be graded.

OHIO.—I am thinking of qualifying for a teaching position. It seems to me that there is a real need for good teachers. However, I am not a college graduate, and as many of the better schools require their instructors to have a degree, I hesitate to launch myself on a career in which I must be content to rate as second class, at least. I am 42 years old and a degree looks impossible now. I taught school five years before I took up nursing and I believe I could teach nurses without an A.B. or B.S.

NEW JERSEY.—My one great desire now is to make this a Grade A hospital and a Grade A nursing school by affiliation to a general hospital. I shall try a short time longer, and if unsuccessful I feel that I must apply for a position in a Grade A school. (25 average patients—12 students. Hospital gives only a 1 year course in obstetrics.)

INDIANA.—Before I entered training I did not have a high school education, but since I graduated I have tried to make up for it, and have taken work at night school, under private instructors, and by correspondence. I am still taking work by correspondence, and this winter I am taking a four-hour credit course at the college here.

California.—Until I opened this private sanitarium I was employed in a general hospital where nurses, both graduate and practical, work 10½ hours a day, and receive respectively $90 and $60 per month with board, room, and laundry, and one day off each week, and usually half of the holidays. The course in nurses' training here requires 28 months and two years of high school. Now, here is the *joker:* In this same institution is an art teacher teaching patients basketry and the like. She receives $125 per month, rooms in officers' quarters, has every Saturday afternoon and Sunday off, works (and plays) eight hours a day. She completed her course in training as an art teacher in six months, and had no high school at all, so when aspirants ask my opinion on their becoming nurses, I say absolutely not, and I am a trained nurse too.

Illinois.—A hospital superintendent should have a working knowledge of business methods. I am confident that many hospitals need and want as superintendent women who have health, business ability, and some understanding of medical and nursing problems. The position appeals to me because a busy hospital keeps one alert mentally. One needs some knowledge of all professions, crafts and trades. One is in touch with the newer methods of nursing and medicine. When the private duty nurse must slow down and cut her salary in life, the superintendent is increasing her salary. My living expenses are normal only. I have saved consistently for many years. All interest has been reinvested.

2. How Superintendents Tell About Their Work

Even the extraordinary complexities of hospital and training school work do not lessen the enthusiasm of those who give "impassioned service."

New York.—Training schools for nurses are wonderful places. People outside can never realize the opportunities and advantages these young women receive. To watch a young person of 18 years of age enter our school, and to watch her develop and be trained into an efficient young woman at the end of her training, is most satisfactory.

INDIANA.—As your hospital progresses you feel that you are building and growing a part of it.

WISCONSIN.—I like the contact with the students because I am vitally interested in the growth and development of young people, and in preparing them to adequately fill some "job" (not position) which will contribute toward better living, better nursing, better womanhood.

MISSOURI.—Before taking up administration I was a nurse instructor, and I must say I think I derived more real happiness from this work than anything I have ever done. The contact with the girls, the watching of unfolding personality and character, the real service given (helping young girls with little background to get a start) was true pleasure. I always felt that my work was more play than work, and that I hardly deserved the salary because I never felt weary.

However, like a great many people the commercial aspect had something to do with my change to administration. Teachers have very little chance of advancement, either monetary or otherwise. I was teaching in a school of 200 student nurses, had charge of the school with three assistant instructors, and received $1800 per year salary. My room was a hideous green shade with an assortment of furniture. The grounds were filled with flowers and many of the offices were given flowers every day, but the classroom was always overlooked. Of course, we had flowers because we helped ourselves after twilight hours, and a little later grew a little garden full of our own. The instructors had no office—a small corner was reserved in the huge mustard-colored classroom for the four of us.

Of course, if I had been self-sacrificing I would have overlooked all these trifles, but I was not. So I took up administration and at least have had a small suite of rooms with a bath of my own, and much more consideration. I have been able to make the lives of my instructors fairly happy. We have a fine school and I still teach a little.

ILLINOIS.—I enjoy my work. I have no trouble in securing efficient instructress and supervisors. We work harmoniously together, which makes our work a pleasure.

RHODE ISLAND.—This is a mental hospital. We have a flourishing nursing school which we are constantly trying to improve. I feel that we are making a definite and much needed contribution to nursing, and that there is a great deal yet to be done. I am working with congenial, progressive people. Living conditions are excellent.

NEW YORK.—I have spent sixteen years in institutional work, charge of ward, operating room, supervisor's assistant, superintendent of hospital and superintendent of nurses. I have saved money every year since my graduation. I have lived comfortably, dressed well, had sufficient recreation, including two trips to Europe, one to the Bahamas, and yearly trips to Canada. I have a yearly income of $1,000 from my money invested, which I have saved since my graduation, and five thousand dollars insurance. I have always been interested in hospital work and nursing, and have never regretted my choice of a profession, but I did not care for private duty.

From my observation I would say that a nurse earning $1200 a year and maintenance in a hospital position is better off at the end of the year than the private duty nurse.

VERMONT.—After 23 years of hospital experience I am still wondering at the Providence that gave me a job which I so enthusiastically love to carry on.

MASSACHUSETTS.—Always learning something; keeping in touch with young people and progress; a good comfortable home with full maintenance (I did private duty for five years and know its uncertainties); a chance to get the newest in nursing magazines and books where the hospital must keep these before the students always; the satisfaction of being able to help more people; the consciousness that one must go ahead and progress along all lines in order to help in the community; and the business end interests me too. We have men only on our board—no doctors, no women.

NEW YORK.—For a number of years I did training school work, and I find that the executive work of a small institution is much more interesting and not as nerve-racking.

WISCONSIN.—It is easier in a large hospital than in a small place.

MISSOURI.—There is probably no one who really enjoys this work more than I do.

MASSACHUSETTS.—My present job is in a small hospital (150 beds) and consists mainly in furnishing supplies and propitiating the medical staff on one point or another. There is no interne, and the maintenance of proper clinical records, as well as their housing, falls to the lot of the administration. The former superintendent was also director of nurses. I am not, and the task of separating the two positions in the public (and private) mind is requiring great persistence as well as care. I think we are succeeding, but the process is proving conclusively to me that my main interest is in the nursing part of the game. The head nurse on the ward seems to me to be in the crucial position, dealing directly with the patients, helping or handicapping the physicians, as well as the administration, and (by no means least) shaping the habits and hands of the nurses of tomorrow.

The most satisfactory thing I ever did was night supervising; next to that, running a floor, although supervising graduate nurses is disheartening in the extreme! I hope in the course of another year to be back (?) as a head nurse or floor supervisor, having proven in four years that I can do a job like this, but do not want to.

I am enjoying the independence attendant on the position; contact with as fine a group of men and women (as directors) as I can imagine; and the ability to bring things to pass, creation of an out-patient department and social service; equipment of a dietetics laboratory for the school of nursing; landscaping of hospital grounds; change in name of institution; arrangements for vacation; and house for student nurses. I do not mean to give the impression that I am having a dull time. I am too far removed from patients and students, that is all.

New York.—Administrative work is much more to my liking than actual nursing. Financially I am much farther ahead and have had many more advantages and opportunities.

Maine.—I think any young nurse would do well to have charge of a small well-equipped hospital before taking a more responsible position in a larger one. Personally I know that I am much better fitted for another position now than I was a year ago, due to my experience here, though I know that this statement will be contradicted by many who do not know just what a small hospital under the proper sort of a surgeon really has to offer.

Ohio.—This is a small hospital (15 beds) in the country, population 1200. The work is interesting and fascinating. We do considerable surgical work. Although the city is only 45 miles from here, with its many large, well-equipped hospitals, we are very proud of the work done here, and the wonderful results of our work. We have several good surgeons in the small surrounding towns, and as I just finished training in November, 1926, I have gained much experience in my present position. The hospital has done very well in the past year and plans have been completed to put a large addition to the hospital in the early spring.

PENNSYLVANIA.—There has always been great injustice shown towards the woman executive. A woman builds up on a substantial foundation but always with a check valve of cautious economy imposed by men trustees. When the institution has expanded in its capacity for increased service, in its popularity with the public, in its wholesome influence upon the community, the question seems to be raised in the minds of the management, should we not pass on to a man's control, and this often when a woman has mortgaged her health in her impassioned service to the institution. Why is a woman often replaced by a man whose salary exceeds hers by several thousand dollars? Why must a man have the privilege of maintaining his family at the expense of the institution, while a woman can't even have her mother live with her? Why is he allowed to spend only a few hours in his office every day while women are expected to be in the office every hour of the day? He is free to go and come as he pleases at the expense of the institution. The reasons are many for the passing of the old reliable woman incumbent from the field where she wrought to make the present day hospital possible. Contrast the freedom of the nursing Sister with the non-sectarian hospital. They have ability and are rarely interfered with.

3. Graduates Versus Students

The wide divergence of opinion shown in the following quotations may be due to fundamental differences of attitude. It seems fairly obvious that an all graduate service requires skilful leadership. Granted that, might it not prove more desirable for many institutions than student service?

PENNSYLVANIA.—In 1925 there was a full graduate nursing service here. This was not considered desirable from a nursing standpoint, because of frequent changing of service and less interest shown. The financial outlay was greater than with pupils. The hospital has added necessary equipment and organization. A building for Nurses' Home and classrooms has been built, and a class of 12 admitted in October, 1927. (40 average patients.)

KANSAS.—I prefer students because graduates are here today and gone tomorrow.

KANSAS.—We would rather have student nurses because this is a small hospital, and there are times when we have only a few patients. Graduate nurses do not seem to like it, and leave, and we often have to make changes. When we have pupil nurses we can keep them busy with theoretical work, and they stay longer even though we do not have the success at present that we used to have when we had a surgeon here who has left.

CALIFORNIA.—I think the reason for frequent change on the general duty staff is due to the fact that the majority of nurses applying for floor duty are transients, and simply put in time to suit their convenience.

CALIFORNIA.—The graduates, after they have done special work for any length of time, seem to find it very difficult to adjust themselves. I find that the young graduates are more willing to do general duty than the older ones, and cover the work better and with more ease.

CALIFORNIA.—The general run in graduate help on floor duty:
1. No special interest, hours and salary only objective.
2. From lack of supervision, uses a "short cut" method in taking care of her patients and rather resents being asked not to throw linen on the floor, to change bath water frequently when giving a bed bath, etc. Setting up trays properly, etc.
3. Frequent changes, transient.

CALIFORNIA.—I have found in my experience with graduate nurses that they lack the ability to adapt themselves, not, however, due to lack of being efficient in training, in the actual care of the needs of their patient or patients, but of being able to understand their patient (and relatives sometimes) and having the personality to handle the situation agreeably to all. In institutions among other nurses, especially undergraduates, they are sometimes overbearing. It seems the lack is caused by undeveloped personality rather than improper or insufficient training.

KANSAS.—Due to reorganization of our school we have had a force of graduate nurses. They all are from different schools, have different methods, all have finished their student nurse days and do not care for supervision and corrections necessary to adjustment. Naturally, it would be easier to have students trained to my own methods.

NEW YORK.—If hospital authorities would pay graduates at the rate of six dollars per day or night, I feel that there would be no shortage of nurses for general duty, as many nurses prefer general to private duty, but find it impossible to live on the salaries paid.

New York.—The student nurse is less apt to be careless in technique, gives better cooperation in regard to hospital regulations, is less extravagant with hospital linen and supplies, and with the help and advice of an experienced supervisor gives her patients care equal to that of the graduate. Student nurses work together with less friction.

Kansas.—Student nurses quite frequently take more responsibility and are more economical with foods, linens, supplies, etc.

California.—Student nurses are more cooperative and conscientious.

Kansas.—Student nurses are usually eager to learn modern methods, more interested in progression of technique, may be shifted according to house demands, and are more stable.

Graduates on general duty are demanding, exacting and shifting.

California.—Student nurses are much more familiar, of course, with the routine of our hospital. Aside from this, however, they are much more appreciative of constructive criticism and supervision. Of course, some graduate nurses are equally eager to learn.

Kansas.—Some of the graduates are very good conscientious girls, but my doctors here ask for my students if their patients want special care for a few days. They think the students are more careful, steadier, and pay more attention to business. We have had so much trouble with graduates coming in and causing some uprising in our training school. Our place is so small and the girls are so closely in contact with each other. They talk shop talk and things they pulled while in training, or how different their school was to what they have to put up with. I find that the majority of special duty nurses always find fault, always complain of their luck.

CALIFORNIA.—I find greater satisfaction in employing only graduate nurses. Patients themselves have more confidence, and work can be assigned and there is no break in the service or changing of nurses due to the interruption of classes, etc. The nursing care is of a higher character.

WASHINGTON.—My experience with graduates has been a very happy one. All of the girls who have been sent out from the central registry in our nearest large town have been splendid types of women, trustworthy and dependable. I could not leave the hospital with a pupil nurse or an undergraduate, and have the same feeling of security that I have when I leave a graduate. In a small hospital of this kind a great deal of responsibility is placed upon the floor nurse. That is why I prefer graduates.

CALIFORNIA.—Another nurse and I own and operate a twenty-bed hospital, and in order to do it satisfactorily our duties are decidedly varied in character and our hours very uncertain. We employ only graduate help and they have regular hours. My associate and I try to keep regular hours, but emergencies are always arising which demand our attention.

It might be of interest to your Committee to know that in the five years we have been carrying on this work we have never had any difficulty in getting graduate nurses, both on general floor duty and as private nurses.

CALIFORNIA.—Floor duty called "just general" has the stigma attached to it of being used only as a "filler" when other work is unavailable. Every nurse who applies for it expects to have too much to do, and hopes she can "get away with it" for a while. General duty should be dignified. The name should be changed. It sounds like the old "general servant." Nurses should be told that you consider that they are doing real nursing, and hold just as dignified a position as any one else on the hospital staff. Floaters should be employed to relieve rush times. They should have an eight-hour day, and one day off per week. They should have better housing than that of students. What is the use of graduating if you cannot attain that much? Besides, the student ought to see something in the position of the graduate that she wants, not something she scorns. Neither should she scorn the care of patients.

There is only a shortage of good nurses, courteous, well-bred, kindly women, not necessarily college women. College sometimes makes the elbow stick out farther, and the nurse dissatisfied for lack of intellectual stimulus. Ill-bred, discontented nurses should be dismissed if remonstrance fails. They are like bad apples in a box. Hospitals should spend less money on elaboration in building, and more care when purchasing expensive equipment. More attention should be focused on costs of other departments. Nursing costs look big because they used to be so little. Nurses' homes can be much less elaborate, and the inmates happier in training and also when they join the working women of the world if there are enough of them to do the work. At present we educate them to think they are superior to other women, and do not treat them accordingly when they graduate.

Effort should be made to show the student something ahead of her, good remuneration, better than other workers because people should and can pay for what it costs other people more to do—nursing must always be an effort for the sensitive and they are the most successful. If we can show any advantage in nursing, there will be no shortage. The old time "idealists" seem to have forgotten that $25 a week sounded like a very attractive fortune when no other woman was getting it. We heard a great deal about it, too, in the towns they came from.

Hospitals need better business management, doctors, business training. They are too personal in their judgment and reckless about other people's money. The atmosphere of "rush" in hospitals has always been as foolish as the old policy of killing the well to heal the sick. We must seek system, and secure an adequate number of workers. Nurses have always filled in all the holes, kept the thing going when others failed, and have reaped the usual reward for such well-meaning but unthinking competence. Patients have suffered from our unnecessary excitement. Clever women in charge, much more conscientious about detail than the male administrators, have lost prestige by trying to please everybody with insufficient assistance, and wearing out in the process. Doctors and management grew to think we were doing nothing unless we looked haggard and had our hair falling down and caps crooked.

California.—The only difficulty we find in engaging graduate nurses for floor duty is for the night work. We generally have to take what we can get rather than what we want. This is not so of day duty. Positions in the surgery are very easily filled.

California.—I believe that the thought of night duty prevents many from entering institutional work—that insufficient consideration for night workers exists in most hospitals, and that the hours are too long.

California.—It seems that a good number of the hospitals that employ graduate nurses for general floor duty offer a salary range of $80 to $90 per month, which is very little more than the practical nurse or an untrained attendant gets. It seems to me that in this day and age the salary for good graduate nurses for floor duty should be at least $100 per month. The practical nurse can get from $75 to $80 if she does good work, and can get $25 for private cases per week. Maids can get from $60 to $75. The requirements for the registered nurse are high, and the responsibility heavy for the conscientious nurse.

Wyoming.—In this hospital we like our general duty nurses and find them efficient, as we are able to choose. The Board here pays good salaries, $100 per month, which is better than the usual $75 to $80. Also we have a single room for each graduate, and the Nurses' Home is a desirable place to live.

Illinois.—Student nurses, decidedly, under careful supervision. They are more adjustable, have more uniform technique. We employ graduate nurses for general duty only when necessary, and hope to increase our enrollment of students to give adequate care to the patients, because we feel it is more satisfactory in every way.

4. Separate Dining or Sitting Room for Specials

Apparently the relationship between special duty nurses and the other workers in the hospital is not always a happy one. Has the writer of the first excerpt found the answer?

California.—We take particular pains to teach and help all new specials that come into the house and consequently we have a very friendly feeling among the specials and our floor nurses. In other words, the "Golden Rule" is practised twenty-four hours each day, and it has been months since a complaint, either from patients or the staff, has come to me.

Washington.—Our pupil nurses have certain ideals held up to them. Intimacy with "Specials" may or may not improve our pupil nurses' ideals.

Wyoming.—In most training schools we find the graduate nurses from different schools, each with her own individual peculiarities and methods of training, each thinking her training school the best, and about one-third, I find, inclined to talk to the pupil nurses about how things were done in their training schools.

I also notice that the special nurses are very extravagant with the hospital supplies; and at various times I have asked them if they were allowed to do in their own training schools as they were now doing, and invariably they answer in the negative, and are unable to give any reason why they should do differently in this hospital.

I am sure that, if the trained nurse would do and act in other hospitals as she is trained to do while in training, graduate nurses doing special duty nursing would be more appreciated.

KANSAS.—I think it better to keep the special nurses separate from those in training because of the conversation of some special nurses at table.

I think that nurses do not care for institutional work, as general duty on a floor, because they are under supervision, while on special cases out in the country, etc., they are more independent.

ILLINOIS.—I do not like the graduates and students together too much, as the graduates talk about things the students do not need to know.

WASHINGTON.—Because some of them discourage the students by their remarks.

WYOMING.—A separate dining room is greatly needed because of criticism about administration.

KANSAS.—Nurses board out of the hospital. Prefer this, as they are not always agreeable about board.

CALIFORNIA.—There is less gossip and criticism when kept separate.

CALIFORNIA.—We need separate sitting rooms for specials to prevent congregating in halls and offices smoking.

5. Group Nursing

There is no apparent agreement as to the meaning of the term group nursing and naturally, therefore, no very general agreement as to its desirability.

California.—Generally speaking, the student nurse can care for more patients than the private duty nurse, because of the reaction of the patients. When a private nurse is employed, the patients so frequently demand a great deal of care not essential to their recovery, but because they like the personal attention. Usually, though not always, they do not expect a student nurse to devote so much of her time to them.

Kansas.—Our student nurses (or general floor nurses) can care for only three or four patients. They have complete care of patients assigned them, are on duty nine hours, so must relieve each other. Specials spend more time, are slower to cover work with patients, spend part of the time entertaining patient.

California.—Special nurses could care for at least three patients, as they would have a definite assignment to these patients, with no interruption of classes. They could not take care of more, for the demands of the patient when taken care of by a graduate are more demanding than of a student, for they feel they are "paying for" graduate nursing service.

Kansas.—Our patients rarely want special nurses. They go out remarking about their good care. Our nurses are five-year combined course students, and we are getting intelligent, pleasant girls that give thorough, efficient service. We even have gall-bladder cases and thyroids among our faculty people who could pay, who do not desire special nurses. We do not favor it, as our nurses receive very much better privileges of training.

ILLINOIS.—A graduate nurse doing twelve hour duty has entirely too much time on her hands, unless the patient is acutely ill. She could easily care for two or even three patients, and I believe both patients and nurse would feel better satisfied. I am heartily in favor of definitely regulated hours for nurses, but the system of having one nurse for one patient, particularly a convalescent patient, for twelve hours, is not right. We are planning to try group nursing.

Student nurses are more interested in their work. They are under constant supervision, and their work is graded, which gives them an incentive to endeavor to improve.

Our only experience with graduate nurses for general floor duty is during the vacation season. We find it very unsatisfactory, and have great difficulty in securing well-trained nurses for this type of work.

ILLINOIS.—We have on one or two occasions tried group nursing (two patients) with much success. However, the question of salary came up, some of the graduates feeling that they should be paid $2.00 for the additional patient. Later we tried it with a clear understanding beforehand that the nurses should charge the regular rate for one patient for one day, and it proved very satisfactory from every standpoint.

CALIFORNIA.—A convalescing average patient does not need or want constant attention, therefore the "special" has little or nothing to do after the morning care is given. She could very easily take care of two such patients to the satisfaction of herself and them.

CALIFORNIA.—I think a regular paid staff of registered nurses for group nursing with an eight hour day would conserve nurses and time and supply the demand in a very satisfactory manner. I believe group nursing should be supplemented with hourly nursing.

KANSAS.—People who employ a "special" want all of her time; they may not need it but they would not be willing to share her with another patient. Those who do not employ a "special" seem well satisfied with floor duty service and would rather have it than a part-time "special."

6. Miscellaneous

"Knowledge is power and it always fascinates brains" might be a good slogan for recruiting student nurses from the upper level of high school graduates.

MASSACHUSETTS.—Since I have reorganized this hospital, secured an all-time *competent instructress* and a Superintendent of Nurses, the training school has increased to capacity and we have a waiting list.

We have a very good type of student. With a very few exceptions all are high school graduates; some have an additional business course.

INDIANA.—Our training school, when first organized, was giving a four year college course and only high school graduates could qualify. There were many students who wanted to take a nurse's training but did not care for the college course, so we started a three year course and admitted students with one year of high school education. Last fall we had many more applicants than we could take and so this year we have raised our educational requirements to four years of high school, and expect to get all the students we can take.

CALIFORNIA.—I should like a training school for nurses, provided it could be affiliated with a University or Junior College where students could have the better advantage of science and training. Student nurses, providing the hospital is located where advanced "advantages" can be secured for the student. Otherwise the burden upon the hospital is more than it can financially carry, unless it is endowed, or is a general hospital that has county aid or appropriation.

New Hampshire.—I like the administrative work but find the training problems much harder than they were 10 years ago. The girls who enter today are too young and irresponsible.

Washington.—I would like to make a few remarks that may seem irrelevant but which, from my viewpoint, are really not. I'm vitally interested in nursing education and this is the second small hospital (150 beds) I have had charge of. But I really think the best of my information was gathered in the public schools, first as Red Cross instructress, later while presenting the work in the parochial and some of the high schools as instructor and superintendent of nurses.

Most of the senior classes in all high schools have an A and a B section. Invariably when you ask the B section (usually composed of undernourished children with adenoids, tonsils, poor teeth, and all the rest of it) if they are interested in nursing, the answer comes promptly "Yes, I'd like to be a nurse." Why? "Well, it's hard but it gives you" and then in their various ways they tell you it improves their social standing, they make more money, they do not have to finish high school, and the grades do not have to be so high to enter a nursing school. Heaven help the mark! The work of all others that requires a broad-minded, thoroughbred, intelligent young woman with high ideals and stamina enough to stay with them, made the resort of the incompetent, for that is just what it has become, with few exceptions. As one truly brilliant high school student replied to my question about choosing nursing, "I respect you and I got a lot out of your classes and this has been an eye opener to me, but I'll never choose it as a profession. All the dummies in our school that can't get a teacher's certificate go in for nursing."

When we make a bid for the A division of the seniors of the high schools, and have intelligent teachers interested in nursing, in our own classrooms, we will not have the "Specials" reading Snappy Stories and looking into vacancy, while a patient is lying in the bed with a cold "proc" or drinking from a half glass of water that has been standing on the table for hours. Nor will our student nurse disdain her profession if she has a sufficient knowledge of the structure, working, disease and cure of the human body, which means a good knowledge of anatomy, physiology, pathology, and materia medica. This should be given by a thoroughly trained woman who has gotten it in a college laboratory. Knowledge is power and it always fascinates brains. Bid for the A division of the high school and present your subjects in the classroom clearly and scientifically by a competent woman, and it will diminish your troubles.

PART 2

A FEW OF THE IMPLICATIONS

The rest of this book contains comments and suggestions concerning some of the implications of the data in Part 1. No exhaustive discussion has been attempted, partly because the Committee has been impressed by the need for haste in making the findings generally available, and partly because the results seem to have such serious significance that the Committee is not yet ready to discuss them in any but frankly tentative terms. It is eager in its hope that the various groups concerned with the nursing problem will proceed to thoughtful consideration of the findings, and will early acquaint their representatives on the Grading Committee with their conclusions.

CHAPTER 18

WHY BE CONCERNED?

Why should we be alarmed by the prospects of overproduction, or distressed by the continuing influx of poorly prepared nurses to the profession?

If nurses belonged merely to one of the useful occupations rendering personal service (like barbers, manicurists, cooks, waitresses, restaurant owners, and the like) they might well be left to the inexorable workings of economic law.

It is because there is inherent in nursing something far higher than the ordinary concept of useful personal service to the sick; and because nursing is not only making contributions of inestimable value to curative and preventive care, but has actually become a social necessity, that the need for guiding and protecting its development seems paramount. Perhaps there is no better way of explaining this viewpoint than by inserting at this point a paragraph, written by a nurse, which goes far towards bringing to those outside of the profession some understanding of what nursing may mean.

"One cannot hand the art of nursing out to anybody. The tools of nursing are many of them simple enough, but the range of sources from which they are drawn must be very wide, and their uses perfected by long and arduous effort. Senses and perceptions must be trained to their finest adjustments. Behind that quick sure touch, that fine and delicate manipulation, must be months of

toil and practice, experiment and failure, as well as progress. Behind that sure judgment lie long stretches of experience and careful study of persons and situations; of comparison of methods and results. The relation between patient and nurse is a peculiarly intimate and vital one, and it should contribute richly and constantly to our knowledge and understanding of our art. It should be preceded and accompanied by carefully directed study of the interdependence of mind and body; of those psychological truths which can serve in some measure to guide us in the conduct of helpful human relationships. Every branch of nursing stands in need of just such serious and scientific study of the problems inherent in its particular sphere. Emphasis has been laid in nursing always on the development of skill in technique, and that is essential, but equally so will be found training of these other kinds, if we are to prepare nurses adequately for the infinitely varied and complex needs which are inherent in the work awaiting them."

(Mary Adelaide Nutting, R. N.: A Sound Economic Basis for Schools of Nursing. Page 357.)

CHAPTER 19

FACING THE ECONOMIC FACTS

Nursing is an idealistic profession, but that fact does not render it immune to economic considerations. Except in the Sisterhoods, the Spirit of Nursing is in perpetual conflict with the economic fact; and whenever economic conditions in nursing begin to be unhealthy, it is the damage to the Spirit of Nursing which shows first evidences that something is wrong. If nurses are intelligent in their desire to maintain the best of what nursing stands for, they will probably do well to make a careful study of the laws of supply and demand which apply not only to nursing, but to other professions as well.

1. What People Want They Pay For

One of these laws may be stated as follows: *Under healthful conditions the number of workers in a profession bears a close relation to the amount of adequately paid work available for them.* In other words, there is no civic virtue in enticing hundreds of new recruits into a profession unless there is some work in sight at which they can earn a living after they get in. It is not enough to say, "Humanity needs them!" Wages in the United States are good, the standard of living is high, what the public wants it rather adequately manages to get. If humanity wants nursing, it will pay for it, just as it pays for automobiles; and if it does not want nursing, it will not buy it. Therefore, it would seem wise (unless some definite promises can be secured for ample and long term subsidies) for the nursing and medical professions to begin at once an energetic inquiry not merely into "How much nursing would it be good for people to have?" but "How much and what sorts of nursing is the public ready to buy?"

According to the figures shown in Chapters 2 and 3 of this report, the growth of nursing schools and nursing graduates has been startling and unchecked. More than a quarter of a century ago the medical profession began to make a careful study of its field. Perhaps unconsciously, but directly as the result of its efforts to improve the quality of its graduates, it reduced the number of colleges by half. It is still actively and conscientiously employed in limiting new recruits to the profession to young men and women of high quality in sufficient numbers to provide adequate medical care for the expected population at each decade, but not to result in a flooding of the medical market. Is it reasonable to suggest that nursing might well follow the same policy?

At the present time there are apparently three nurses to every two physicians in the United States. Except in some rural districts and in a few specialties, physicians almost unanimously report that there is no shortage of nurses in their localities. The typical physician reporting in this study had, on the day he answered the questionnaire, three patients who needed special nurses and two who got them; but the third patient was not the victim of a nursing shortage. According to medical testimony, the third patient went without a nurse because he did not want her enough to pay her price. The physicians who provided the material which has gone into this study are a selected group. They represent that part of the medi-

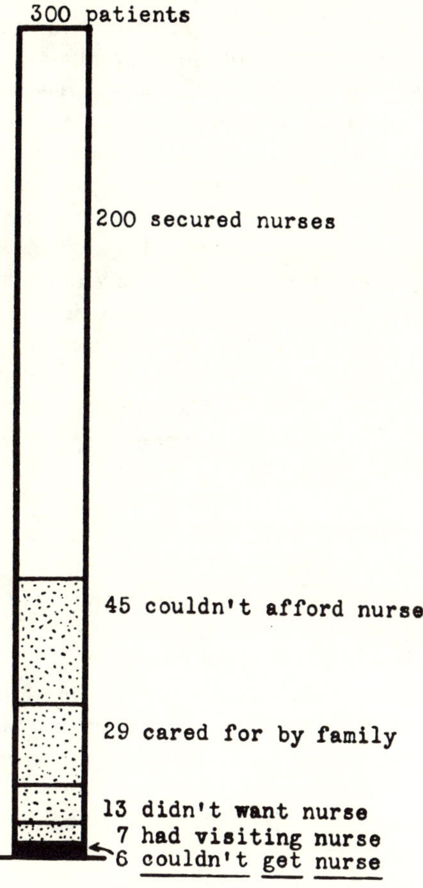

Diagram 59. On the average, each 100 physicians had 300 patients needing special nurses on the day they answered the questionnaire. Of these 300 patients, 200 secured nurses; while only 6 wanted a nurse but could not get one

cal profession which is particularly interested in nursing problems, and that means the part which most frequently has occasion to employ special duty nurses. If in this report the average physician had only three patients who needed special nursing care and only two who were willing to buy it, it seems reasonable to believe that the average for the whole profession would be even lower.

Registries for private duty nurses report serious country-wide unemployment. Physicians report an ample supply of nurses. Yet there are only three nurses to every two physicians at the present time. What then is going to happen in 1965 when, according to the extremely conservative estimates in Chapter 3, there will apparently be nine or ten nurses for every two physicians? Can the physicians treble their use of special nurses and persuade their patients to pay the cost?

2. Where Can the Graduates Go?

More than half the nurses are in private duty. If there were some obvious opening for nurses in one of the other fields, might the increased production be taken care of? Here, perhaps, is the real answer to part of the problem, but it needs qualification. Every one is agreed that there is need for more public health nursing; yet, as was shown in Chapter 6, for every public health nursing position filled in the month of March, 1927, there were five applicants. There is no shortage of applicants for public health nursing. There is a lack of applicants properly prepared to do public health work, but the shortage is one of quality, not quantity. Moreover, even in this field there is real question of how many new workers can be absorbed. Public health salaries are low as it is. Public health nurses, so far as one can judge, are apt to hold on to their positions rather tenaciously, and do not step aside to make room for newcomers.

No estimates are available at present, but it would seem rather important that the nursing profession attempt some evaluation not only of how much public health nursing the country might beneficially receive, but of how many new nursing positions *with salaries attached* are likely to be created each year. Is the public so eager for public health nursing that it will buy more of it and at the same time not try to cut down on the amount of money it is spending for salaries for the present workers? Until the nursing profession has some answer to this question, how can it tell whether or not it should be seeking many thousands of new workers? Five applicants for every position, even though they be poorly trained, must, it would seem, inevitably have some effect upon keeping present salaries perilously near the minimum level, below which self-respecting professional women will decide that they cannot afford to go.

In institutional work there would appear to be a definite shortage, but is it one which can be looked upon as the solution for disposing of the horde of new workers? Apparently, almost all hospitals are seriously understaffed. Many of them have no graduate nurses at all for the care of their patients. Here, one would say, is the great untilled field for nursing. Perhaps it may be. If the nursing profession can persuade hospital authorities that the trained nurse is better for the care of patients than either the student or the attendant, there perhaps may be the solution of where the 60,000 graduates of 1965 can go.

The estimates given in Chapter 3 are conservative. Mathematical statisticians will see, on glancing at Diagram 6, that the logarithmic curve used there to predict the numbers of graduates each year in the future might, with almost equal fairness, have been so calculated on the basis of the existing data that the annual crops of graduates in the future would be much larger than the estimates as given. Instead of a graduating class in 1965 of 60,000, the estimate might perhaps, with equal validity, have been for 80,000 or 90,000.

Moreover, the computations of total nurses actively engaged in the profession for each year in the future have been based upon records supplied by superintendents of nurses for past graduates of their schools. It is known that these records have failed to include reports for large numbers of married graduates who have left the profession only to return later. It seems to be a phenomenon of American life, not peculiar to the nursing profession but to be seen in every field, that married women are increasingly keeping on with their professional activities. It is impossible at present to estimate how great this tendency now is or how rapidly it will continue to grow, but it seems safe to say that the numbers of nurses in active practice each year in the future would be enlarged considerably over the estimates as given in Chapter 3, if it were possible to predict how many of the married nurses will each year return to active professional practice. They would be even more increased if estimates were included covering nurses coming into the United States from other countries.

It is not desired to exaggerate conditions, but it is believed that there is at hand ample warrant for calling attention to the possibility of serious overproduction in the nursing profession and raising the question which must be faced: "How are we going to provide adequate paid employment for nurse graduates?"

3. SUMMARY

To summarize what has been said in this chapter:

a. The fact that nursing is an idealistic profession does not render it immune to the working of economic law. If nursing is to retain its high idealism, it must make sure that its members are free from undue economic pressure.

b. Therefore, nursing must consider ways and means for insuring that the number of graduate nurses admitted to the profession shall bear a close relation to the amount of adequately paid work available for them.

c. The medical profession has long faced this problem. It exercises strict control over the number and quality of new workers admitted to its ranks.

d. In nursing no such control exists. The result is, apparently, that there are already more graduate nurses available than there is paid work for them to do. Evidence of this has been secured:

   From physicians
   From nurse registries
   From public health organizations
   From hospitals
   From the nurses themselves

e. While many positions for nurses remain unfilled, there is no lack of applicants. The shortage is not in quantity, but in quality.

f. Conservative estimates indicate that, if present trends continue, the overproduction of nurses will become extremely serious.

g. The question which must be faced is:

"*How are we going to provide adequate paid employment for nurse graduates?*"

CHAPTER 20

THE HOSPITAL AND THE SCHOOL

The student nurse is worth money! Nursing is probably the only profession where students are eagerly sought because of their economic value; and this fact accounts probably for the best and the worst characteristics of nursing education. It is because the student is of real economic value to the hospital that nursing education furnishes one of the few examples of the much preached, but rarely practised, educational maxim: "We learn to do by doing." Probably most of what is best in nursing education today has been made possible by the fact that the hospital has found it profitable to place the actual patient care in student hands.

Nursing has suffered and is suffering today, however, for exactly the same reason that it has profited. The amazing growth of schools of nursing, which have multiplied their number 143 times within the past fifty years, has come about not because the public wanted more nurses, but because the hospitals wanted more students. The profoundly disturbing estimates of numbers of graduate nurses from now until 1965 are doubly significant when it is realized that to check the rapid growth of nurses implies not only a conviction on the part of the nursing profession that such a check is necessary, but an almost wholesale change of policy on the part of hospital administrators.

1. Cheap Student Labor

Hospitals run training schools for two reasons. The first reason is that it is cheaper to run a poor school than it is to employ graduate nurses. Hospital trustees and administrators, however, have for so many years regarded themselves as public benefactors because they have been conducting schools of nursing that it is going to be a surprising and unpalatable suggestion when they are told that from some of them such educational service is not only no longer needed, but no longer desired. It is rather pathetic to listen to the occasional sincere, but not especially thoughtful, representative of a hospital training school argue for lower state standards of registration, on the ground that his hospital cannot afford to conduct a school which will meet the minimum state requirements; and then to watch his confused indignation when it is suggested that his hospital give up the school entirely and care for its patients with graduate nurses. Such a hospital man, be he administrator or trustee, is apt, with apparently perfect sincerity, to state that his hospital is losing money in conducting its training school; and within the next five minutes to admit that the reason the hospital wants to run the school is that graduate floor duty nurses cost too much. It is an extraordinary thing, but it seems to be a fact, that hospitals regard the suggestion that they pay for their own nursing service as unreasonable. They have been receiving free service from students for so many years that they regard it as an inalienable right.

This is not true of all of them, of course, but it comes painfully near to being true of most of them. Witness the cost accounting studies purporting to show the cost of nursing education, which have charged salaries of head nurses and supervisors, and even sometimes the cost of upkeep for the nurses' home, to education, as though, if no school existed and all the work done by graduate nurses, there would be no need for any supervision or any place for nurses to live! There is great need for a good cost accounting study which will show the true contrast between student labor and graduate labor, but when it is made it is to be hoped that the theoretical value placed on student labor will be decided not upon some imaginary charge, but upon what it would cost the same hospital to replace the eight hours a day of floor service which each student now gives by another eight hours of floor service rendered by graduate nurses.

Nursing education—if it is of high grade—is undoubtedly expensive, and it is going to be more expensive as time goes on. There is real question whether the ordinary hospital can possibly afford to conduct a high grade nursing school. It is a fortunate thing, perhaps, that the Supply and Demand figures indicate that there is no longer any reason for any hospital to conduct a school solely because it feels that more nurses are needed. That time has apparently gone by.

2. Hospitals Prefer Students

The second reason why hospitals conduct training schools—and this probably applies to most of the large and famous schools, as well as to many small ones—is that it is easier to handle the nursing service of a hospital with student nurses than with graduate nurses. This is an extraordinary thing! Who can imagine a bank, for example, openly preferring to staff its offices with utterly untrained students, teach them all it can in three years, and as soon as they have learned the rudiments of banking, discharge them all and seek a new supply of untrained students to take their places? Or who can imagine a public school system placing all its schools in the hands of normal school students, letting them teach as long as they stay in normal school, but the moment they receive their diplomas, telling them: "There is no place for you in the public school system. We run our public schools on student labor. You go out now and support yourselves by being governesses!" Yet that is very nearly what most of the best hospitals in this country are saying to their own graduate nurses.

If this method were adopted wholesale, it would bring disaster to our business world. Any one who is interested can demonstrate this by turning to the occupational figures in the United States Census, and making a few simple calculations. For example, for the single year 1920, assuming that other occupations copied the methods prevalent in our best known hospitals of changing one-third of their workers each year and replacing them with young women 18 or 19 years old—

> if one-third of the women who were saleswomen, teachers, bookkeepers, store and office clerks, stenographers, and factory workers or others engaged in the "manufacturing and mechanical industries" had been discharged and replaced by young women 18 and 19 years of age from outside those occupations—

Then, in this one year, the draft would have taken every girl in the United States of those ages. None would have been left in school or at home or on the farm or in any other industry. Every girl, white or colored, 18 or 19 years old, would have been employed in one of the occupations listed above, and there would have been vacancies for 147,344 more.

As was shown in Chapter 16, 76 per cent of the superintendents of nurses who were asked the question reported that, if given a free hand, they would prefer to have their patients taken care of by students, rather than by graduate nurses. Many of them seem to feel that students are keener, more alive, more loyal; that they lose something precious as soon as they enter the nursing profession as graduates. If this is true, it is serious. There would seem to be something radically wrong in the educational methods of these hospitals if, after they have had the education of a student for three years, they would honestly prefer to start the training process all over again with raw material, rather than to avail themselves of the services of their own product.

However famous the hospital and however great its contribution to nursing education—and as was pointed out in the opening paragraph of this chapter, the contribution of many hospitals is of incalculable value—nevertheless the fact remains that most hospitals conduct training schools either because they can save money by doing so or because they think they can avoid trouble by doing so. They run the school with the express purpose of getting cheaper or more satisfactory labor. As was shown by the tables in Chapter 16, practically all the hospitals with nursing schools in this country expect the students to carry the entire nursing load. Even where graduate floor duty nurses are employed, there is reason to believe that they are not always supplied for the purpose of supplementing student labor, in order that the students may be given a better education, but are rather used for the nursing service of newly built wings of the hospital until such time as the training school can be expanded to carry the extra load.

3. How are Students Chosen?

This fact—that schools are run not primarily to educate graduate nurses, but primarily to serve the administrative needs of the hospital—results in an almost universal and thoroughly natural tendency for hospitals to admit applicants to the training school on the basis of whether or not they are likely to be good student material; good material, that is, for use in the hospital. The tradition of the hospital training schools is such that every student who enters is subjected to almost continuous supervision, in (to the outsider, accustomed to the loose supervision of college or business office) almost incredibly minute detail. For three years practically every act of the student's waking life is known, checked, and controlled. This course, perhaps, is necessary when it is remembered that the lives of patients are in the hands of these relatively inexperienced and very immature young women, but it has one result that is not fortunate. Because supervision of the hospital training school is so exceedingly strict, it becomes possible for the school to admit as students many young women who will be useful hands and feet in the hospital wards, but who are not at all safe prospects to go out into the completely unsupervised graduate activity of private duty nursing after the hospital is through with them.

When we examine the educational records, we find that practically 40 per cent of all nurses have never had more than two years of high school, and 11 per cent have never gone beyond grammar school. For private duty nurses—those who are going into the home and specialing in the hospital—the records are even lower. Nor are these low figures merely the results of low educational standards in earlier days. Of graduate nurses who have entered the profession within the past five years, at least one-sixth have never been beyond the first year of high school. If the proportion still holds for 1928, it will mean that something like 3,000 of this year's graduates will be so poorly educated that they would have difficulty in getting positions in a good department store.

Among the older nurses lack of high school education may not be so serious a matter, but as we look at the young people of today we must ask ourselves whether the modern girls who are dropping out of grammar and high school before finishing the course are, in most cases, girls whom we really want to have taking full responsibility for life and death in the sick-room. There are many splendidly conscientious women in these inadequately educated groups, but character alone is not enough when a patient is in danger. If it were, we should have no need for trained nurses at all and could rely upon the thousands of devoted relatives for care in illness. The fact that the people who most love the patient demand a trained nurse for his care indicates that they want something beyond high principles and self-sacrificing devotion. They want keen intelligence, good educational background, and sound nursing training and experience.

It seems to be a fact that hospitals can utilize as members of the student body (strong, young, subservient, and kept under strict supervision) young women of rather low grade. The hospital is always tempted to admit such women in order to get the great volume of its work done.

The willingness of some hospitals to admit young women of doubtful character and low intellectual capacity is so well known that in some places the public assumes that all nurses must be of that type. The principal of a famous high school for girls, in one of our largest cities, is quoted as having stated in an educational meeting that his school had always been puzzled to know what to do with the feeble-minded or incorrigible cases. He went on to say that the problem had been most happily solved by sending the girls into hospital training schools where the discipline was excellent and the girls were well taken care of! Another illustration of this attitude is found in the following letter, which is genuine—only the names have been changed. The letter was written to a Red Cross nurse by the well-educated assistant principal of a famous high school for girls:

"Dear Miss ———:

"Lillie Haynes, of Section 561, has set her heart on being a nurse. She is colored. Is there any opening for her? What are the requirements? Where can she apply? She is a hopeless failure in her studies, but I think she would do well in nursing."

It is unfortunate that the public sometimes regards the nursing school as a sort of respectable reform school, where its mental or disciplinary cases can be sent. When a girl won't mind her mother, is beginning to stay out late on the streets at night, refuses to go on with her high school work, and in general becomes a family problem, not infrequently the school authorities say to the mother: "Why don't you put your daughter into a hospital training school? The girls are kept under very careful supervision there, and the discipline is just the thing she needs." All too frequently the hospital, in its eagerness to secure students, will accept the problem girl. Since the training school hospital depends largely on student labor, and since the students are kept under strict discipline, the hospital not infrequently carries that problem girl all the way through her student course and graduates her with the seal of its approval. It gives its official sanction, that is, to a woman whom the public school was not willing to continue in association with its own students. Not infrequently the hospital is responsible for sending out into the profession a nurse whom it is entirely unwilling to employ even on special duty within its own walls.

4. What Becomes of the Low Grade Graduate?

Each year the school looks over its graduating class and selects one or two of its brightest students for supervisory work in its own wards or operating rooms. It then sends the rest of the class out as graduates, to find their own salvation. The result of this attitude, which looks upon the school primarily as a means of securing student labor and pays little attention to the quality of the work which its graduates are doing, is that educational standards tend to be low. Not only that, but when the hospital accepts students who have had only one year of high school training, it either accepts them when they are very young (there is more than one hospital where girls of sixteen are being left alone on the night ward or in the delivery room, to carry full responsibility!) or else, if its age limit is high, it has to accept girls who have been very slow in going through or who have left school several years before and have, therefore, dropped out of the habit of study. The poorly educated student is apt to be young or immature, and incompetent to carry the life and death responsibilities which are to be laid upon her shoulders.

When the graduating class go out and begin hunting for work, the other hospitals and health groups look them over and make alluring offers to those who have the best background. The graduate nurse of good family and good education can practically make her own choice as to whether she will accept a position in one of the better institutions, or go into public health, or into private duty, but the young graduate of today who lacks breeding and background, who has had only one or two years of high school, has no such choice. There are only two things she can do. She can go into private duty in the home and in the hospital, or, as a last desperate resort, she can go into general floor duty (usually in some other hospital!).

The result of this process is that students who were safe in the hospital only because the hospital has developed its extremely strict system of supervision are the very ones who are forced by present conditions out into private duty where there is no supervision at all. Many of these workers could probably continue to be reasonably safe and useful on the hospital floors, with proper supervision, but they are positively dangerous when set adrift in the free lance fields of private duty. There is no need to argue this point. All one has to do is to turn back and read the testimony of patients in Chapter 11. Most readers will agree that many of the nurses described in those brief stories should, in the first place, never have been admitted to hospital nursing schools; and, in the second place, should never have been permitted to undertake the heavy responsibilities of the unsupervised private duty nurse.

5. How Control the Schools?

If readers consider seriously the figures in Part 1 of this report, they must begin to ask themselves: "*How many nursing schools are really needed?*" "*How can educational standards for the profession be raised to meet the public need?*"

and, "*How can hospitals already struggling under heavy financial burdens possibly afford to give up or to limit their schools?*" The answers are often more difficult than they sound. If there are too many graduates, for example, it may sound rather simple to say: "Let us raise the requirements for admission and by so doing automatically cut down the number of students, and at the same time raise their quality." But, as Diagram 53, on page 382, shows, the almost universal effect of raising requirements for admission is not to decrease the number of applicants, but to increase them. The desire for education is becoming so great in present-day America that the most effective way for a school to increase its supply of students is to announce that none but the best prepared will be admitted.

Another solution for decreasing the annual numbers of nurses being graduated from nursing schools in this country is the simple one of saying: "Abolish all the small schools." Here again the answer is not so helpful as it sounds. In the first place, while it is probably true that many of the small schools are producing low grade and inadequately educated nurses, they are not the only offenders in this regard, nor are all of them guilty. There are, here and there, small schools the graduates of which are women of whom any profession might well be proud. They are receiving something in those small schools which apparently the large school cannot give. Smallness in itself is probably not an educational crime.

The second difficulty with the suggestion that the over-supply of nurses be controlled by eliminating all the small schools is that from the point of view of plain arithmetic the solution will not work. Diagram 60 illustrates this difficulty. The diagram shows two columns. The first column represents all the nursing

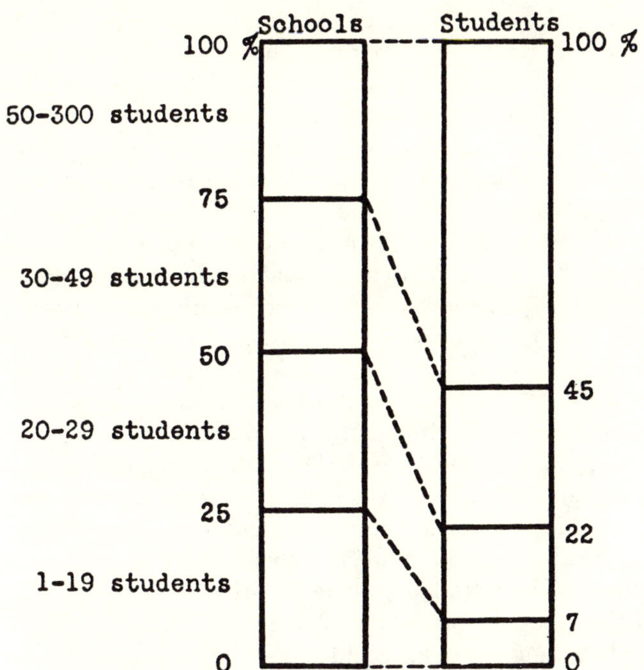

Diagram 60.—Per cent of nursing schools in the United States having 1 to 19 students, 20–29, 30–49, and 50 students or over; and per cent of all student nurses in the United States who are enrolled in each of these groups of schools

schools in the United States.* It is divided into fourths according to the numbers of students in each school and shows that one-fourth of all the schools in this country have 1–19 students, the next fourth 20–29 students, the next fourth 30–49 students, and the top fourth 50 stu-

* The figures on which this diagram is based were secured by tabulating the data for 1,500 schools contained in the 1927 list of Schools of Nursing Accredited by State Examiners, published by The American Nurses' Association, 370 Seventh Avenue, New York City.

dents and over. The second column represents all the student nurses in this country, and the dashed lines between the first and second columns indicate the per cent of all student nurses who will be found in each quarter of the schools. If, by some extraordinary feat of legislation it were possible to wipe out of existence all nursing schools with less than 20 students, the total number of schools would be cut down by 25 per cent, but the decrease in nursing students would be only 7 per cent. Similarly, if all the schools having less than 30 students were put out of business, this drastic reduction of half the schools in the country would result in cutting out only about 22 per cent of all the students.

There are probably many hospital and nursing administrators in the larger schools to whom the idea of giving up the school would seem almost sacrilegious, yet it is the 25 per cent having 50 students and over who are largely responsible for the threatened overproduction of nurses. Their students alone constitute 55 per cent of all the student nurses in this country.

These figures would seem to raise the question: "Have hospitals any social justification for running any but very high type schools in the face of an apparent overproduction of nurses, not all of whom are reasonably acceptable to society?"

If some of our large and highly respected hospitals would frankly face the issue and proceed to experiment with methods for providing full graduate nursing, on a self-supporting basis, and at a price which the average patient can afford to pay, they would be making a most important contribution to every one in the hospital field. The problem will have to be solved. It almost certainly can be solved if the famous hospitals will take the lead.

Is it an unreasonable thing to suggest that the famous hospital ought seriously to consider placing at least part of its nursing service in the hands of skilled nurses? Hospitals are always under serious financial pressure. They need help in meeting their heavy burdens. But should that be taken as sufficient justification for jeopardizing the future of the nursing profession through an overproduction of nurses. The Grading Committee has the deepest sympathy for hospital administrators who are struggling to render an important public service under serious financial handicaps. It believes that every legitimate aid should be given to secure public support for hospital service. It has gone on record, however, as holding strictly to two principles:

1. No hospital should be expected to bear the cost of nursing education out of funds collected for the care of the sick. The education of nurses is as much a public responsibility as is the education of physicians, public school teachers, librarians, ministers, lawyers, and other students planning to engage in professional public service, and the cost of such education should come, not out of the hospital budget, but from private or public funds.
2. The fact that a hospital is faced with serious financial difficulties should have no bearing upon whether or not it will conduct a school of nursing. The need of a hospital for cheap labor should not be considered a legitimate argument for maintaining such a school. The decision as to whether or not a school of nursing should be conducted in cooperation with a given hospital should be based solely upon the kinds and amounts of educational experience which that hospital is prepared to offer.

6. SUMMARY

This chapter may be summarized as follows:

a. Nursing is probably the only profession in which students are sought because of their economic value. This is at once the strongest and the weakest point in its educational system.

b. The reason why nursing schools are so extraordinarily effective is that, in contrast to other vocational schools, the students are given real responsibility. They are expected to meet professional, and not amateur, standards. This is because their services are worth money, and the work they do would have to be paid for at professional rates were the students not available.

c. On the other hand, the reason why the number of schools and graduates is out of all proportion to the public demand, and why thousands of graduates are yearly thrust into the profession with a totally inadequate social and educational background, is, again, that students are economic assets to hospitals. Most hospitals, apparently, run schools not in order to produce graduate nurses for public service but in order to secure student labor for their own patients.

d. The arguments for conducting schools are twofold: First (except in the best schools), to save money. It is cheaper to run a poor school than to employ graduates. Second, to maintain a permanent and docile staff. Students stay for three years and accept strict discipline.

e. Because most hospitals run schools for their own advantage, they admit some students suitable for their own needs but not suitable for graduate nurse responsibilities. Most of these women, who should never have been admitted to the profession, go into private duty where they are particularly dangerous because they cannot be controlled or supervised.

f. These low grade products of low standard schools compete with the high grade products of high standard schools. They aggravate an already serious unemployment situation.

g. Hospitals regard nursing education as their private concern. They will find it difficult to adjust to the proposition that it is not. Yet the impending overproduction of graduate nurses and the public demand for different types of graduates must force that realization upon them.

h. The nursing profession must face three questions:
   1. How many nursing schools are really needed?
   2. How can educational standards for the profession be raised to meet the public need?
   3. How can hospitals, already struggling under heavy financial burdens, possibly afford to give up their schools?

i. While a general raising of entrance requirements is almost certainly essential, the probable result will be, not to reduce, but to increase the number of student applicants. This will raise the quality, but will not solve the question of overproduction.

j. The suggestion has been made: "Abolish all the small schools!" This would not solve the problem, because
   1. There are some small schools which are producing high grade graduate nurses. Smallness in itself is not an educational crime.

2. Most graduates do not come from small schools. They come from large ones. The quickest way to curtail production would be to begin at the top.

k. Some of the largest schools are doing an excellent educational job. Others are not. These facts would seem to raise the question: "Have hospitals any social justification for running any but very high type schools in the face of an overproduction of nurses, not all of whom are reasonably acceptable to society?"

l. Hospitals will need to learn how to nurse their patients with graduate staffs on a pay basis. The problem is extremely difficult, and involves serious administrative and financial adjustments. If a few of the best known and most highly respected hospitals will undertake to lead the way in experimenting along this line, they will be making an important contribution to every one in the hospital field.

m. The Grading Committee has gone on record as holding strictly to two principles:

1. No hospital should be expected to bear the cost of nursing education out of funds collected for the care of the sick. The education of nurses is a public responsibility.
2. The fact that a hospital is faced with serious financial difficulties should have no bearing upon whether or not it will be connected with a school of nursing. The decision should be based solely upon the kinds and amounts of educational experience which the hospital is prepared to offer.

CHAPTER 21

THE PREPARATION OF STUDENTS

1. Why are Some Physicians Happier than Others?

Surgeons are more apt to be happy about the quality of nursing service their patients receive than are the physicians in other specialties. Neurologists and psychiatrists, on the other hand, are apt to be exceedingly unhappy about it. Pediatricians comment on the lack of well-trained nurses for the care of children, and especially for the care of children with contagious diseases. Obstetricians testify that while there are many good obstetrical nurses, the supply is low compared with demand. Most nurses apparently are not well prepared for obstetrical service, and those whose education along this line is lacking are apparently genuinely afraid to try it.

Practically all physicians insist that *for their own cases* they need, above everything else, young women of good breeding and attractive personality, with high professional standards, making for close cooperation with the physician; with such keen intelligence and quick perception that they can note changes in symptoms and report them accurately; and with a thorough nursing education in a high grade nursing school, which will have prepared them to practise intelligently and skilfully the art of bedside nursing. Physicians whose patients are almost uniformly hospital cases are apparently more apt to secure special nurses of these high types than are those physicians who most frequently rely upon nurses sent by commercial or central registries to home cases.

The preparation of nurses bears a direct relation to the special interest of the hospital. In hospitals where most of the work is surgical—and there are apparently many such—it is natural for the graduates to be interested in surgical cases and to be better prepared to take care of them than to take care of cases of other types. Students who have had practically no undergraduate experience in psychiatric nursing are apt to share the popular fear of mental cases. The best bred and most intelligent girls in such hospitals are naturally attracted by the surgeons to the surgical cases and are not attracted by mental nursing, because they know so little about it. The increased emphasis upon the importance and interest of psychiatric nursing, however, and the outstanding success of those high grade young women who have taken special training in this field, would seem to offer sufficient evidence that the demand of psychiatrists for women as well prepared and of as high social and intellectual standards as those available in the best hospitals for surgical nursing, is not an impracticable dream, but is one which could be met were proper courses in psychiatric nursing available.

Similarly the obstetrician, the pediatrician, and the medical men in other specialties report a scarcity, not of nurses in general, but of nurses properly educated and trained for service in their particular fields. Probably more and more hospitals will need to face the fact that the training which the student nurse receives while in school should be determined not primarily by the administrative needs of these hospitals, but rather by the needs of the physician and the patient for whom the nurse will work after she leaves school.

2. Preparation for Private Duty

A frequent criticism which the medical profession makes of the private duty nurse is that she "picks and chooses" her cases. She either frankly registers against certain types, or more adroitly manages to avoid taking calls which do not appeal to her.

Apparently the real reason why the nurse refuses to take a case is often that, unconsciously, perhaps, she is afraid of it. She never met a case like that in the days when she was in training, and naturally enough she hesitates about taking full nursing responsibility now. Although conditions are rapidly improving, there are still probably thousands of nurses who have never had any undergraduate experience in taking care of contagious diseases, or of mental cases, or of T. B. Many nurses were trained in hospitals primarily for adults and know little about children. Some have had no real experience in obstetrics. Some of these unevenly trained nurses go into private duty in the home or specialing in the hospital; others go into the hospitals on general floor duty. In either field they are apt to find the work excessively difficult because they were never given adequate preparation for it.

Perhaps one of the greatest complaints on the part of physicians and patients is that while they have no difficulty in securing competent private duty nurses for work inside the hospital, they are sadly handicapped when they try to secure equally competent nurses for home cases. The superintendent of one of our largest and most famous hospitals recently remarked that none of the graduates of its school went into private duty. He asked, "Why should they when there is so much more interesting and attractive work for them in the institutional and public health fields? Why should any ambitious and well-educated girl go into the home when she doesn't have to?" It seems to be a fact that home cases are generally regarded as far less desirable than hospital cases, and for rather obvious reasons.

Hospitals are not like homes, and the undergraduate training which the student receives in the hospital cannot readily include supervised experience in the particular technique necessary for handling home cases. For example, how many training school hospitals are able to give special supervised experience in how to handle relatives or to get along with servants? How many teach the student how to improvise from the ordinary utensils found in the home the equipment which is so lavishly provided in the modern hospital? How much experience does the student get in giving complete bedside care to men patients? Recently a gentleman who had been taken ill while visiting in England, and again later in this country, remarked that the English nurses took care of him as though they were nurses and he was a sick patient, while the American nurses, although fully as well trained and as competent, seemed never able to forget that they were females and he was a male. Could a way be found to teach students the proper way to give the intimate personal care to male patients which may be required of them as graduate nurses?

Another difficulty with the home case is that the nurse is frequently required to work in close contact with unknown physicians who not infrequently use unfamiliar methods. In the hospital she always has had the head nurse or the superintendent of nurses to whom she could go when the problems of adjusting to the demands of the physicians became too difficult for her to handle alone.

In the home the problems are far more difficult, and she never has any older nurse at hand to whom she can turn for counsel. In the hospital, when life and death decisions had to be made, there was always the wiser and more experienced nurse to whom the student could turn for guidance. In the home she must carry full responsibility. No wonder she is often afraid.

Probably another reason for the reluctance of nurses to take home cases is that 56 per cent of her nursing days in the home will be on twenty-four hour duty, whereas in the hospital only 12 per cent will be on twenty-four hour duty. In other words, in most parts of the country twenty-four hour duty has practically gone out of the modern hospital. Most students graduating today not only have never been on twenty-four hour duty, but they know that hospitals disapprove of it, as definitely bad for the patient. When the student is graduated and starts private duty, she finds that more than half of the home calls are for twenty-four hour service. Moreover, twenty-four hour service in the home has a bad reputation; and apparently with considerable reason. We know of nurses who on twenty-four hour duty have been obliged to sleep on the ironing board or on top of the set tubs, and it seems unfortunately to be equally true that occasionally a nurse has been obliged to leave the case because of unwelcome attentions from some male member of the family. However rare these instances may be, they surely furnish sufficient basis to make any careful young nurse hesitate when she is asked to go to a case in an unknown family under the direction of an unknown physician.

These few instances perhaps are enough to indicate the fact that the young girl who has just been graduated from training school faces the prospect of private duty with trepidation. Moreover, as she comes out from the training school she is actually in all too many instances poorly educated for the work which she is about to do. She knows only the work of her own hospital and she is not prepared to face the many perplexing problems which the future will inevitably bring. Physicians and patients suffering from the inadequate preparation of these nurses for service in the home are saying to the hospital training schools, "We do not like your product."

3. Preparation for Public Health and Institutional Work

Public health administrators are continually talking about the shortage of nurses for their work, yet if our findings are representative there are about five applicants for every nursing appointment in the public health field. The difficulty is not one of numbers. It is one of quality. The criticism of applicants for these positions is that many of them are not high school graduates, and there is an increasing tendency in public health work to make graduation from high school a minimum requirement for nurses who are to carry the responsibility of work in the homes. The second criticism is that many nurses do not seem to regard the patient as a human being—they lack "the public health viewpoint." If at the present time nearly one-fifth of all nurses are engaged in public health work, and if, as seems probable, the proportion is rapidly growing, should not the schools of nursing make some real attempt to raise the entrance requirements sufficiently so that their graduates will have a reasonable hope of being accepted by the public health field? Should they not also seriously consider ways and means for bringing home to the student while she is still in training a realization of the fact that patients are not just sick people in hospital beds, but are members of families with a great, complex background of human interests and problems which the nurse and physician must try to understand if they are to render good nursing and medical care?

Apparently most hospitals make very little attempt to base the training in the hospital upon a careful study of what the students are going to do after they get out. If we compare the course of study with the fields into which the students actually go, we find little agreement. What the hospital trains for is ward service in institutions, and to some degree supervisory service in institutions. Of the 24,389 nurses actually employed, from whom we have received reports this year, only 23 per cent are in the institutional field; 19 per cent have gone into public health; and 54 per cent have gone into private duty, which, of course, includes private duty in the home and what is called specialing in the hospital. In other words, less than one-fourth of all the nurses are going into institutional work, and three-fourths are going into other fields. Yet the hospital partially trains for the one-fourth and pays very little attention to the needs of the other three-fourths.

While there are exceptions, it seems fair to say that most training schools give full training in the technique of general floor duty in their own institutions. Many do not prepare for different techniques and conditions which the students will later encounter if they go into general floor duty in other hospitals. The hospital gives a little experience in administration and teaching, but this is usually because it hopes to secure workers for its own staff. Most of the schools do not give any definite basis for public health work. More important still, although most of the graduates from training schools are going out into the free lance field of private duty, particular preparation for this field is almost unknown.

Many training school hospitals are recognizing their responsibility for educating nurses to meet the needs of the community, by seeking affiliations for their students, so that the students may be better prepared for their life work than the local hospital alone can make them. Because training schools are supported from hospital funds, hospitals think of them as private enterprises which are no one's else business; and not only are rather inclined to resent state control or outside criticism, but acknowledge very little responsibility for meeting outside needs. Consequently, the broad-minded school which attempts to secure this affiliation sometimes does not find it easy. The different hospital schools do not belong to any general organization. Each hospital is an independent unit, and it is inclined to grant affiliation to its neighbor not in order to serve its neighbor or the community, but in order to get its own work done. This does not make for socially minded cooperation.

4. The "Basic Course"

Many school administrators will say, "A good basic training in hospital bedside nursing is sufficient, no matter what field the graduate enters." Evidence that, *in the form in which it is now given*, this is not true, is furnished by the protest now being raised against the results of the present system.

Much of even the "basic course" depends on chance. As was shown in Chapter 16, very few hospitals give their superintendents of nurses a free hand in supplementing student service with graduate service. Almost all hospitals are understaffed. They are trying to carry more work than can possibly be handled adequately by the number of students enrolled; and this has two serious results. The first is that, although students may be taught techniques of fine bedside nursing, they shortly learn that in times of heavy load they are not really expected to practise those techniques in their full exquisite detail. When there are more patients than a student can possibly take care of properly, she learns that it is no use to report that fact to the office. The superintendent, being helpless so far as assigning additional nurses to the floor is concerned, and not feeling free to criticize the management of the hospital to the student, is obliged to ignore such pleas for help; and the student who insists that she cannot carry the load is quickly made to feel that she has offended.

It does not take a bright student long to realize that what she has been taught is the theory of bedside care, but what she is expected to practise on the wards is always a compromise between theory and necessity. Students of poor moral fibre quickly learn to neglect the less obvious aspects of bedside care and to specialize on the things which show. Students of fine moral fibre may be forced to do the same thing, because they literally cannot give adequate care in the hours allowed or even in the overtime hours to which many of them are so generally accustomed; but the high grade student rebels internally against the hypocrisy of a hospital which teaches her how patients should be cared for, which refuses to acknowledge that lower standards may ever be necessary, and which at the same time is not willing to spend the extra money necessary to provide enough workers so that its own patients can be given something approaching the type of care which the school pretends to stand for.

The second educationally pernicious aspect of this perpetual sacrificing of the student to the daily needs of the hospital is that, where work has to be done and where there are only students to do it, it is frequently necessary to assign a particular student to work with which she has already had sufficient experience.* Students are kept in the operating room, for example, for weeks and sometimes months longer than they should be, not because they are poorly trained nurses who need more operating room experience, but because they are already so exceedingly skilful that the hospital thinks it cannot afford to let them get away. Similarly, in other departments it is found over and over again that the assignment of students to certain duties is determined not by the needs of the student, but by the needs of the patients in the hospital.

It would be a sad thing indeed were student nurses ever to acquire the attitude of mind which says, "I am more important than the patient. I must not be sacrificed just because a patient needs me." In other professions students are not ashamed frankly to be seeking their own educational advancement. In nursing such an attitude is unthinkable; and it is to be hoped that the time will never come when student nurses will be more interested in their own welfare than in the welfare of the patients under their charge. To the student the patient should always come first; but to *somebody* the student ought to come first! Except in those few schools—

* For detailed testimony on this point the reader is referred to the Report of the Committee for the Study of Nursing Education; Dr. C.-E. A. Winslow, chairman; Miss Josephine Goldmark, secretary. Macmillan Co., N. Y., 1923.

almost all of them connected with universities—where the education of nurses is a project separate and distinct from the administration of a hospital, and therefore under separate educational direction, with power to act, there is no one in the whole school of nursing to whom the education of the student is of paramount importance. Superintendents of nurses are deeply interested in their schools. They are capable of great sacrifices for their students; but the fact remains that wherever the position of superintendent of nursing service and principal of a school of nursing is held by one person, she must, and probably should, give first attention to safeguarding the welfare of the patients in her hospital, and she must over and over again sacrifice the education of the students to that end. Not until schools of nursing are controlled by some person or persons whose chief responsibility is educational, and not administrative, can the nursing profession hope to secure graduates with thorough basic nursing education.

5. SUMMARY

The chief points made in this chapter are:

a. Practically all physicians agree that they want as nurses for their own patients young women of good breeding and attractive personality, with professional standards making them willing to follow medical direction; able to observe symptoms and report them accurately; and sufficiently skilled to give high grade bedside care. These requirements imply the need for young women of good family, high grade intelligence, quick perceptions, and thorough nursing education.

b. Surgeons are better satisfied with the preparation

of nurses than are other specialists. Neurologists, pediatricians, obstetricians, are often not satisfied. Physicians feel that the education of the nurse while in school should have a direct relation to what they may need of nurses after graduation.

c. It is much easier to secure good nurses for hospital specialing than for home duty. This is partly because home duty is often difficult and unattractive and partly because hospital schools give very little preparation for home nursing.

d. Public health and institutional nurses report that while there are many applicants for employment in those fields, most of them have had no adequate preparation for the work; and in many cases the applicant's preparatory schooling has been so inadequate that she could not profit by post-graduate nursing courses.

e. Even the so-called "basic course" is inadequate in many cases because not every student gets an equal share of the different nursing experiences which in theory she should have. Assignments to different services are often governed not by the needs of the students but by the needs of the hospital.

f. To the student the needs of the patient should always come first. But if the hospital school is to be a real school and not merely an administrative asset, there should be at least some in authority to whom the needs of the student are more important than the needs of the patient.

CHAPTER 22

THE SHORT COURSE NURSE

Physicians agree that from the point of view of the patient, the private duty nurse costs too much. They are considerably more impressed with this difficulty, apparently, than even the patients themselves; although, of course, the patient questionnaires frequently deal with the same problem. The medical profession has for several years been keenly concerned with the cost of nursing care and, as a result, many suggestions have been made for lowering the cost and so bringing nursing within the reach of the average patient. Perhaps the commonest suggestion, and one which has been made frequently by physicians in this study, has been that of trying to secure a "short course" or "basic" nurse.

The testimony in Chapters 8 and 9 has been rather surprisingly uniform and emphatic in its criticism of the so-called "practical" nurse. Contrary to the impression held by many nurses, it is not true that physicians generally are employing practical nurses for their own patients. Most physicians not only are actually employing R.N.'s but definitely prefer R.N.'s. Their experience with practical nurses, while occasionally happy, is, for the most part, so extremely unsatisfactory that, as one physician said, "One comes to feel that all so-called 'practical' nurses ought to be deported!"

The comments on the undergraduate nurse are in some cases even more vitriolic than those relating to the frankly untrained. The criticisms for both groups may be summarized under the four words

IGNORANT—INCOMPETENT—UNCOOPERATIVE—COSTLY

Many cases have been reported to the Grading Committee of practical nurses who are charging more than the standard price for R.N. service. For the entire study the reports show that the typical practical nurse costs only $1 a day less than the typical R.N. Physicians are almost uniform in their protest against the types of practical nurses usually available and against their excessively high charges.

1. Specifications for the Short Course Nurse

It is not wholly easy to understand why rather a large number of physicians who have had experience with the practical nurse and who are frank in their condemnation of her methods seem to feel that a new group of semi-trained workers would somehow avoid the undesirable characteristics of which they complain in the present supply.

When the physicians describe the "basic" nurse, the plan seems to be about as follows:

a. They would like to secure girls of fine breeding with reasonably good minds and—this is especially emphasized—a large amount of tact.
b. The girl should have had at least one or two years of high school.
c. She should be sent to a hospital which is willing to take her for a 12 or 18 months course.
d. After finishing the course, she should concentrate on private duty in the home.
e. She should specialize in 24 hour service.

f. She should be willing and competent to handle the more important parts of the house work.
g. She should never charge more than $25 a week.

The specifications in different communications vary, of course. One physician suggested that these girls be recruited from newly arrived immigrants, another suggested that the graduates of these courses should never be allowed to charge more than $15 a week, but the general outline seems to run about as listed above.

2. Questions Others Ask

When these plans were discussed with hospital and nursing school administrators on the one hand, and with housewives and other employers of domestic labör on the other, many questions were raised.

a. Will girls of the breeding, intelligence, and tact indicated be content to undertake this type of work?
b. If it is true that practically any respectable girl with one year of high school education can find some registered nursing school to which she can be admitted, why should she choose to enter a school which is not registered? (It is not generally recognized that the basic admission requirements for the R.N. are, in many parts of this country, only one year of high school.)
c. If, by working from 28 to 34 months with all expenses paid, a girl can get an R.N., why should she enter a 12 or 18 months course which will not lead towards the R.N.? (Apparently most girls enjoy their experience in nursing school. Nursing students are no longer the overworked drudges of a generation ago. Life in the nursing school is

fascinating and when it costs the student nothing to remain for the full term, it is difficult to see why she should be so foolish as to leave earlier.)

d. Why should a girl accept training which will not lead to the R.N. when she must know that, by doing so, she definitely places herself on a servant level? (Even young women whose parents have been household servants realize the advantages, socially speaking, of an R.N., and one of the present problems in the nursing profession is that it promises so much social prestige to some of the frankly less desirable types.)

e. Suppose the short course girl were actually produced, would she be more in demand for home service than the practical of today? (Most physicians and most patients want intelligent and thorough nurse training. Would they be satisfied with anything less good than they can get now?)

f. Would the short course product be attracted by 24 hour duty? (The modern servant is no longer willing to accept any position where she works a total of more than 8 hours a day. Employment bureaus definitely state that cooks and housemaids must have a period of three hours off every afternoon and must not be expected to work beyond eight o'clock in the evening. These are not exceptional requirements but are apparently becoming standard for most types of household workers. If the short course girl is drawn from the same social class as the household servant, will she not be even more insistent than the well-bred R.N. upon short hours and high pay? Why should she do 24 hour duty unless she has to?)

g. Will a girl of this type be interested in doing general housework? (Employment agencies report that it is increasingly difficult to provide competent household servants to undertake general housework even when conditions are favorable and there is no one ill in the family. Is there any reason to assume that relatively low grade girls will be more cooperative and eager to help out in housework in times of family crises than the skilful cook or housemaid?)

h. Why should the girl in question limit her wages to $25 or less a week? Why, in fact, should she charge any lower price than she can succeed in getting? (Outside of the largest cities where charges are considerably higher, the wage rate for cooks and housemaids seems to be $60 or $65 a month with board, lodging, and laundry. Is there any reason to suppose that short term practical nurses, drawn more or less from the servant class, would be willing to maintain their own rooms, as must be done in most private duty, pay their own laundry, and buy most of their food, maintain telephone connections, and charge less than they could earn elsewhere? When it is remembered that the ordinary scrub woman charges $4 plus her 10 cents carfare for an 8 hour working day, it is difficult to understand why any one should assume that the semi-trained servant girl nurse would cheerfully work three times as long for less money.)

3. A Few Conclusions

After reading some of the reports of physicians and nurses, a member of the Grading Committee remarked that apparently the chief difficulty in private duty was because, side by side with the gentlewomen whom we think of as nurses, servant girls *had* been allowed to enter the profession. "The mercenary spirit," "the negligence while on duty," "the impudence," "the overbearing attitude towards servants," and the various other characteristics of which frequent complaint has been made, are to any employer of domestic labor unfortunately all too familiar.

It is not believed that the difficulty in private duty is that most nurses are too well-bred or too well educated. There is, of course, the occasional nurse from a good family and with a high school or college education who has an unpleasant personality, but one gains the definite impression that most of the serious criticisms directed at private duty service are based upon the experience of patients and physicians with the servant girl element in the profession, and not with the rank and file.

In talking with hospital administrators it has seemed increasingly clear that very few hospitals are anxious to run short courses. The hospital loses money on the completely untrained student. It is only after a few weeks and sometimes after several months that the new student becomes sufficiently familiar with hospital routine so that she is an asset and not a liability. It seems probable that very few hospitals would be cordial to the proposition that they should carry the brunt of introducing students into hospital technique and then, at the very time when they are beginning to pay their way, should let them go and take on a new group of untrained young women. It is the third year of the student service which makes the hospital want to run a training school, not the first year.

One is inclined to believe that hospitals do not generally look with favor upon establishing 12 month or 18 month courses. It would also seem that unless entrance requirements in regular nursing schools are almost uniformly raised to high school graduation (and while this is probably desirable, it is undoubtedly some years in the future), comparatively few young women can be persuaded to enter the short term courses.

Evidence has already been presented in this report to indicate that students are definitely attracted by high entrance requirements and not by low ones. It does not, therefore, seem probable that any great increase in cheap labor would be secured by a campaign for short term courses for practical nurses.

There is reason to doubt whether the product would be satisfactory. Apparently there is general agreement that at least two years of eight hours a day of service on the floor are necessary in order to prepare graduate nurses for bedside care. The common criticism of graduate nurses is that even with these long hours of practical bedside experience, they are inadequately grounded in bedside technique. It would seem logical to suppose that the student who has had half or a third of the amount of bedside experience would prove unsatisfactory to the physician's needs.

There seems no reason to assume that the short term nurse would charge any less than the present practical nurse. One is inclined to believe that the fact that hospitals were sponsoring such graduates would be used by them as an argument for charging as much or more than the registered nurse now charges.

Finally, one would question whether there is any good reason for seeking to increase the number of semi-trained, relatively incompetent, inadequately educated young women in a field which is already oversupplied with material of that sort. It is an unfortunate fact that many low grade women have been admitted to the nursing professions and are actually registered and practising. The problem would seem to be, "How can such women who are already in the profession be placed under some form of guidance so that they can be an asset and not a danger to the community?" There seems no strong argument in favor of increasing this social burden.

The problem of the cost of nursing care is an extremely serious one. To the average patient with a long illness the expense is often excessive. It would not seem, however, that the solution is to keep on with present methods of distribution by attempting to lower the standard of living for nurses. The problem must be squarely faced and better methods of distribution somehow devised so that the cost of nursing care can be lowered to the patient while the standard of living for the individual nurse can accord with that of other professional women. There must be possible solutions for this problem which will work out to the mutual satisfaction of the nurse, the patient, and the physician.

4. SUMMARY

This discussion can be summarized as follows:

a. Physicians are even more emphatic than patients in stating that the private duty nurse costs too much. Patients also, however, often stress this point.

b. Physicians and patients are agreed in their dislike for most so-called practical and undergraduate nurses. They ordinarily avoid them when they can.

c. Some physicians seem to feel that a new type of

practical, semi-trained, or short course nurse might be produced who would solve the cost problem, while avoiding the defects of present practicals and undergraduates.

d. The picture they draw seems impracticable. It calls either for women above the servant level to accept, without special reason, conditions which servants will not tolerate; or for women at or below the servant level voluntarily to forego opportunities for personal advancement.

e. Some solution must be found for the excessive cost of nursing service. It is believed that this solution will come not through adding more incompetents to an already overcrowded field, but rather through devising new methods of distribution, so that the cost of nursing care can be lowered for the patient, while at the same time the standard of living for the individual nurse can be maintained at a reasonably adequate level.

CHAPTER 23

THE FREE LANCE NURSE

There are no bars to private duty nursing! In public health nursing or institutional nursing there is always some one to interview the candidates and decide whether or not a given applicant should be admitted to work with that organization. It is true, of course, that the decisions as finally made in both of these fields seem occasionally not to have been particularly wise, but the fact remains that public health and institutional nursing have the power to keep out undesirable applicants if they wish to do so.

The profession is helpless to protect private duty. Any one who wants to call herself a nurse can enter the private duty field in competition with all the others in it. It is true that there are certain laws for the registration of nurses but apparently there is not one of the 48 states with the sort of legislation and inspection which would insure that every person who calls herself a nurse shall have had at least a few months in a school of nursing.

Because there are no bars to private duty—because it is a free lance occupation open to all comers—there are at work as private duty nurses today:

a. Some of the finest women in the profession, who select private duty because they love it.

b. Many young girls who have gone into private duty not because they love it, but because they are attracted by the high initial earnings.

c. Most of the women who are not eligible to public health positions or institutional supervisory jobs.
d. The free lance individualists, who avoid any form of group activity because they want to be their own masters.
e. The incompetent, the stupid, the graduates from schools so poorly run that they are not in fact schools at all.
f. Graduates of correspondence school courses in nursing.
g. So-called "practicals," students who failed or were expelled from training school; low grade women who see in private duty a chance to raise their social standing and who, in some cases, have never been in a hospital; women who have been maids in hospitals and have picked up a smattering of nursing technique.

1. Free Lance Nursing

What happens to the young graduate who goes into hospital specialing or home private duty? In the first place, under present conditions, she is very young, often not more than 21 years old. Looking back at their own histories, how many of the readers of this report feel that they could safely have been let loose into the work-a-day world at the age of 21, as completely independent beings without any form of supervision or guidance? Yet that is what happens to these extremely young and immature women. They have been under strict discipline for three long years. Then, in a day, all discipline is removed and they are completely divorced from every type of supervision. They are thrown out into a field in which there is intense competition for work, and in which, as has just been pointed out, they will come in contact with nurses of every conceivable grade, from the wise, wholesome, beautiful private duty nurse whom everyone reveres, down to the unspeakable drab who figures on the front page of the yellow newspaper and soils the profession every time she touches it.

The young graduate goes into the private duty field without supervision and without leadership. She goes into an atmosphere of work when you please, rest when you please, live where you please, do as you please. If she does poor work, there is no penalty. If she does good work, there is no reward. She stops learning at the point where other professional women are just beginning to learn. During the first few years she can, if she wishes, earn surprisingly large amounts of money. She is strong and healthy, and physically attractive. She is fresh from training and therefore up to date in her methods and careful in her technique. Physicians and hospitals like to employ her, and if she is willing to work full time, she may earn $2,500 or $3,000 a year for a while. She has not yet begun to worry about old age, and is under constant temptation to use the greater part of her earnings for clothing, theater, and many vacation trips.

For the first few years she has a wonderfully good time. Sometimes it goes to her head. There is no one to warn her of the dangers she runs. She begins to grow careless as to her technique; she does not read the nursing magazines; she does not attend the meetings of her professional groups; she may perhaps begin to be a trifle arrogant and difficult to work with. Little by little she becomes less desirable as a nurse, and her calls begin to fall off.

Private duty nursing under the soundest conditions is

a most irregular life, making heavy demands upon the health of its workers. Even the nurse who tries sincerely to work steadily, to render good nursing service, and to keep professionally alive, begins to find after a few years that she is no longer an effective physical machine. She is obliged to take extended periods of rest between her cases. Her annual earnings begin to decrease, and she is well started upon the long downward road of private duty, where no matter how earnestly she tries to retrieve her fortunes, she grows less able to carry the work, and less desirable in the eyes of patients, physicians, and hospitals, and her capacity for earning decreases every day she lives.

The picture is rather appalling to those who see the fresh young girls going out full of high hopes and desire for service, and know the pitfalls which await them. The amazing thing is that there should be as many thoroughly worthwhile private duty nurses as there are. Thrown into a branch of the profession in which almost every influence is against them, there are, nevertheless, thousands of private duty nurses who have continued to grow in their profession; who have not only lived up to the high ideals which were fostered by their training schools, but have developed steadily in sanity and spiritual strength. They triumph over great odds because there is something in them just too fine to be killed!

2. The Nurse and the Physician

Even worse than the constant economic pressure is the psychological pressure under which the nurse lives; and this is particularly severe in the case of the high grade private duty nurse—the one who goes into the field because she loves it. She works as an isolated unit, and she is a lonely person. If her work is heavy, she loses touch with the other nurses in her field; and that means that she is almost wholly dependent for her human contacts upon two people—the physician and the patient.

The real nurse enters the private duty field with high ideals of team play. She wants to have her own particular group of physicians, and if she is fortunate and works with the same physicians on case after case, she and they grow to know each other, and to work together as a well organized team. Sometimes the surgeon and the head nurse in the operating room develop that mutual understanding, that finely coordinated team play, to such an extraordinary extent that they hardly need talk at all. Each understands the other almost without words.

In private duty, team play something like that of the operating room, but with less speed, and more time for professional discussion and consultation, sometimes develops between physician and nurse. To the physician it is a rarely satisfying thing to have a nurse as an intelligent coworker. It is good to share in the kind of friendship which develops when two people have fought side by side, hour after hour, to save a human life. But to the private duty nurse such a relationship is more than satisfying. It is the very heart of her professional life.

The physician is the only person who has any intelligent understanding of what she does, because he is the only one who sees her work. If she is so fortunate as to be working with a physician who is really interested in his patient; who is eager to listen to the nurse's report of changes in symptoms as she sees them; who will take the time to ask her about the nursing care she is giving, and to suggest how she may make it better, the nurse is fairly radiant with professional pride and happiness. That kind of a physician is apt to be generous in his acknowledgment when she has done especially good work. He tells not only the patient, but perhaps telephones the hospital and the registry, and in so doing he is being something more than kind or just. He is making a definite contribution to the nursing profession, because he is showing that he, as a physician, respects the private duty nurse, and he is emphasizing the need for a high standard in bedside nursing.

All too often the finely sensitive, conscientious nurse has no such medical leadership to guide her. She is called from case to case, from physician to physician. Sometimes she has to work for the wrong kind of physician. His visits are hurried. He does not know this new nurse, and doesn't particularly care to. She will only be on the case a few days, and is therefore hardly worth bothering with. If she ventures to ask a question or make a suggestion, he decides that she is trying to "practise medicine," and he freezes her on the spot. Occasionally one hears a physician say things to a nurse that no servant girl would tolerate. If he talked to his cook that way, she would leave, but the nurse bites her lip and goes on with her work. Although the physician almost always is responsible for having the special nurse on the case, the type described seems almost to resent her presence after she has come. A physician of that kind is definitely dangerous, because he represents the medical profession to that nurse. Is it any wonder if she comes off the case with three convictions—first, that he has no respect for bedside nursing; second, that he has very little interest in the welfare of his patient; and third, that she does not want to work with him again?

Nurses respect physicians. They take their opinions seriously; and the private duty nurse especially is almost wholly dependent upon the members of the medical profession for her own self-respect, and for the respect of her associates. If the medical profession is really anxious to have the members of the nursing profession respect bedside nursing and take it seriously, they are the logical people to bring such a change about. In public health work and institutional administration, each nurse is surrounded by a jury of her peers. She respects her work because others tell her it is worth doing. She grows professionally because she is always comparing what she does with what other nurses in her line are doing.

In private duty there is no such healthy professional competition, because special nurses are free lance workers, and do not have any opportunity to compare their skill. There is only one professionally equipped observer to note whether a private duty nurse's work is good or poor, and that is the physician who is in charge of the case. The attitude of the nursing profession towards the value of bedside nursing is probably directly dependent upon the attitude of the physicians who are the only competent judges present when it is being given. The physician who believes that the nursing curriculum should give more emphasis to bedside nursing can make his plea effective if he shows that he himself respects bedside nurses at least as much as he respects nurses in the other two fields of public health and hospital administration.

Perhaps the most helpful contribution which the medical profession could make at this time would be to demonstrate its conviction that sick-bed nursing is worth while. If every physician would ask each special nurse for her credentials, and show that he feels it important to choose well qualified people; if he would take the time to discuss with her the kind of nursing care his case needs; if he would call for detailed reports on what she has observed; and hold her to a high standard of observation and recording; he might have to exercise some patience, but he would be a tremendously effective means of raising the quality in private duty. And, finally, if every physician would make a special effort to report upon those outstanding cases where the work of the bedside nurse was an important factor in saving the patient's life, nurses in public health and hospital administration would begin to regard bedside nurses as their equals, and the result would probably be definitely beneficial to all concerned.

3. What is the Matter with Private Duty?

The economic aspects of private duty have been dealt with at length in Chapters 12 and 14 and will be touched upon again in a later chapter. It seems clear, from the many pieces of evidence presented, that private duty nurses are suffering from three great handicaps.

The first is that there is apparently already a serious overproduction of nurses and this overproduction is felt first in the private duty field because more nurses go into private duty than into either of the other main fields.

The second difficulty is that private duty is open to all comers. The fine bedside nurse who honestly prefers private duty to any other field because she likes to give individual care to sick patients is obliged to face competition of a type unknown in either of the other fields. She has to struggle against a wave of popular dislike and suspicion for which she and others like her are in no way responsible. The sins of the low grade free lance practical or registered nurse must be shouldered by all nurses in that branch of the profession. For the good nurse, this is hard to bear.

Finally, free lance work in any profession is almost inevitably hard on its workers. The freedom is alluring, but the free lance worker pays for that independence of action by lowered income, irregular employment, and extreme professional loneliness.

4. SUMMARY

This chapter may be summarized as follows:

a. There are no bars to private duty. Any one can enter regardless of whether or not she has ever had any preparation for nursing. The profession has no machinery for the protection of the high grade private duty nurse.

b. The result is that the young graduate going into private duty nursing finds herself working shoulder to shoulder with women of all degrees from the highest to the unspeakably low.

c. Private duty is difficult and demoralizing. The young woman who enters it directly from nursing school leaves a strictly supervised, highly sheltered life, for one in which she has neither guidance nor protection. It is an amazing fact that with such forces arrayed against her there are so many eminently worthwhile nurses to be found in the private duty field.

d. The relations of the nurse to the physician are particularly important in private duty, because since the nursing profession offers her no supervision or professional stimulus, the only help she can get is from the physician on the case. His attitude towards the nursing care of the sick patient must inevitably affect her own. Physicians, therefore, are in a position to contribute greatly to the importance which nurses attach to bedside nursing, if they will make a point of discussing nursing problems with the private duty nurses on their cases.

e. Three things are wrong with private duty:
   (1) There is an overproduction of nurses. This results in unemployment problems which are especially acute in the private duty field, since the field must absorb all workers who cannot secure either public health or institutional positions.
   (2) Private duty is a free lance occupation open to all comers. Good nurses suffer from the competition of women far below their level in breeding and intelligence, professional ethics, and nursing knowledge and skill.
   (3) The free lance worker in nursing, as in other professions, inevitably pays for her cherished independence of action through lowered income, irregular employment, and extreme professional loneliness.

CHAPTER 24

WHAT NURSES·WANT

Nurses like nursing. They are glad they are nurses; they want to take care of sick people and make them well; and they want to keep other people from ever getting sick. That is the fundamental note which is struck in report after report received by the Grading Committee. Nurses are proud of being nurses. They are proud of their profession.

There are also, however, certain other facts which seem to be indicated by the thousands of bits of testimony which are summarized in this volume. Nurses do love nursing, but they want nursing to be, in so far as possible, a profession, and the things they stress when they talk about the economic conditions under which they work are apparently those things which other professional workers take for granted:

Reasonable hours
Adequate income
Constructive leadership
Opportunity for growth

1. Reasonable Hours

Among private duty nurses by far the commonest complaint, the chief reason given for wanting to leave that part of the profession, is the unreasonably long hours. The twenty-four hour day has practically disappeared from modern hospitals, but it still is found more frequently than any other in home duty. For special nurses in the hospital twelve hour duty is generally accepted. Outsiders, in thinking of the twenty-four hour day and the twelve hour day for private duty nurses remark upon the obvious fact that the nurse is not kept busy for the entire period of her working day. Twelve hours, they say, actually mean three or four hours of hard work and the rest is just sitting around and resting. Twelve hour duty is supposed to have two or three hours off each afternoon for the nurse's recreation. When speaking of twenty-four hour duty they say that the nurse gets four hours off every day and at least six or seven hours of sleep at night, and they feel, many of them, that the protest of the private duty nurse against the twelve hour and the twenty-four hour day is unreasonable.

The nurse herself makes two replies to criticisms of this sort. She says, in the first place, that while in theory twelve and twenty-four hour service includes fairly generous amounts of free time, actually the cases on which such assured rest is most essential are the very ones where the nurse is least likely to get it. The sicker the patient, the less rest there is for the nurse. If a patient is too ill to be left without a responsible person in charge, the nurse cannot take her afternoon hours off; and if the patient is ill enough to need care at night, frequently this means that the nurse will be disturbed seven, eight, or nine times during the night hours.

Physicians are often careful in trying to protect their nurses, so that if the patient becomes so ill as to need day and night care, they tell the family that instead of having one nurse for twenty-four hour duty, another nurse should be secured to help. The difficulty is, however, that physicians are not always able to judge whether extra help is really needed or not, and in cases where the patients are finding the financial pressure of illness already extremely serious a physician naturally hesitates to increase the burden by adding $7.00 a day to the cost of nursing. A psychiatric nurse recently reported that she had been on twenty-four hour duty with a home mental case for seven months. She said, "I shall have to give up the case soon, because I am getting worn out. You see, I have to sleep in the same room with the patient, and since he has a homicidal tendency, it is necessary for me to keep the door locked so as to be sure that he cannot get at the other members of the family. Every time he turns over I wake up." It is no wonder that nurses hesitate about accepting cases of this kind, and yet a case of the type quoted, which lasts for months and sometimes years, involves the family in such exceedingly heavy expense that the prospect of two or three nurses for each twenty-four hour shift seems more than they can stand. One sympathizes with the patient, the family, and the nurse.

The other reply which the private duty nurse makes to the suggestion that twelve and twenty-four hour service do not actually involve that number of hours of hard work is: "Even so, I have no time left which I can call my own." While there are exceptions, it seems to be true that most nurses would honestly prefer to work hard for eight hours a day and then be free to do what they wish with the remaining time, than to sit around wasting time on a twelve or twenty-four hour service.

In public health the eight hour day, with a half day on Saturday and a full day on Sunday, is so generally accepted that any deviation from that rule arouses comment. In institutional nursing the ten hour day is common, and the eight hour day is rapidly being accepted for all workers except special duty nurses. There are no other professions and very few other occupations in which a twelve hour day is the accepted standard for workers. Many professional people work long hours, but they do so because there is work to be done which they want to carry through. They do not work twelve hours or more a day simply because some one else orders them to do so. The tendency towards short hours in industry is too strong to be ignored. To the outside observer the astonishing thing is that even twelve hour duty has lasted so long.

From the point of view of the patient, who needs some competent person—not necessarily a nurse—to take charge of the family in time of illness, twenty-four hour service seems essential. This report does not pretend to offer a solution for meeting the difficulty. Yet the evidence is overwhelming that before long private duty nurses will be unwilling to work for more than forty or fifty hours a week, except in cases of genuine emergency. No amount of scolding will make any difference in this trend. It is inevitable; and the problem would seem to be to discover ways and means by which patients can be given as much nursing care as they really need at a reasonable price, and yet the short working day and a reasonable working week be provided for the nurses who give that care.

While it is not safe to predict exactly how this reorganization is to be brought about, that it is inevitably coming seems safe to predict. It will imply, of course, something more than merely keeping on with the same sort of service for shorter periods. It would seem probable that for most nurses the choice will lie between the present scheme of being on private duty for twelve or twenty-four hours at a stretch, caring for only one patient and having comparatively little to do during many of those hours, or, on the other hand, being on duty for eight or ten hours, caring for several patients, either in different homes or in the hospital, and being active all the time. The short versus the long day is, for most people, apparently a question of the busy versus the leisurely day, and workers have to choose whether they will take their rest time during working hours or whether they will get their work done first and rest independently afterwards.

The problem of the responsible adult for home service during the hours when skilled nursing care is not needed still remains to be solved. It seems probable that in many cases relatives must face the necessity of carrying this burden for themselves. Whether employment agencies will be able to supply competent servants to take charge in times of such emergency seems doubtful. It might be possible to secure untrained workers from the great groups of middle aged, penniless women who, because of lack of professional training, are unable to earn their livings in other ways; or it may be that in the nursing profession itself there will be found groups of workers, either inadequately trained or else physically unable to carry the strain of severe nursing cases, who would be willing to take on twenty-four hour duty for, say, five days a week, if they could be relieved by some one else from the same registry for the other two days. The Grading Committee does not pretend to know the answers to these problems, nor does it recommend any of the foregoing solutions. It does, however, feel that no good can come from a refusal to face the fact that private duty nurses of high grade are leaving that branch of the profession in large numbers and that the chief reason for their doing so is because the twelve hour day seems to them impossibly long. There is no reason to expect that they will change their minds. There is much reason to suggest that the problem of hours must receive serious consideration, and some adjustment must be found if nurses of that type are to be retained in private duty.

2. Rest Periods

The subject of hours includes not only the hours worked in a given day, but the number of hours worked consecutively between days off. In public health and in institutional nursing there are certain rest periods provided for every week. These rest days are sometimes ignored in the actual institutional administration, but the nurse is supposed, at least, to have them at regular weekly intervals. In private duty the nurse is supposed to stay on the case until the need for her is over, and the number of rest days she has depends upon the length of her cases. Many nurses seem to specialize on one and two night cases and are unable to secure assignments to anything which lasts as long as a week. Other nurses go for three, four, or five weeks at a stretch without a single day off. The nurse who reported to the Grading Committee that she was still on a particularly bad cancer case where she was on her feet most of the day for twelve hour duty, that she had been on that case for seven weeks and had not had a single full day's rest during the entire period, offers a concrete illustration of why so many nurses report nervous breakdowns. At the end of such a case the nurse is free to rest (provided she has saved enough money to live on) for as long as she wishes before she takes another case; but it has been found true in other occupations and undoubtedly holds true for nursing that one day's rest every week is a very different thing from seven days' rest after seven weeks of work. The more frequent break is necessary if the nurse is to retain her health and vigor.

In practically all other occupations the employers grant a day or a day and a half of rest every week as a matter of course. This time is given to the worker, not out of generosity to him, but because industry has found that the staff works better during the next six days if it has rested on Sunday and that one day's rest in seven means a definite saving in dollars and cents to the company.

In talking about this problem, nurses say that patients would not be willing to have their nurses relieved for one day a week. It is probably true that many patients would object to this suggestion, but there is no reason why they should expect professional service to accept conditions no longer tolerated by domestic service! Patients have already learned that the modern cook expects invariably one afternoon off a week, and recently the tendency has grown for her to insist upon two. Moreover, patients in hospitals on ward service are accustomed to being taken care of by anywhere from three to seven or eight different nurses in the course of twenty-four hours. While patients might not particularly enjoy letting their nurses have a day off once a week and accepting for the same price an equally competent substitute from the registry, it would seem probable that they must make up their minds to some such adjustment if they hope to secure the services of high grade nurses. More and more the nurse is learning that, like other professional people, she must secure somehow not only reasonable working hours, but adequate rest periods at regular intervals if she is to continue as an efficient and active worker.

3. Adequate Income

While many institutional positions are underpaid, it nevertheless seems to be true that the chief difficulties in institutional work are not those which have to do with salary. The floor duty nurses in most hospitals receive $90 or $100 with maintenance, and the salaries increase for supervisory and administrative positions, so that all the evidence gathered by the Grading Committee indicates that the workers in the institutional field earn more, save more, and borrow less frequently than the workers in public health or private duty.

Public health salaries would seem to be considerably less adequate, for while the actual amount of cash received by nurses of equal training in institutional and public health is approximately the same, the institution provides maintenance, and the public health organization does not. It seems probable that public health salaries will need to be increased in the near future.

The income of private duty nurses, however, is definitely less than that for nurses in either of the other fields. While there are some high earnings, half the nurses in private duty earn less than $1,300 a year. Some earn only $400 or $500 a year and are living on savings or gifts from relatives. For industrious nurses, earnings in private duty are apt to be higher immediately after graduation, and they decrease as the nurse grows older, more tired, and less in touch with nursing practice. In public health and institutional work the nurse may look forward with confidence to increased pay as she becomes more proficient. In private duty all nurses are supposed to charge the same amounts, regardless of whether or not they are efficient. There are no money rewards for high grade bedside nursing skill.

The suggestion is frequently made that private duty nurses should not consider themselves badly paid, because in many places the public school teacher receives no more than they do. It is difficult to get adequate figures on public school salaries. In the few cities for which such figures are available and for which comparative private duty figures have been gathered, it is found that the public school teachers start somewhat higher than the private duty nurses and that their pay increases almost every year thereafter until they have reached levels many hundreds of dollars above what the private duty nurse receives. These figures for New York City, for example, show that in 1926 the average private duty salary (which is higher in New York than in most other cities) was $1,380. A fourth grade school teacher in New York City starts her work at $1,500. Five years later she is earning $2,000; ten years later she is earning $2,600; and when she reaches her peak after 13 years of service she is earning $2,800 and continues there until she finally retires on a pension. These figures are for the automatic increases which the New York City fourth grade school teacher receives. They do not indicate that she has done anything to improve her position except to grow older on the job. The suggestion that private duty nurses are as well off as public school teachers leaves out of account the relatively permanent tenure of the teacher's position, the automatic increases in pay, the opportunities to earn increased money during the long summer vacations, and the very frequent provision for a pension or annuity when the teacher becomes too old to work.

The amount of money the typical private duty nurse earns is pitifully small, and in addition the nurse works under the serious handicap of never knowing from day to day what her income will be. Public health and institutional nurses have regular salaries. Private duty nurses live from hand to mouth. The private duty nurse must live, during periods of idleness, upon the money which she is able to extract from patients during periods of work. This system is hard, not only on the nurse, but on the patient. It seems no more reasonable for the patient to pay the entire cost of a nurse's idle time than it would be for firemen or policemen to depend upon securing from people whose homes have actually burned or householders whose goods have actually been stolen the money upon which they expect to support themselves and their families throughout the year. There should be some method by which the upkeep of a nursing service ready to save lives in times of domestic emergency could be borne by many people, instead of by the few who are least prepared to carry the extra financial burden.

4. Free Service

In considering the annual income of private duty nurses we should also realize that the private duty nurse gives an astonishing amount of free nursing service. Like the physician, the nurse often has difficulty in collecting the money due her. One of the frequent complaints of the special nurse is that although her calls often come through the hospital, the hospital collects its own fee in advance, but makes no attempt to help the nurse collect her fee. Home cases, also, not infrequently cheat the nurse out of her earnings. Last summer a private duty nurse in one of the western states was on four cases in succession—all secured through her own hospital and under the care of reputable physicians—for which she has not been able to collect a cent. Three of the patients have completely ignored her. The fourth gave her a check for $6.00 which proved to be bad. She writes, "One of my doctors has offered to lend me $6.00 until I can get a case which pays. But I don't want to borrow from even my doctor. I want to be paid for my work!"

In addition to the cases where the nurse fails to collect her fee, there are many others where she renders no bill, but voluntarily gives free nursing care. The typical private duty nurse works about eight months a year, of which seven months are for pay and one month out of every twelve is given in some form of charity service. The typical private duty nurse gives $175 worth of free nursing service every year. Some of this service, to be sure, is given to relatives and neighbors, but so far as the nurse's annual income is concerned, nursing service, however generously given, is charity service if it is not paid for. Relatives who would not dream of asking the school teacher daughter to leave her classes or the stenographer daughter to stay at home from the office, call without hesitation upon the private duty nurse, not for one day, but for weeks and sometimes months of high grade professional service without pay. A public health nurse who was recently asked why she had left private duty confessed, "I had to, in order to get away from my relatives. I love them, but I simply cannot afford to take care of all of them in their numerous illnesses, free of charge. Now that I belong to a regular office, they do not dream of suggesting such a thing!"

Not all of the free days are given to relatives. Private duty nurses take many calls from patients who are too poor to pay. Like the medical profession, the nursing profession may well be proud of its generous contributions to charity through personal service. Unlike the physician, however, the nurse who gives such service cannot make up for it in any other way. She cannot, by working longer hours, earn enough to offset her charity service, because charity with her means not one hour, but twelve hours a day. It is a full time proposition. Moreover, since her charges are on a fixed scale, she cannot give charity service to the poor patient and then charge a double fee to the rich patient in order to break even. Such an additional charge would be considered unethical. The typical private duty nurse who earns $1,297 a year and still manages to give $175 worth of free nursing service is one of whom both the nursing and the medical professions may well be proud.

5. Constructive Leadership

The best example of constructive leadership in nursing is that offered by the public health group. When the public health movement started, it shortly became clear that student nurses would not be able to handle the many varied problems involved in public health nursing, and the whole system was built up on the proposition that graduate nurses should be employed. The graduate nurse who is employed on a regular salary and who has the privilege of quitting her job if she does not like it cannot be handled with the same despotic abruptness which characterizes the control of student nurses in the hospital. The director of a public health nursing organization stands or falls according to the skill with which she is able to handle the graduate nurses on her staff. The result is that whenever public health nurses get together and talk shop they almost invariably begin to stress problems dealing with staff education and supervision. They recognize that constructive leadership is a technique to be studied and practised with all the skill which the supervising staff can give.

In institutional nursing there are already to be found many examples of effective staff leadership. There are a few hospitals which are taking the graduate general duty problem seriously, are seeking to secure high grade graduate nurses for this service, and are consciously developing the techniques of administering such a staff. This movement, however, is still so new that comparatively little space is as yet given on convention programs, when institutional problems are discussed, to ways and means for securing happy and cooperative activity on the part of graduate floor duty nurses.

Private duty nurses know even less of what supervision means. They are familiar only with the old type of training school discipline, and to many private duty nurses the suggestion that supervision and staff leadership are the things which she needs and which would make her happiest is an alien thought which she cannot grasp. The supervisor should be the friend and leader under whom staff members delight to work. She should be one who illuminates their problems for them and provides the professional support they need. Most women in other professions take supervision so much for granted that they will not accept a position of any responsibility unless they can be assured that some form of supervisor, director, or committee is ready to stand back of them.

The private duty nurse faces almost daily extremely difficult professional problems. Except where she is so fortunate as to be working in close cooperation with a wise and sympathetic physician there is no professional person with whom she can discuss these problems. Although she is often young and inexperienced, she is supposed to handle without any help problems which the high grade public health nurse would immediately bring to her own supervisor. It is the opinion of students of this problem that two of the important forward steps for the nursing profession will come when superintendents of nurses begin to study seriously the technique of administering graduate floor duty service in hospitals and when, through registries or some other source, private duty nurses are provided with the friendly and constructive leadership they so definitely need.

6. Opportunity for Professional Growth

In reading Chapter 13 one is impressed by the reference made by public health and institutional nurses to their own professional growth. "I am learning something new every day. A good hospital is a wonderful place to work in." The institutional nurses particularly stress the advantages of their positions because of the close contact with medical men who are growing in their own profession, the ever-changing problems, and the opportunities to develop new nursing techniques. In contrast to these reports come the stories of private duty nurses, as shown in Chapter 15, which repeatedly say in one form or another that because of the long hours and the irregularity of employment the nurse has found herself unable to take courses, read books, or mingle with her professional associates.

In public health and institutional nursing the amount of money a nurse earns bears a definite relation to her increased value as a nurse. In private duty, as has been pointed out earlier in this chapter, there are no rewards for increased skill. It may sound mercenary, but it seems to be a human characteristic, that most people feel professional respect for those who are receiving large salaries and find it hard to respect either themselves or others if their pay checks are small. In private duty the quality of workmanship would probably increase, and almost certainly the pride in being a bedside nurse would greatly increase, if methods were provided for giving adequate professional and financial recognition for extremely high grade service. When nurses can become famous because of their bedside technique, and when their salaries can increase correspondingly, it seems fair to predict that much of the existing dissatisfaction will disappear.

7. SUMMARY

The discussion in this chapter may be summarized as follows:

a. In spite of their many criticisms of the conditions under which they work, one fact has impressively stood out in the course of these studies. It is that nurses like nursing.

b. They want nursing to be a profession, and they are seeking the four attributes which are characteristic of other professions. They are:

Reasonable hours
Adequate income
Constructive leadership
Opportunity for growth

c. By far the commonest complaint against private duty is the unreasonably long hours. Twenty-four hour duty is still common in home cases. Most hospitals have abolished twenty-four hour duty and substituted twelve hour duty for special nurses. In either case the nurses declare that the hours are too long.

(1) If the case is difficult rest hours must be given up because the patient cannot be left alone, and there is no regular provision for providing expert nursing care while the regular nurse is resting.

(2) If the case is easy the nurse must waste many hours while she is on duty. This is extremely unsatisfactory to her, and often irritating to the members of the patient's family, who want her to fill in the time with non-nursing duties.

(3) Nurses feel that it should be possible for them to have some life outside of the sick room. The twelve hour day, whether on easy or difficult cases, makes such life impossible.

d. There is no question that for sick patients in the home, the problem of securing the continuous care of a responsible adult—not necessarily a nurse—is serious. The Committee is not yet convinced that the nursing profession should carry the responsibility for solving this problem any more than should the medical profession. It is a question which is naturally of great concern to the members of both groups, as well as the general public, and should be discussed by them all.

e. Shorter hours for private duty nurses are inevitable. This would seem to be true no matter what patients or physicians think about it. Good nurses will not continue to stay in any field where the twelve hour day is expected of them, except in cases where there is a genuine temporary emergency.

f. In institutional work the eight hour day is rapidly becoming generally accepted. In public health work it is definitely and almost universally accepted.

g. It is becoming clear that methods must be devised for insuring a short working day to private duty nurses. This may perhaps be done through hourly nursing in the home or group nursing in the hospital, where the nurse works hard for eight hours and takes her rest after the eight hours are through, rather than taking rest and work irregularly throughout a twelve hour period.

h. Private duty nurses not only want a shorter working day, but a shorter working week. They want to be assured of one day's rest in seven. This assurance is now almost universal for public health and institutional nurses, except in times of emergency. Methods must somehow be devised for making sure that in private duty there is also some definite provision for rest periods at frequent intervals.

i. Institutional salaries, while not high, seem to be better than those in other fields. Public health salaries are probably too low. In institutional and public health work, however, the principle is recognized of increased pay for increased efficiency.

j. In private duty salaries are lower than in any of the other fields. The amount of money earned bears no relation to the quality of service rendered. The worst and the best nurse get the same pay. Nurses are apt to receive more in the first few years after graduation than they will receive later, no matter how much better nurses they may have become in the meantime.

k. The typical private duty nurse gives about one month out of twelve to free charity service. She is unable to make up for this free service through working over time, or through larger fees to wealthy patients.

l. In public health and in institutional nursing there is a definite arrangement whereby staff nurses are under group leadership, so that the quality of their work is constantly being improved, and so that they are afforded professional stimulus. In public health, in fact, the technique of staff leadership is taken with great seriousness. In private duty there is no device by which the special nurse can discuss her professional problems with any one. Young women, lacking constructive leadership, often fail to live up to the promise they gave while in training.

m. In public health and institutional staff positions there is constant opportunity for professional growth. Nurses may advance from one position of authority to another. They are expected to keep on learning as long as they are active in the profession. In private duty, there is no such opportunity or stimulus.

n. It will mark an important development in the nursing profession when, first, superintendents of nurses begin to study seriously the technique of administering graduate floor duty service in hospitals; and, second, when, through registries or some other source, private duty nurses are provided with friendly and constructive leadership.

CHAPTER 25

THE DISTRIBUTION OF NURSING SERVICE

While nurses and physicians often disagree when they are discussing nurses' problems, it has seemed to those making this study that this disagreement was mostly a matter of different emphasis rather than a fundamental difference in principle. Physicians are naturally not as intimately acquainted with nursing economics as are the nurses themselves—they talk from a different standpoint.

1. What Do the Physicians Want?

In the first place, the physician is not really interested in how many hours the nurse works. He may talk about wanting a 24 hour or a 12 hour day because he is afraid that under the shorter working day his patient will not get a square deal. When the physician talks "hours," he is not thinking about the nurse—he is thinking about his patient.

He has to think about his patient. The patient is the physician's responsibility. The physician's job is to make that patient well, and everybody who works for that patient—the *x*-ray man, the laboratory worker, the druggist, the nurse, the patient's relative—belongs to a team which has to work together in a well-organized group, under the leadership of the physician. The nurse obeys the physician's orders, not because he is a man, or because he went to medical school, but because he is the captain on that particular case. He is legally responsible for everything that happens to the patient; and responsibility means the right to give orders and be sure that they will be obeyed.

The physician would not object to short hours, providing his patient were properly cared for. If he could be assured that his patient was satisfied, he would probably be glad to see all nurses on an 8 hour day. But nurses can not have medical approval for short hours unless they are able, somehow, to devise a scheme which will benefit the patient as well as the nurse.

What do physicians want?

First, they want to be able always to get a nurse if she is needed. They do not want to have to wait for half a day, or call up a dozen different registries. Physician after physician writes to the Grading Committee: "The reason I use the commercial registries is because they never leave me in the lurch. They always send me someone." One writes, "I'd rather use the hospital registries because I much prefer to employ competent graduate nurses on all my cases. But I find that often the only way I can get any one at all is by taking the women sent out from the commercial registries."

The physician wants to be able to get a nurse whenever the patient needs one—whether it is a week-day or a Sunday or a legal holiday; whether the case is in the city or the country; whether the case is surgical or pediatric, or mental, or contagious. He asks—and he has a right to ask—that there be some way in which every patient of his who needs a nurse can get one.

Second, he wants some method devised whereby the cost of nursing service can be reasonably within the patient's reach. When physicians talk about limiting the nurse's fees, they are not doing it through any dog-in-the-manger attitude. It is not really that they want nurses to be poor! It is rather that they feel that the middle class patient ought not to have to pay $50 or $60 a week for nursing. What the nurse earns is none of the physician's business; but what the patient pays is his business.

Third, the physician wants to be sure that the nurse to whom he delegates so much responsibility for the patient's care is competent to carry that responsibility. He wants to be sure that the nurse will play the game squarely—that she will follow his orders not only in the letter, but in a high grade professional spirit. For mildly ill patients he wants mostly a friendly, kindly nurse who can fit into the family situation, and who knows how to make her patients comfortable. But for the desperately ill patient he wants to be able to count upon getting a nurse who knows the disease and the technique, who is skilled in asepsis, who can observe and report symptoms, and who keeps her head and knows what to do in an emergency. He has need for nurses of all different degrees of skill and ability—they can all be kept busy. But the physician wants private duty nurses to be so organized, under such intelligent leaders, that the nurses who are sent out will be selected to fit the case; so that he can count upon their being able to do their particular jobs well.

Finally, physicians want the nurses to keep up to date. They want the older nurses to learn modern methods, so that physicians will not have to teach them simple nursing procedures which younger nurses are automatically learning in the hospital.

The physicians—to summarize what they are saying—want very nearly what the nurses want; only they use different language in talking about it and they are thinking from the point of view of the patient and not of the nurse. They are willing that the nurse should have a shorter working day, if that means that the patient will benefit. They would be willing and glad to have the nurse earn a larger annual income, if at the same time the fee to the patient could be smaller. Physicians all over the country are beginning to talk about hourly nursing and group nursing—to save the patient's time, to save the nurse's time, to increase the nurse's earnings, and to decrease the patient's bill.

Physicians want nursing to be better organized and administered. And they want the nurses to keep up to date. The returns indicate that if the needs of the patient are kept in mind, the medical profession may be counted upon to stand solidly behind the nurses in their concerted endeavor to secure:

Reasonable hours
Adequate income
Constructive leadership
Professional growth

Physicians have one bitter complaint which is stressed over and over. They say that they cannot always get the right kind of a nurse at the time when they need her. They can get nurses for day time hospital cases, but they report serious difficulty in getting competent nurses for home cases, for night service in the hospital or home, for 24 hour cases, and for many of the special types of sickness, such as maternity, contagion, mental, and G.U. They write: "It is easy to get good surgical nurses, but hard to get nurses good for anything else." Physicians especially report difficulty in finding competent nurses for patients who happen to fall ill on Sundays or holidays. Here, in fact, seems to be the basis for the frequently stressed belief that nurses have some sort of a trade union where, as one physician expressed it in his letter, "They have banded together to refuse cases on holidays."

This is, of course, just the opposite of the facts. Special, or private duty, is a free lance occupation. The nurses not only do not belong to unions, but most of them do not belong to any effective group organization. Some of them do not even keep up membership in their district associations, and those who belong are often lax in their attendance. The registry exercises very little control over free lance workers, and as a result the physician cannot get a nurse on a holiday because, since there is no central organization, there is no one to assign days on duty. If the private duty nurses all want to go home at Christmas, there is no one to suggest that holidays should be taken in turn and that the nurses who go home should be sure that there is some one left to take the calls which come. Probably a large part of the existing irritation which physicians, many of them at least, are feeling so strongly against the special duty nursing group, arises from the fact that special duty is a free lance occupation.

2. Nurses Should Take Turns

The worst sufferers from the free lance organization of private duty are the private duty nurses themselves. One is impressed with the fact that the distribution of cases seems to be largely left to chance and the result is that many apparently unfair situations arise.

Some nurses are surprisingly successful in avoiding home cases. If we assume that the hospital case is ordinarily more attractive to the nurse than the home case, it hardly seems fair that some nurses should be able to spend most of their time in the hospital, while others are obliged to take mostly home cases because they cannot get hospital duty. It seems rather a curious professional situation which permits the attractive jobs to be regarded as the private property of relatively small groups.

Night calls are almost as numerous as day calls. Most nurses do not like night duty. Some of them cannot stand it for long periods at a stretch, because they cannot sleep in the day time. Here again one is puzzled by the fact that apparently many nurses are able to escape night duty almost entirely, while others are obliged to accept it regularly, although they do not want it. Night duty, of course, has to be done. Some nurse has to take it. Could there not be some fairer arrangement so that the undesired night calls could be distributed among all the available nurses, and each one would carry her share, but no more? If nurses were organized into cooperative groups, under skilled and sympathetic leadership, it would seem as though a more equitable division of such desired and undesired assignments might be made, and every one, including patients and physicians, as well as nurses, might be happier.

If a nurse has money on hand, she definitely plans to take a few days off after every case. She likes her week-ends and her holidays. She likes to go shopping. She has to plan for shampoos and for visits to the dentist. Some nurses frankly say that at the close of every case they plan to take several days off and that when they do so, they simply refrain from notifying the registry or the physician that they are free. No one questions that the nurse ought to have some time to herself, but it often works hardship when the nurses choose their own rest periods, because these are apt to happen simultaneously. It is an unfortunate patient who comes down with pneumonia the day before Christmas.

Here again the present system seems to be unfair. The nurse who is young and attractive and who, because she was graduated from the local hospital, has strong local connections, can usually keep about as busy as she wants to be. She does not hesitate to take Christmas and New Year's and Easter, and all her week-ends if she can. The nurse, however, who has come from some other city, or who happens to be in disfavor with the local registry, or who is a little old and not quite so attractive, and who has become more serious about the necessity for earning and saving money, feels that she cannot afford to refuse any case, and that she must be on registry all the time if she is to make enough money to live on. It is that nurse, therefore, the less fortunate nurse, who is obliged to take the undesired calls. She is the one who has to give up her holiday. She rarely can count on a week-end for herself.

In any other profession where working on Sundays and holidays is required, the assignments are so distributed that each member of the staff takes an equal share. He is on duty perhaps one Sunday out of every four, or if he has to work on Christmas, he gets New Year's off. This is true even among elevator boys and household servants; and it would seem that it ought to be possible for nurses to organize themselves into groups so that these undesired calls would be more equitably distributed. No nurse would mind being on call on Christmas or New Year's or Easter occasionally if it did not happen too often, and the consciousness that she was being a good sport and helping out some sister nurse by taking an undesired assignment, ought, it would seem, to make her willing to cooperate in such a group. Some such simple arrangement would do much to lighten the burdens of private duty nurses, and it would be vastly appreciated by physicians and patients who need skilled nursing service over the holiday.

Most cases are short cases, and some of them are very short. There is some reason to suspect that these cases are not divided equally among all workers, but that certain nurses specialize in the long time cases, and others, often against their will, specialize in the extremely short cases. There is no machinery by which the assignment of new cases bears any relation to the sorts of cases the nurses have previously had. There is no scheme whereby the nurse who has been working for 45 days without a rest can be assigned several 1 and 2 day cases, or the nurse who has been doing nothing but 1 and 2 day cases for weeks be given a long time case for a change. Under the present arrangement, apparently, nurses must take what they can get, and the nurse who happens to be in high favor with some particular physician whose cases are apt to be long is practically assured of the long time employment; while again, the stranger to the city or the older nurse who is a little rusty in her technique, or the one who for some reason or other is a little unpopular with the head of the registry, may be obliged to fill all her time with the extremely short, unlucrative, and nerve-wracking work.

3. The Out-of-Town Nurse

A superintendent of nurses in a large hospital in New York City remarked recently that she had no particular difficulty in securing graduate nurses for floor duty. She said, "Nurses are so eager to come to New York that all I have to do is to put an advertisement into the American Journal of Nursing and I can take my pick of out-of-town nurses who are glad to come for floor duty in order to get a footing in New York City."

The out-of-town nurse needs to have some such standby as an institutional job if she is to come into any big city. If she comes as a free lance private duty nurse, she is rather apt to have a hard time. The local nurses naturally enough are inclined to be none too cordial because they often have a hard enough time to get sufficient employment for themselves, and they feel that the outside nurse is adding to their difficulties. Hospital registries favor their own graduates, and while many of them admit outsiders to the registries, they are frank to say that they give the more desirable calls to their own people. The central registries, in some cities at least, are comparatively weak organizations which work more or less in competition with the local hospital registries. There seems to be no reason why the central professional registry could not be an impartial, strong organization, which would care for all reputable and well-trained nurses fairly, regardless of whether they are locally trained or not; but the development of such strong and modern registries calls for money and thought, and while hopeful experiments are being tried, there are as yet few central registries which have begun to approach the brilliant possibilities which lie in the future.

In every large city there are numbers of commercial registries. Some of them are excellent. Some of them are unspeakably unethical and dangerous. The out-of-town nurse runs a serious risk when she comes to a new city and goes to a commercial registry, yet in many cases that is the only resource for her. It would seem that the development of central professional registries, dealing skilfully and impartially with all qualified nurses, would help enormously in protecting the nurse from out-of-town or the older nurse who has lost her original connections with the hospital and medical world.

4. The Registry

Most physicians secure their nurses through hospital registries. The hospital registry is rather frankly conducted for the purpose of securing specials of the type the hospital desires, which usually means specials from its own alumnæ to take care of cases within its own walls. The hospital registry apparently pays very little attention to meeting the needs for nursing in other institutions or in homes. Moreover, as was shown in Chapter 4, the control of the hospital registry is only a minor activity for the busy hospital administrative staff. (Does this fact account, perhaps, for the unwillingness of nurses to take home cases?)

Running a registry is a difficult technical task, and there are very few hospitals in this country which will ever feel able to pay a specialist in employment problems to conduct the registry for them. Even with the district and club registries there is no evidence that the registrars have been given encouragement or opportunity for special training in the technique of personnel work. The result is that the physician and the patient who call either the hospital or the central professional registry have great difficulty in securing prompt and efficient service. Nurses who enroll with these registries are ordinarily given very little supervision or help and often find it difficult to secure enough work through the registry to keep them busy.

From a business point of view the commercial registry is frequently better run than either the hospital or the central registry, but there the high professional ideals for which the others stand are often lacking, and the commercial registry not infrequently caters to a type of nurse who is below the grade which the good physician demands for his patient. Moreover, since the commercial registry usually collects 10 per cent of the nurse's pay as commission, it naturally urges its clients—whether registered nurses or the so-called "practical" variety—to charge as much as they think the patient will give. The result is that not infrequently the conscientious registered nurse, charging $6 a day, finds herself competing with practical nurses who are charging not $6, but $8 or $10 or $12. Every time the physician or the patient calls a commercial registry, he runs the risk of getting a commercially minded nurse!

If the professional central registry could become a central nursing force for service in each community, under skilful and wise direction, it would seem probable that many of the difficulties of which physicians, patients, and nurses at present complain could be rather rapidly solved. Until the registry is made into an effective organ, the physician will continue to call one hospital after another, he will need always to have his own notebook with his list of favored nurses, and he will from time to time be forced to turn to the commercial registry in a last attempt to get some kind of a nurse, whether good or not, for the desperately ill patient.

5. Hourly Nursing

The registry returns indicate a serious condition of unemployment among private duty nurses which apparently exists in all parts of the country, and if the estimates given in this study for the future production of nurses hold true, it is inevitably bound to become worse.

Registrars in case after case have pointed out that hospitals are graduating such large classes that the number on the waiting list hunting for jobs is far beyond the number which can be profitably employed.

There are two solutions to the problem which this unemployment condition raises. One is to reduce drastically the number of nurses who are allowed to enter the profession. Another solution is to devise new ways in which nurses can be employed. The returns from physicians and patients seem to indicate rather clearly that with the present method of 12 and 24 hour service, the call for nursing service has about reached the saturation point. Apparently very few patients who are really eager to secure nurses at prevailing rates and at prevailing hours are going without them. There is reason to believe, however, that many people who are now entirely without any nursing service would be glad to pay for service on an hourly basis. Everywhere there are probably many mothers of sick children who do not feel that they can pay $7 a day for a 12 hour nurse but who would gladly pay $2 a day to have a nurse come in and give certain of the more difficult treatments. Probably there are large numbers of chronic cases in every community for which some nursing service is needed daily and for which the relatives or the patients would be glad to pay a $2 or $3 fee for a short period of daily care and yet would feel wholly unable to employ a full time nurse.

Nurses and physicians are already talking about the possibility of building up this hitherto unmet need and thereby giving more employment to nurses, while at the same time supplying a type of nursing service which would be genuinely valued and readily paid for by the community.

Some hourly service is already to be found in every large city. But the word "hourly" needs careful definition since there are apparently many different types of service which are labeled by that name. Some hourly nursing is done independently. The nurse has her own office. She works under no one's direction. There is one hourly nurse in a large city who picks her cases and will not go to the home of any one whose name does not appear in the Blue Book. Some hourly nurses work for a small group of physicians, carrying out special treatments at their orders. Others specialize in one form of treatment only. There is one hourly nurse who is said to make an excellent living with yearly trips to Europe on a practice which consists solely of colonic irrigations. Some nurses are employed by beauty parlors for the purpose of giving colonics.

For the independent hourly worker there is no standard as to price. She sets her charge for the treatment according to the amount that she thinks the patient can pay. There are other hourly nurses who are sent out by registries. The registry fixes the price and the nurse goes for two or three hours at a time, usually to relieve a regular nurse during her off-duty periods.

None of these types is apparently what thoughtful nurses are beginning to describe and recommend to the profession under the heading "hourly nurses." The modern definition of hourly nursing implies apparently that the nurses are on regular salaries, employed throughout the year, that they are selected because they are good nurses and know how to give good bedside care and how to make their patients comfortable. Some of them are selected because they are especially good on certain more difficult parts of the technique such as skill in asepsis, or skill in observing and reporting symptoms. They belong to a regular staff on eight hour shifts. The organization administering the hourly service is open day and night and assignments to night duty or holiday duty are taken in rotation by different members of the staff. The patient pays the organization and does not pay the nurse. The nurse's salary comes in as a regular check at the end of each month.

Hourly nursing which accords more or less with this description is already being conducted in different centers. In some cases it is under the direction of a visiting nursing association. In other places it is controlled by a nurses' registry; and in some instances the control is under a joint board representing both types of organization. The specific characteristics in each case vary, of course, from the scheme as outlined above, but the general picture is approximately the same. Such hourly nursing is new and can not be said to have demonstrated its full value and possibilities. It is clear, however, that it is something with which careful experiments should continue to be tried.

6. Graded Work for Graded Pay

Most people like to think that they are not keenly interested in the amount of money they can earn. They like to believe that they are primarily interested in serving humanity and that the pay check is an unimportant incident. It seems to be true, however, that even for those who are unquestionably highly idealistic in their attitudes toward work, an increase in salary gives a real thrill. In general, people respect those in their profession who earn more than they do and they feel something close to pity for those among their colleagues who are known to be earning less.

It is probably true that one of the most stultifying characteristics of private duty is the fact that the least experienced, most unskilled nurse on the registry is allowed to charge exactly as much as the most skilful nurse. Patients resent this fact almost as much as nurses do. Patients repeatedly say that it seems unfair to them to pay exactly the same amount in cases where nurses were unsatisfactory as in cases where nurses have, they believe, saved the patient's life.

It would seem entirely feasible for registries to establish some system by which the nurses enrolled would be classified according to experience and ability and would be given an opportunity to work up from group to group as they proved their worth. It would seem fair for registries to establish a scale of charges according to the degree of skill of the nurse. There is every reason to believe that patients and physicians would be better satisfied with registry service if, when they called the registry for a nurse, they could be given a choice so that they could secure a low-priced, semi-skilled nurse or a high-priced, highly skilled nurse, according to what they felt was needed and what they were willing to pay for. Such a scheme of graded service and graded charges, with ample opportunity for the nurse to rise from group to group as she demonstrated her value, would seem to offer professional stimulation to the nurse and at the same time to meet a real need on the part of physician and patient.

7. Registries of the Future

Reforms do not come through miracles. Somebody has to work for them. Moreover, good things are not brought about just by hating what is bad. Administrative reforms come through finding out what is wrong, getting groups of workers together, talking over possible solutions, and then trying them out, one after another, until some experiments are found which work.

If private duty nurses will get together, work together, and join in experimenting with the different solutions which are now being urged, they can remake their jobs and the process will be rapid. Moreover, if in their talking and thinking and experimenting they keep the sick-in-bed patient steadfastly in mind, and work to help the patient as well as to help themselves, they will before long discover that the medical profession—or the intelligent main body of it at least—is willing to help. Physicians already are talking about hourly nursing, group nursing, and registries. It will not take long, if the nurses really want medical cooperation, to secure it, and secure it heartily.

Probably, if the private duty nurses want to save time and do an efficient job, they will be wise to call upon the medical, institutional, and public health fields for help and advice. Most of the reforms which private duty nurses want are already matters of course in institutional and in public health nursing. What institutional and public health nurses have, private duty nurses can almost surely get. The big advantage which private duty now has is its personal independence of action. The big problem for private duty nurses is how much of this cherished independence of action they are willing to give up, in order to get the other things they want.

It may be profitable to compare private duty as it is now organized with the way it might be if it adopted the standards almost universally accepted for other professional women and already largely accepted in other branches of the nursing profession. Suppose that private duty nursing were run as other professions run their work. Then we should see private duty nurses joined together in centrally organized groups under intelligent and friendly leadership. The calls for private duty would be received by the central organizations, and the assignments of work would be given out according to the strength and capacity of the members. All nurses would be on annual salaries. They would be carefully selected for their jobs on the basis of whether or not they were competent to take adequate bedside care of sick patients. They would work eight hours at a stretch.

The headquarters office would be open day and night, year in and year out. Hard jobs and easy, long and short, day and night, city and country, would be equitably distributed among the members of the staff, so that each nurse would carry her fair share, and no patient would be sacrificed. Nurses and calls would be fitted together so that, except for special emergencies, each nurse would be sent out on the work she could do best, and the inexperienced nurse or the less skilful nurse would get the simpler calls, while the especially experienced or most skilful nurse would get those calls which demand the highest degrees of nursing ability. Courses, clinics, and demonstrations would be planned every year so that nurses who had failed to have certain types of training while they were still in school, or who were rusty in their techniques, could bring themselves up to date and so make themselves more valuable to the organization. As each nurse thus became more experienced and more valuable, her annual pay would be increased and her nursing assignments would be correspondingly more important. Attached to each central group would be an advisory board of nurses and physicians and patients. They would not interfere with the details of administration, but they would help in formulating policies.

If such a central group of nurses could be adequately organized and established, one would then have something similar to the professional organizations of women outside. Nurses would be working under conditions similar to those which other people take for granted. They would work together in a professional atmosphere, they could discuss the problems of their cases with their group leaders and with other members of the staff. When they did especially good jobs of nursing, there would be some intelligent person who knew what that work had implied and who could give the professional appreciation which all of us need. And when the Grading Committee next asked the question, "Do you plan to stay indefinitely in private duty?" the answer would become a definite and unqualified, "Yes!"

8. SUMMARY

The discussion in this chapter may be summarized as follows:

a. In discussing the four attributes of professional work for which nurses are asking, the reader should remember that the physician is not, and probably should not be, primarily concerned in securing proper working conditions for nurses. If nursing is an independent profession, as its members believe, the details of working conditions should be settled by nurses and not by members of outside professions.

b. Readers must, therefore, realize that the discussion

of members of the medical profession is, and probably should be, based upon concern for the welfare of the patient rather than the nurse. The patient is the physician's responsibility.

c. Physicians want first to be able to get a nurse whenever one is needed; second, to bring the cost of nursing service within the reach of the patient; third, to be sure that the nurse is competent to give the kind of care the case demands; fourth, to have nurses keep up to date so that the patient will receive the benefit of the most recent advances in nursing knowledge and techniques.

d. If the needs of the patient are kept in mind, the medical profession may be counted upon to stand solidly behind the nurses in their concerted effort to secure

Reasonable hours
Adequate income
Constructive leadership
Professional growth

e. Much of the criticism of private duty nursing seems to arise from the fact that there is no mechanism by which nurses can take turns. Home cases, night duty, week-end and holiday duty, and short cases are all relatively unattractive to nurses. Under present conditions graduates of local hospitals who are young, pleasing, and in favor with the hospital and medical people are able to avoid practically all calls of this sort. Out-of-town nurses, older nurses, nurses from small schools without registries, or those who are out of favor with the hospital or medical authorities, are almost obliged to specialize on the less desired calls. It would seem that some mechanism might be devised so that attractive and unattractive assignments could be shared equally by all competent nurses on the registries and so that no particular group would be unduly favored or penalized.

f. Running a registry is a difficult technical business. Most of the hospital and central professional registries are conducted by people who have had no special training in personnel management or placement problems. It is believed that if central professional registries could be established on a thoroughly business-like basis, with broad ethical outlook, many of the present difficulties in private duty would disappear.

g. Under present conditions it seems to be true that the field for private duty is no longer large enough to absorb the nurses who wish employment in it. The profession should consider the possibility of enlarging its field by cultivating a demand for short time or hourly nursing service. It is believed that the provision of such service would not materially decrease the demand for full time nurses but would expand the possible opportunities for employment by reaching the patients who are at the present time going without any nursing service.

h. It is believed that hourly service, if it is to succeed on a broad scale, should be carefully organized and supervised.

i. In most professions the payment received bears a direct relation to the value of the work done. Workers regard salaries as indices of ability. It is suggested that registries might increase their effectiveness to patients, physicians, and nurses if they would establish graded service on graded pay, so that the choice of a nurse might be made in the light of the kind of nursing service needed and the amount of skill which the patient is willing to pay for. Nurses should be encouraged to move from lower paid to higher paid groups as their value to the patient increases.

j. It is believed that if registries could be developed into well-organized professional centers for the adminstration of local private duty, patients, physicians, and the nurses themselves would all benefit.

CHAPTER 26

THE HOSPITAL AND THE GRADUATE NURSE

The amazing growth in the numbers of nursing schools and graduate nurses and the threat of overproduction for the nursing field are the logical result of the way in which nursing education has been organized. Nursing schools were developed to take care of the sick in hospitals. It is only recently that there have been enough graduate nurses available so that graduates could be used for this purpose. Even now it is probably true that if every graduate nurse in the United States were doing bedside nursing in the hospitals, there would be only about one nurse to every three patients, which is below the best standards. The supply of nurses is increasing so rapidly that if, say, three-fourths of the hospitals today really believed that a trained nurse is better than an untrained or semi-trained nurse, and if they could raise funds in order to employ such nurses, the supply of students from the other one-fourth would probably be ample to keep up with the increasing demand. But this condition has come to pass only within two or three years.

1. How it Started

Hospitals began using students not in preference to graduate nurses, but in preference to attendants. The motive was probably excellent, and it is easy to see why the tradition has been established in the best hospitals of this country that student service is the normal and efficient type of service to seek for. Now that graduate nurses are available, hospitals are going to ask, "Why should we change? We know students to be efficient. We are unaccustomed to graduate nursing staffs, and we hesitate about changing our methods. Graduates would cost more. Why should we change from an inexpensive method which works to a more expensive method about which we know little?"

Superintendents of nurses would probably at the present time agree with hospital administrators in this point of view. They have always thought of high grade hospitals as being run with student service. They have not known any other standards. Very few of the superintendents of nurses are primarily educators. If they were, they could not hold their present positions, because the superintendent of nurses must be, first and foremost, a skilful administrator. The success with which patients are cared for in her hospital can be measured directly by the speed with which they get well. The success with which students are educated in her hospital can be measured only by the indirect evidence of their skill as nurses years later when they have left the hospital and gone out into the field. Naturally, practically all superintendents of nurses are administrators of nursing service first and foremost, and while they are sincerely interested in the education of students, most of them have only slight acquaintance with modern educational philosophy and methods and are conducting their schools along much the lines in which they themselves were taught years ago. Many of them are not college women and have never come in contact with professional schools other than nursing schools. Since they know no other form of education, they have had little reason until recently to question the essential rightness of the scheme.

It is worth noting that nursing education is one of the comparatively early forms of vocational education for women in this country. It was rather an extraordinary thing for women in the 1870's, '80's, '90's to develop almost single handed so complicated an administrative organization as the nursing service of a hospital. When one remembers the attitude of society towards professional women in 1880, it is easy to understand how some of the nursing traditions which seem out of date today (of fighting for principles, but avoiding explanation or argument; of respecting the opinions of all males, but proceeding to go straight ahead in the work which needed to be done, regardless of those opinions) were founded. There is some evidence to indicate that the early struggles of pioneer nurses were not so much to establish and promote *education* as to demonstrate that skilled nursing care was better for sick patients than unskilled. They, like every one else who thought about it at all, probably assumed that the nurse who had spent some months in hospital nursing would be equipped to be self-supporting in hospitals and homes thereafter, but there seems to be comparatively little discussion in the early days as to what sort of experience in the hospital and what sorts of supplementary teaching were needed in order adequately to prepare women for their future nursing activities. In those days—the early seventies and eighties—general education had not progressed very far in its conscious philosophy. Even if the pioneer nursing educators had sought help from the public education group, it is probable that they would have been disappointed. Moreover, why should any one seriously have questioned the validity of educational methods which were producing such good results? That the results were surprisingly good is demonstrated by the very quality of the women who grew up under the old régime.

2. Nursing Education Now Under Fire

Most people think of hospitals as founded on the work of the student nurses. This is not wholly true. Of the 7,416 hospitals in the United States in 1927, only 2,155 have nursing schools. The other 5,261 are dependent for their supply of trained nurses upon the product of the 2,155. These facts are illustrated in Diagram 61.

It is true that the hospitals with training schools are, for the most part, the large general hospitals. Those without training schools are either very small hospitals or else state institutions. It is interesting to note that even when the large state hospitals are included, the average number of beds in hospitals without training schools is 76, as compared with an average of 186 beds in hospitals with training schools.* Hospitals which do not have schools usually have most of their work done by attendants or practical nurses, with an occasional graduate nurse in charge. The graduate nurses are, of course, the products of the schools, so that the situation is that 70% of the hospitals are dependent for whatever graduate nursing they secure upon the educational product of 30%.

There are now so many hospitals and so many schools that there are not enough high grade, well-bred, thoroughly equipped nurse teachers and administrators to run them all. The result is that all too many are in inefficient hands. A glance at the tables in Chapter 16, showing the education of superintendents of nurses, will illustrate this point.

* These figures are taken from the Journal of the American Medical Association for March 12, 1927.

Because there are so many nursing schools, it has been possible for daughters of good families who wish to be-

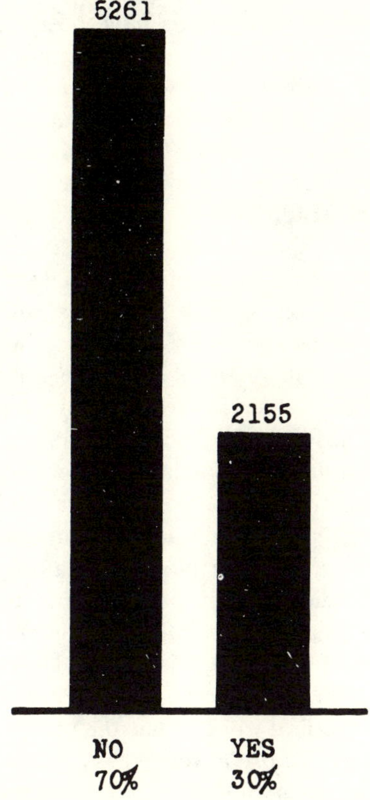

Diagram 61.—Of the 7,416 hospitals in the United States, only 2,155 have nursing schools. The other 5,261 are dependent for their supply of trained nurses upon the product of the 2,155

come nurses to select which of the schools they will enter. The result has been that schools, with very little to offer the prospective student in the way of real education, have allowed young women of inferior capacity and background to enter, because that has been the only way in which some of these hospitals have been able to secure enough students to do the work. Much of the popular criticism of the nursing profession would seem undoubtedly to have arisen because of the presence of these large numbers of low grade women for whose entrance into the profession the hospitals are directly responsible.

The hospital tradition which, as we have seen, was at first reasonable enough, that all work must be done by students; the success of the students in doing it; and the actual conviction on the part of hospital authorities that there would be neither sense nor justice in paying good money for the employment of graduates if students could be secured instead; has resulted in a general feeling on the part of many women now in the nursing profession that bedside or floor duty nursing is a "student's job," and the result of this attitude has been that when hospitals seriously desire to secure high grade graduate nurses for general floor service, they are blocked because of the hesitation of most women of the type they want, to enter a field which is not considered desirable for the graduate nurse.

Another result of the tradition that a large and successful hospital will, of course, depend upon its student nurses for all hospital work is that the practice of employing special nurses for private cases has grown to widespread proportions. This is wholly natural. The superintendent of nurses is given to understand that she must handle all the nursing in the hospital with her student group. Since most hospitals are seriously understaffed, and since the superintendent rarely has the privilege of employing additional graduate nurses when needed, the almost inevitable result has been that she has eased her burden by encouraging such patients as could afford to do so to provide their own nursing care. Here is perhaps one of the chief reasons for the present popular belief in many circles that no patient is really safe in a hospital unless he employs his own special to take care of him.

3. Graduates Versus Students

Chapter 19 has reluctantly but emphatically voiced the conviction that hospitals must begin to utilize greater numbers of graduate nurses on general floor duty. There will be two outstanding reasons why this suggestion will be received with considerable hesitation on the part of thoughtful hospital administrators. They will question how they can possibly run their hospitals on a basis which would require the regular payment of graduate nurse salaries to all nurses who take care of patients. While some hospitals with schools are in the habit of saying that the school costs them more than it would cost to run the hospital on graduate service, very few of them actually believe this statement. For most hospitals the problem of instituting complete graduate service would seem at first to involve heavy expenditures.

The second reason why the suggestion will cause much discussion in hospital circles is the almost universal conviction on the part of superintendents of nurses that students are better nurses for hospital service than graduates.

The early fight to demonstrate the superiority of *trained* nurses in bedside care is not yet won. Hospital philosophy now accepts whole-heartedly the proposition that graduate nurses are needed in the operating and delivery rooms, at the heads of schools, in charge of the nursing service, and rather generally as superintendents of the smaller hospitals; but the proposition that the graduate nurse is really better than the student, or even than the attendant, for the actual giving of bedside care cannot yet be said to be accepted. Even nurses themselves will often be found unconvinced on this point. It is, then, not surprising that hospital authorities, physicians, and patients are also unconvinced!

As was shown in Chapter 16, most superintendents of nurses prefer students to graduates. This is partly because students are young, strong, and docile. It takes less tact to govern them, because the students do not dare to argue or rebel. Although traditionally the discipline of a nursing school is severe, students accept and even rather enjoy it, because it is part of the dramatic setting of "learning to be a trained nurse." Students accept the strict discipline for three years because they know that it is in the nature of an initiation which will finally open the door to freedom.

The superintendent who tries to treat a graduate nursing staff as though they were a class of student nurses finds shortly that she is losing some of her best people and that her administrative troubles mount high. The technique of staff leadership which has been worked out with such care and attention by the public health nurses—who had to learn how to do it because they could not rely on student nurses and were obliged somehow to get along with graduate nurses or give up the whole plan—is as yet almost unknown in hospital nursing administration. Without it no graduate floor service would be expected to be smoothly successful.

With a few outstanding exceptions the superintendent of nurses is a busy, worried person. She carries enormous responsibilities, and if anything goes wrong in the nursing service the penalty is severe. It may mean the killing of a patient. She has autocratic power over her students, and at the same time is often almost powerless outside. Conditions for the nursing service are laid down, and, so far as she is able to see, there is no hope of changing them. Feeling particularly impotent so far as making any fundamental alteration in the nursing system is concerned, and having unquestioned power within the system, it is natural for superintendents of nurses to prefer students to graduates, because students will do what they are told to do without argument.

It is an open question whether the superintendent of nurses is actually as helplessly bound as she is apt to think of herself as being. There is a generally accepted belief, apparently, that trustees, medical men, and hospital superintendents are beyond the reach of argument and reason. Sometimes there are specific cases quoted which seem to give a basis for such conclusions; but more generally the superintendent admits, when questioned, that she has not discussed some of the more pressing of the educational and administrative problems with her board because, "They would never understand!" The fact that many hospital boards of trustees know nothing beyond the surface facts concerning the schools which they are supposed to be running is sometimes not so much their fault as the fault of the unduly reticent superintendent of nurses.

4. What Do Superintendents of Nurses Think About General Duty Nurses?

Superintendents of nurses make certain specific criticisms of graduate staff nurses. They say that graduates come from different schools where each has learned a different technique. Many of them have learned these techniques by rote and have no intellectual background which would enable them to understand why different ways of doing the same thing might be equally good, or even better, under conditions in a new hospital. It is necessary to teach these graduate nurses the techniques the hospital wants, and many of them find it difficult to understand or accept new methods.

Student nurses stay for three years. Graduates can leave on a week's notice. It is necessary to provide the graduate with working and living conditions which are reasonably attractive to her, or she will not stay; and it is often extremely difficult for the superintendent of nurses, with no control over the hospital budget, to provide such satisfactory conditions. In many hospitals the turnover among graduate general duty nurses is excessive.

Graduate nurses must be paid salaries. Salaries are usually between $90 and $100 a month, plus maintenance. The suggestion to a hospital board that a full staff of graduate nurses be supplied at this figure would seem to many superintendents of nurses so inevitably doomed to failure that it would hardly be worth attempting. At present as long as respectable hospitals can get students at the prevailing low rates without losing caste (for in many hospitals the cost of purely educational activities is negligible) they will naturally cling to their "schools" and avoid graduate staffs.

It would seem, from the material already presented in this report, that the day is now at hand when many of the 2,155 hospitals with nursing schools must begin thinking in terms of wide employment, or almost complete employment, of graduate general duty nurses; and when the other 5,261 hospitals, which are now relying primarily upon practical nurses or attendants, will find that patients will refuse to enter their doors unless an adequate graduate nursing service is available. The problems of maintaining a graduate staff, both in their financial and administrative aspects, will undoubtedly cause much discussion in the near future.

Many superintendents of nurses testify that when they are able to secure graduate general floor duty nurses these women are apt to be below the standard grade. They are, some of them, ill bred, poorly educated, and poorly trained. They are recruited from the private duty ranks where years of freedom have left them unfitted to work as members of staffs. They are accustomed to free lance independence and find even kindly direction irksome.

They are slow workers, coming into a situation where every one else is working under pressure. After having had twelve hours a day to lavish on one patient, they find it difficult to adapt themselves to wards full of patients, where adequate care can rarely be given, because there are not enough nurses to do the minimum work well. Graduate floor duty nurses, if they are good bedside nurses, resent such pressure and either work themselves sick or rebel, criticize, and quit. If they are poor bedside nurses, they also resent the pressure, become careless and indifferent, and either quit or conceal the poor quality of their work by various subterfuges.

Graduate floor duty nurses, being older, are not so strong as student nurses. They lack the quickness, resiliency, and receptiveness of students. They break down sooner if the labor is heavy, and they are, therefore, not so convenient to have as workers in a busy hospital.

5. What Do Graduate Nurses Think About Floor Duty?

Nurses who have tried general floor duty are for the most part unenthusiastic about it. They feel that they have lowered their professional status by accepting such work, and this feeling is rather generally shared by their fellows. In some schools the student nurses apparently feel that graduate floor duty nurses are socially and professionally beneath them.

Nurses who have tried general floor duty make the following specific criticisms:

a. "The pay is lower than in private duty." This is probably not true, but it is widely believed. Nearly half of the private duty nurses keep no records and, therefore, have no idea of their annual earnings. Many of them probably greatly overestimate the amount they take in each year. The typical private duty earnings are actually about $1,300 a year. The typical general duty salaries are $1,200 plus all living expenses, which, if the very moderate allowance of $500 is made for maintenance, is the equivalent of $1,700. Under present employment conditions it should be possible to secure an ample supply of high grade graduate bedside nurses for this salary.

b. "Pressure of work is too great." The hospital is unable or unwilling to employ enough nurses or to increase the staff at times of extra heavy load. The result is that the regular nurses are forced to give superficial and inadequate care to their patients. Protests and requests for opportunity to give better care to patients are not favorably received.

c. "Head nurses and supervisors are not carefully enough selected." Well-bred, well educated, and conscientious bedside nurses are often asked to work under the direction of women obviously their social and professional inferiors. The lower the social grade of the woman in power, the more unreasonable and arbitrary she becomes. Sometimes even the superintendent of nurses is reported as belonging to this class. Hospitals which want to maintain good bedside nursing should scrutinize with greater care the quality and qualifications of the people to whom they give authority for administering it.

d. "General floor duty usually requires nurses to live in the hospital." Many nurses wish to live at home or with friends.

e. "The general duty hours are long and irregular, and rest days, although promised, are often denied because of the pressure of work." Pressure of work is the constant complaint for hospitals with schools and for hospitals without. New services are added, wings built, elaborate treatments developed, and record forms devised apparently without any consideration of their effect upon the nursing service. It would seem obvious to any one that, before such changes are permitted, the superintendent of nurses should be consulted and provision for additional nurses made to carry the additional load. But such is apparently not always the case. It seems to be assumed that the nursing service is indefinitely elastic!

f. "General duty as a regular occupation is not quite respectable." There is, to be sure, a growing tendency for ambitious nurses to take a few months of general duty in some famous hospital as a sort of post-graduate course, in order to learn new techniques, and this is considered highly commendable.

To do general duty in an ordinary hospital, however, as a regular and not a temporary worker, at once implies that there is something the matter with the nurse. Nurses who have tried it report that except in a few hospitals they have been made to feel their inferiority keenly. Floor maids and orderlies, student nurses and internes, head nurses, supervisors, members of the medical and surgical staffs, and all other people connected with the hospital, seem to feel that for a nurse to do general floor duty after graduation indicates that she must have failed in the more dignified branches. This criticism does not apply to all hospitals, but it does apparently apply to many.

g. "There is no future in general duty." Increases in pay are infrequent. There are few chances of promotion. The fact that one has done general duty, except as suggested above, for a few months in order to get post-graduate work in a particular specialty, seems to be a handicap rather than a help.

6. Why Are Some Superintendents Eager to Try Graduate Staffs?

Some superintendents of nurses, although perhaps relatively few in number as yet, are genuinely interested in the problems of staff control where all the work is done by graduate nurses. They say that most of the difficulties encountered in handling graduate nurses come from a lack of understanding; that some superintendents of nurses are imbued with the old military spirit and are either wholly unfamiliar with modern staff organization and administration or else are unable or unwilling to learn its principles. Some of them do not seem to realize that there is any special technique which they could study to advantage. It is suggested by superintendents who are particularly interested in the problem that one contribution which public health nurses can definitely make to institutional nurses is the newly developed technique of staff administration, supervision, and education. They feel that as soon as superintendents of nurses learn how to treat graduate floor duty nurses as adult professional workers, instead of pseudo students, most of the general floor duty troubles will disappear.

Many superintendents of nursing of whom this criticism might be made would probably vigorously deny its implications. Supervision in nursing schools is so much less military today than it was 20 years ago that modern superintendents regard themselves, in contrast to those under whom they studied, as almost overly indulgent. They cannot understand the suggestion that their supervision is severe.

Yet part of the time, of course, it must be severe, with a meticulous control of detail far beyond anything required by, say, the public health organizations. In the ward, proper morale demands the expert handling of patients in a group, each one affecting the attitude of the others, whereas in public health nursing, for the most part, the patients may be approached as individuals. In the ward, almost invariably understaffed, every second counts, and bungling technique on the part of one worker may seriously disrupt the schedule for the entire staff. In the ward, moreover, some of the patients are, as a rule, dangerously ill, and therefore the immediate responsibility of the nursing staff is serious. It is almost as though the institutional nurse while on duty lived face to face with a state of perpetual emergency. In an emergency there must be a high degree of effective workmanship as well as swift obedience to orders!

It must take the highest kind of skill and insight, and a fine social philosophy as well, to distinguish between the periods when the nursing staff must be consciously spurred into action, caught up and held at a high pitch of readiness to do exactly the right thing at exactly the right time, and those other periods when no such emergency is at hand and when, if the nurses are to retain their emotional resiliency (which is what makes such efficient functioning possible) they must be made to relax and take their human contacts casually. If she is unable to secure casual and human friendliness among students and graduate nurses during slack and off-time periods, many a superintendent runs the risk of poor supervisory technique. She makes the mistake of believing that relaxation is detrimental to authority.

It is said of certain famous hospitals that the operating room *after the operations are over* becomes almost a scene of gayety. Surgeons and nurses who have been working with the absolute discipline of perfect team play suddenly, when the strain is over, snap back for a few minutes into rather shockingly naughty boys and girls. They may not know it, but this is probably merely another aspect of their efficiency. The violin string snaps if it is held tight too long; and the good player loosens the tension before laying the instrument down. So also the Chief in the operating room, and the Superintendent of Nurses in the hospital, are psychologically wise if they consciously loosen tension between themselves and their subordinates when periods of emergency are over.

The Superintendent of Nurses who wants to hold an intelligent and happy graduate staff must somehow learn what is evidently the extremely difficult technique of constructive leadership in the hospital, with its alternating demands for stimulation and relaxation. It is a subject which will require much thoughtful consideration and breadth of view. She can learn a great deal, evidently, from the experience already on record in public health organizations; and she will need to add to that a fund of further experience to meet the peculiar needs of hospital nursing.

Advocates of graduate general staff nursing claim that the salaries as now paid are adequate to attract and hold high grade bedside nurses. They suggest that the chief reasons for dissatisfaction among general duty nurses are not based on questions of salary, but are more fundamental. In reply to questions as to how graduate staffs may be made effective, they suggest the following principles.

a. Employ *enough* nurses so that patients can be properly cared for. Watch the load of work, and when pressure becomes too great, add more nurses until pressure is over. Not only preach good bedside care, but make it possible.

b. Employ head nurses and supervisors who are at least of as good quality, and if possible a little better quality, than the rank and file. Emphasize the importance of having head nurses and supervisors not only good administrators, but *good bedside nurses*. Encourage them to give informal demonstrations of skilful bedside technique when opportunities offer, so that the staff will realize that the people at the top are proud of being good bedside nurses.

c. Help nurses to realize that it is just as noble to take care of a rich person as of a poor one. Give them pride in understanding the psychology of all patients; and in giving high grade nursing care in private rooms, in semi-private rooms, and in the wards. Try to establish the tradition throughout the hospital that *every patient shall be given as much care as he needs;* that the amount of nursing care shall depend upon the patient's condition, and not upon his pocketbook; and that no patient need employ a special nurse in order to be safe while in that hospital.

d. Offer the prevailing basic salaries for general duty, but in addition permit nurses to live outside if they desire, and give them a reasonable money allowance in lieu of full maintenance.

e. Watch staff nurses, and when feasible, promote them from the staff to head and supervisory positions. Establish the understanding that the door is open to nurses with executive or teaching capacity who wish to climb. Also provide for pay increases within the staff, so that nurses excellent in bedside technique, but not of administrative or teaching types, may still be encouraged and rewarded.

f. Establish an eight hour day, and at least one full day off each week. Except in genuine emergencies do not allow this full day's rest to be interrupted by hospital responsibilities. Try to enforce this rule for every one from the superintendent down.

g. Offer opportunities for study. Encourage the completion of high school work, and the taking of courses in the college and university. Provide for staff conferences and demonstrations. Secure the cooperation of physicians in giving bedside clinics especially arranged for the nursing staff.

7. Some Financial and Professional Considerations

In commenting upon their suggestions, these superintendents of nurses claim that most of the points in the foregoing list call not so much for large expenditure of money as for intelligence, sympathy, and a modern viewpoint.

a. Provision for increases in salary and for the addition of temporary workers during peak periods might be largely offset by the savings resulting from decreased turnover.

b. Moreover, if the general staff could be imbued with genuine pride in bedside care, and given enough time to render such care, the hospital's reputation would grow and its number of pay patients would greatly increase. It is urged that as soon as physicians discover hospitals where private duty patients can receive high grade nursing care from the regular nursing staff, without having to employ special nurses, they will urge their patients to go there. Moderate increases in the regular hospital charge, made to all pay patients which would go far towards offsetting the costs of the more generous supply of staff nurses, could be met without hardship by the patient, if he did not have to pay in addition for the full time services of special nurses.

c. It is pointed out in this connection that while the general adoption of these principles would undoubtedly greatly decrease the opportunities for employment as "specials" among private duty nurses, it would at the same time open up to them a new field, better paid and far more attractive to many nurses than private duty. The outstanding fact in the comments of private duty nurses is that they *love bedside nursing*. The general employment of graduate nurses in hospitals under modern professional conditions such as outlined above would, it is urged, afford broad scope for women now in private duty whose chief interest is not in preventive health teaching, or in administration, but is in the *nursing of sick patients*.

d. The comment is made that while many superintendents of nurses may be distressed at the suggestion that they give up their schools of nursing, and that they place the care of patients entirely in the hands of graduate nurses, such a course might often, in the long run, be more satisfactory for the patient, less expensive for the hospital, better for the future of the nursing profession, and—if she were willing and able to master the technique of staff leadership—considerably less nerve-wracking and more satisfying to the superintendent of nurses herself. This opinion would probably not be accepted by most superintendents of nurses. It represents the combined judgments of the few who have been particularly successful in the employment of graduate general duty staff nurses.

8. SUMMARY

To summarize this discussion:

a. The fact that the largest and best known hospitals take student service for granted as a means of staffing their floors is a natural result of the way in which the profession started. Until recently, graduate nurses were not available in sufficient numbers to carry hospital work. The question has been not whether graduates were better than students, but rather whether students were better than attendants or practical nurses for the care of the sick.

b. The result of the demonstrated value of students, however, is that hospitals will naturally hesitate to change from a student system which gives good service to a graduate system with which they have had no real experience.

c. Most hospitals feel that they would much prefer to have students rather than graduates to take care of their patients. This is partly because it is cheaper to run a poor school than to pay graduate salaries.

d. Even in cases where the schools are genuinely good, and therefore expensive, most superintendents of nurses would prefer to continue with student service.

e. This means that the fight to demonstrate the superiority of *trained* nurses in bedside care is not yet won. There is something wrong with a viewpoint which prefers the services of partially trained women to those who have finished training.

f. Perhaps the chief reason for preferring students to graduates is that students will accept without complaint conditions which graduate nurses will not tolerate.

g. In addition, since graduate floor duty nurses are drawn primarily from the private duty field, they are frequently unfitted to step back into the highly organized, often hectic, professional atmosphere of the hospital.

h. Graduate nurses hesitate to undertake floor duty.

(1) They believe the pay is too low. This is probably not true.

(2) They feel that because of pressure of work and inadequate numbers of workers, it is not possible to do good bedside nursing in a hospital.

(3) Head nurses and supervisors are often of low caliber.

(4) General duty nurses must sometimes live in hospitals. Many nurses prefer to live outside.

(5) Because of too few workers, hours are often long and rest periods irregular.

(6) General floor duty is not respected by other nurses or by physicians.

(7) There is no future.

i. Some superintendents are eager to work with graduate staffs. They feel that the technique of staff administration and leadership can be as successful in the hospital as it is in public health. They make the following suggestions:

(1) Hire enough nurses. Not only preach good bedside care but make it possible.

(2) Select head nurses and supervisors with care. Encourage them to demonstrate their own skill as bedside nurses.

(3) Establish the tradition that every patient shall be given as much care as he needs and that specials are not necessary for safety.

(4) Offer the prevailing general duty salaries but in addition permit nurses to live outside and offer them a cash allowance for maintenance.

(5) When feasible, promote head and supervisory nurses from the staff group. Also provide for salary increases within the staff.

(6) Establish and protect an eight hour day and a five and a half or six day week.

(7) Encourage staff nurses to take college and university courses. Arrange for bedside nursing clinics within the hospital.

j. Superintendents making these suggestions believe that they call not so much for the expenditure of money as for intelligent sympathy and a modern viewpoint. They point out that

(1) Decreased turnover will partly offset salary increases.

(2) Increased size of staff and improved quality of floor duty will mean the reduction in the use of specials. The regular hospital charge to patients might be increased if patients knew that they did not need to employ special nurses.

(3) The reduction in the number of specials would be offset, from the nurses' viewpoint by the greater and more attractive opportunity for nurses in general duty.

(4) Superintendents make these recommendations believing that the change from wholly student service to wholly or partly graduate service would, in the long run, be more satisfactory for the patient, less expensive for the hospital, than running a really good school, better for the future of the nursing profession, and more satisfying to the superintendent of nurses.

CHAPTER 27

NURSING THE COUNTRY PATIENT

The care of the country patient seems to present a series of problems peculiarly baffling. The Committee does not feel that it has as yet collected many data which will be of help in discussions along this line. It does not want to close this book, however, without attempting to summarize the comments most frequently made on the problem of rural nursing, and the suggestions which seem to promise hope for successful experiment and solution.

Probably the schools of nursing most frequently under fire are those in rural districts. There are some schools which have only two or three students, and where the daily average of patients is often not much more. Nurse educators feel strongly that such schools, however well intentioned, are actually dangerous in their results, since they send out as trained graduate nurses young women who cannot possibly have had the breadth of clinical experience necessary to fit them for general nursing service.

Hospital administrators who are responsible for conducting these schools are able, however, to furnish rather potent arguments in favor of continuing the present method. The gist of what they say is that in their communities people must either go entirely without hospital care, or must come to the small local hospitals which are under discussion. They say, that is, that in many parts of the country, even with improved highways and automobile service, the larger hospitals are too far away to meet the needs of the country patient. The hospital, they say, is rendering an important local service.

When it is suggested that the need for hospital facilities is not in itself an adequate reason for trying to conduct a vocational school under the hospital roof, the reply is that even if the hospital were prepared to pay the costs of graduate service, it would not be possible to secure a suitable nursing staff of graduates, because graduate nurses do not want to stay in small country hospitals. Students, on the other hand, will stay. The statement is also made (and this seems more open to question) that the school is making a real contribution because its graduates stay at home and do local nursing. On this point there seems to be wide difference of opinion since the medical profession furnishes rather conclusive evidence that in rural communities there is not enough private duty nursing on a $6.00 a day basis to support graduate nurses. The products of the local schools must either go somewhere else where they can get more cases, or must rely upon donations from their relatives to support them between cases. The argument that the hospital cannot retain graduate nurses, however, seems to carry much truth with it.

In arguing for the school, again, the hospital administrator goes on to say that experience in a small rural hospital, whether as student or graduate, is extremely valuable. Its administrative problems are generalized not specialized, and the nurse, therefore, gets a broad and varied viewpoint. Also, since its patients are friends and neighbors instead of strangers, the nurse learns to think of them as human beings and not cases. The testimony from some superintendents of nurses who are doing administrative work in these very small hospitals seems to corroborate these statements.

1. Why Small Rural Schools Are Criticized

Nurse educators are apt to accept the suggestion that there is something in the country hospital experience which is of real value to the student nurse, but they feel that the disadvantages are so serious as to offset the advantages in that situation. They say that the extremely small school cannot observe high standards in selecting students, since it must draw its students from a relatively small area, and cannot hope to secure those with high educational ambitions. They say that the small rural school of this type cannot possibly afford an adequate teaching staff, well-equipped laboratories, or thorough educational facilities which are essential; that because it is so small it cannot afford a sufficient variety or quantity of clinical experience; that the student does not learn good bedside nursing because she is not given enough of it. Finally, they say that the extremely small rural hospital is often privately owned, under one man's control, and run for personal convenience or profit. Such owners usually know very little about the principles of education, and they cannot be expected to know how to run real schools.

2. Public Health Rural Nursing

When the problem of nursing the country patient is being discussed by public health nurses, they agree that more public health nurses are desperately needed in rural communities. They say that the positions are not very well paid, that since the workers are either alone or in pairs they feel isolated, and that the difficulties and responsibilities which they must carry are considerably more serious than those with which the staff members in city organizations are usually faced. It is hard, therefore, to find public health nurses of the necessary initiative, resourcefulness, and ability to handle people, who will accept rural appointments. Young women of these qualifications are usually able to find city appointments for which the pay is better and the work easier. The public health group in discussing rural problems, goes on to say that perhaps the greatest handicap is that in rural communities it is difficult to secure strong local backing, and careful professional leadership, and that public health without these two forms of support is often ineffective.

3. Private Duty and Graduate Floor Duty

Nurses who are considering either graduate work in hospitals or private duty work in homes, agree that country life is lonely. The nurse is completely cut off from her friends. If she is trying to do private duty she finds living conditions primitive and is often taxed to the utmost to adapt home equipment so that patients will get the sort of care which is possible in well-equipped hospitals. The private duty nurse sent out from the city registry is afraid that she may have to work with a strange physician. Some of the physicians in country districts do not know and do not approve of graduate nurses. She finds that they are sometimes on the defensive because they fear that coming from an up to date training school she may want to teach them something about the care of patients, and she finds this defensive attitude very difficult to deal with. Finally the private duty nurse says that she cannot possibly afford to live in the country, because when she works she cannot always collect her bills, and there is not work enough at any time to make her self-supporting.

Graduate nurses hesitate to accept general floor duty in rural hospitals because the life is lonely. The neighbors are sometimes aloof and unfriendly, and the nurse is expected to live a cloistered existence. Either the staff is short-handed and she is given administrative and nursing duties so numerous and varied that she is under constant strain, or else there is so little to do that the work is monotonous. Cases are few in number, and are apt to be of only one or two types, depending upon the practice in which the owner of the hospital is engaged. Treatments become stereotyped; and the nurse loses the stimulus of new ways, new techniques, and the discussion of new medical and nursing problems. Finally, she says that because the institution is small and the life confining, the personalities of the staff are apt to clash.

4. One Possible Solution

Could these services be combined? The suggestion has been made from several sources, by those who are particularly interested in the rural nursing problem, that a possible solution may come for most of these difficulties by a careful combination of public health and institutional nursing. It is suggested that if there were some way for combining the administration of rural public health work with the administration of the local hospital so that the hospital might become a genuine health center with a unified program for indoor and outdoor service, the effectiveness of the entire health program might be definitely increased.

If nurses could be placed upon the staff who would be

equally competent in hospital bedside nursing, and in rural public health nursing, they might alternate these services so that each nurse would find variety and interest in her work. Nurses would be able to learn the problems of the community in the homes; to follow up the cases through actual bedside service in the hospital; and then follow the patient out again into his home for after-care. This arrangement would bring more patients into the hospital, and would at the same time give a professional center for the public health activities. It should make possible the employment, as superintendent of the joint nursing service, of a nurse who would be highly qualified, and who would be able to provide real staff leadership inside and outside the hospital walls; and it ought to provide legitimate means for so increasing the money income of the hospital that the costs of the larger and improved service could be adequately met.

The Grading Committee has as yet no data upon which to judge whether the foregoing suggestion is practicable or not. It is felt, however, that it is worth while at this time to offer the suggestion for the consideration of the public health, hospital, medical, and nursing groups.

5. SUMMARY

This discussion may be summarized as follows:

a. Nursing schools in rural districts are frequently under fire. Those who administer them say that the small rural hospital is a social necessity; that the hospital could not meet the costs of graduate service; and that the only way to preserve a nursing staff is to secure students, since graduates will not stay.

b. They also say that the products of the local schools serve a felt need as graduate private duty nurses in the community. There is reason to doubt the validity of this argument, since there is evidence to indicate that private duty nurses cannot find sufficient employment at reasonable wages to support themselves in country areas.

c. The hospital administrator states that work in a country hospital whether as student or graduate nurse is professionally stimulating and valuable.

d. Nurse educators agree that the experience has many advantages, but point out that rural nursing schools are apt to admit students with inadequate social and educational backgrounds. They say that the cost of education is too great to be borne by the very small hospital, and that the clinical material furnished by such a hospital is inadequate for bedside training. They point out that the small rural hospital is frequently a commercial proposition, and that the owner or owners are not usually educators.

e. Public health nurses say that more public health work is needed in rural communities. The positions are not well paid; the workers are isolated; and the problems make heavy demands upon the workers. Women competent to fill the positions are usually attracted by city organizations. Perhaps the greatest handicap in rural communities is the difficulty in securing strong local backing and careful professional leadership.

f. Graduate nurses considering private duty in the country speak of the isolation of the nurse; the primitive conditions under which she must work;

frequent conflict with country physicians; and the inability of the nurse to earn enough to live on.

g. Graduate nurses avoid floor duty in rural hospitals because the life is lonely; the duties are either too heavy or too light; nursing treatments are stereotyped; and there is little professional stimulus. The confining life of the small hospital makes for the clash of personalities.

h. It has been suggested that a combination of public health and hospital nursing might offset these difficulties. The hospital might become a health center with a unified indoor and outdoor program. Staff nurses could be selected equally competent in hospital nursing and in public health nursing. By alternating their services within and without the walls of the hospital they might find the variety and stimulus which under present conditions are lacking. The resulting popularity of the hospital and increase in patients, might make possible the employment, as superintendent of the joint nursing service, of a highly qualified nurse able to provide real staff leadership, which would make for the increased efficiency of the service and the contentment of the workers.

i. The Grading Committee is not in a position to state whether or not this suggestion is practicable; but it is believed that it should be given careful consideration by the public health, hospital, medical, and nursing groups who are particularly interested in the rural problem.

CHAPTER 28

THE COMMITTEE GOES ON

The Committee on the Grading of Nursing Schools was fortunate in being organized at a time when the whole nursing profession is apparently awake to its own problems and therefore interested and eager to take advantage of whatever material the Committee is able to gather. The plan for having such a Committee was inaugurated many years before it reached fruition. There is evidence to indicate that had the work been undertaken much earlier, it could not have served the needs of the profession to anything like the degree which is apparently now possible. Had the work of the Committee been delayed for many more years, it would perhaps have been too late to have met the emergency which is apparently now at hand.

One is conscious of nice accord between the work of the Grading Committee and the thinking and planning of the nursing profession at large. When the Director for the Committee first undertook her work, she was alert to detect evidences of pressure from the nurses, who might logically have been expected to use whatever influence they had to sway her judgment along the lines they desired. (It should be remembered that at that time the Director was not well acquainted with nurses.) When month followed month and no evidence of pressure developed, she finally sought out several of the more thoughtful women in different fields and asked them outright why—when so much power for good or harm had been given to the Grading Committee—the nurses were apparently willing to keep their hands off. The answer was, "Because we are so sure of what you will find; and we want you to find it in your own way!"

Not all nurses, of course, could have anticipated the findings presented in the preceding chapters. But it is probably safe to say that each of the more important conclusions reached in this report had already been suggested years earlier, and can be found in print in nursing literature. The difference is that whereas, in the past, the suggestions have been based upon the opinions of a few thoughtful individuals in one or two fields, the present report is based upon the actual experience of many thousands of individuals in many different fields. In the past, suggestions have been colored by the personality of the one who made them. Now they are a composite of the combined judgments and experiences not only of nurses, but also of physicians, patients, and others who are not themselves nurses but who have to deal with them. It is believed that the material presented in this report represents the experience of a sufficiently representative and numerous body of contributors so that it may be safely taken as a basis for action. The Committee is fortunate in being able to present its report to an intelligent and alert body ready to digest the findings and use them wisely.

1. Group Discussion Needed

The semi-annual conferences of the members of the Grading Committee have been steadily increasing in interest and value as it has become possible to substitute a fact basis for previously conflicting bases of opinion.

It is believed that this method of approach will be equally attractive to their professional colleagues. While the initiative in nursing reforms should probably come from nurses, swift progress is impossible without the thoughtful and cordial cooperation of medical, hospital, public health, educational, and patient groups, and it would therefore seem desirable that special conferences be organized among all of them, meeting separately and jointly, for the consideration of the facts in nursing, and the problems those facts raise.

As the author attempted to point out in her brief paragraph of acknowledgment at the beginning of this book, the members of the Grading Committee represent many different groups with many different professional interests at stake. This very fact—that they are a mixed group drawn from different professions, and that they feel strongly on many nursing problems—is probably the reason why the meetings of the Committee have become so stimulating, and their results so valuable. Each member respects the opinions of the others, and no member knows what his neighbor is about to say next! The result is that everyone learns from everyone else. If, then, discussion in a mixed group, representing really thoughtful people with many different viewpoints, can be so worthwhile for a committee, is not the plan worth trying in other situations as well?

2. Further Studies Needed

The Committee is only too well aware that the supply and demand study, as reported in this volume, has left untouched many important questions. Probably every reader as he goes through these pages will ask why certain obviously important questions have been left untouched, and perhaps he will say to himself, "I wonder if some of us couldn't help find the answers?"

This is what the Committee hopes for. There are some problems which the Committee is definitely planning to study. Others it would like to, but probably cannot arrange to carry through. Still others are outside the Committee's field. The need for them is apparent, but they are not strictly the Committee's business, nor can they be properly fitted into the already adopted program.

The Committee will welcome every thoughtfully conducted study which will throw more light upon the nursing problem. This matter has been discussed at various times with the different members, and they have gone on record as sincerely desirous that other organizations will undertake the scientific study of certain of these problems in nursing economics, and will make their findings available to all who can use them. Of especial importance and timeliness would seem to be:

Careful cost accounting studies carried on by hospitals using different methods of administering their nursing services;

Experiments in the organization and administration of central community nurse registries;

Experiments in hourly nursing in homes;

Experiments in group nursing in hospitals;

Studies in graduate floor duty nursing in hospitals with special attention to supervisory problems;

Community surveys to discover the relation of sickness to nursing needs; and the desirable ratio of nurses to physicians and to population;

Experiments among private duty nurses to discover practicable methods for cooperating in order to meet the needs of patients, and at the same time equalize the burden and privileges of all nurses in the group.

3. The Committee's Plans

It would furnish deep satisfaction to the members of the Committee on the Grading of Nursing Schools were they free to continue studying the economic aspects of nursing. They are, however, working on a limited budget and with limited time, knowing that even though they have only begun to touch many of the important aspects in this field, they must nevertheless proceed with their own program as previously adopted. They must from now on lay less stress upon economic problems, and begin a more careful inquiry into the nature of nursing education and the methods by which schools of nursing may be studied and graded. Everything that has been gathered in this first phase of the work is offered to the members of the parent organizations and to all others who are concerned. The Committee itself will now go on, carrying through the rest of its previously announced program.

4. SUMMARY

This chapter attempts to point out:

1. The Grading Committee was appointed at the psychological time. It has gathered very little which is new; but it has, it is believed, in this report been able to supplement the opinions of thoughtful individuals by a firmer foundation of testimony from large numbers.
2. The Grading Committee—a mixed group with strong and varying professional interests—has found group conferences of increasing value. The

suggestion is made that their colleagues in the various professions represented on the Committee would also find such cooperative discussion groups of interest and value.

3. The Grading Committee has left untouched many problems which it cannot, or should not, include in its own program, and yet which obviously need careful and expert study. The Committee is eager to see such studies carried on. It has listed a few for which there seems to be particular need. Others will suggest themselves.
4. In this book the Committee offers everything that has been gathered in the first phase of its work to the parent organizations it represents and to all others who are concerned with nurses. It will now proceed with the next project in its program.

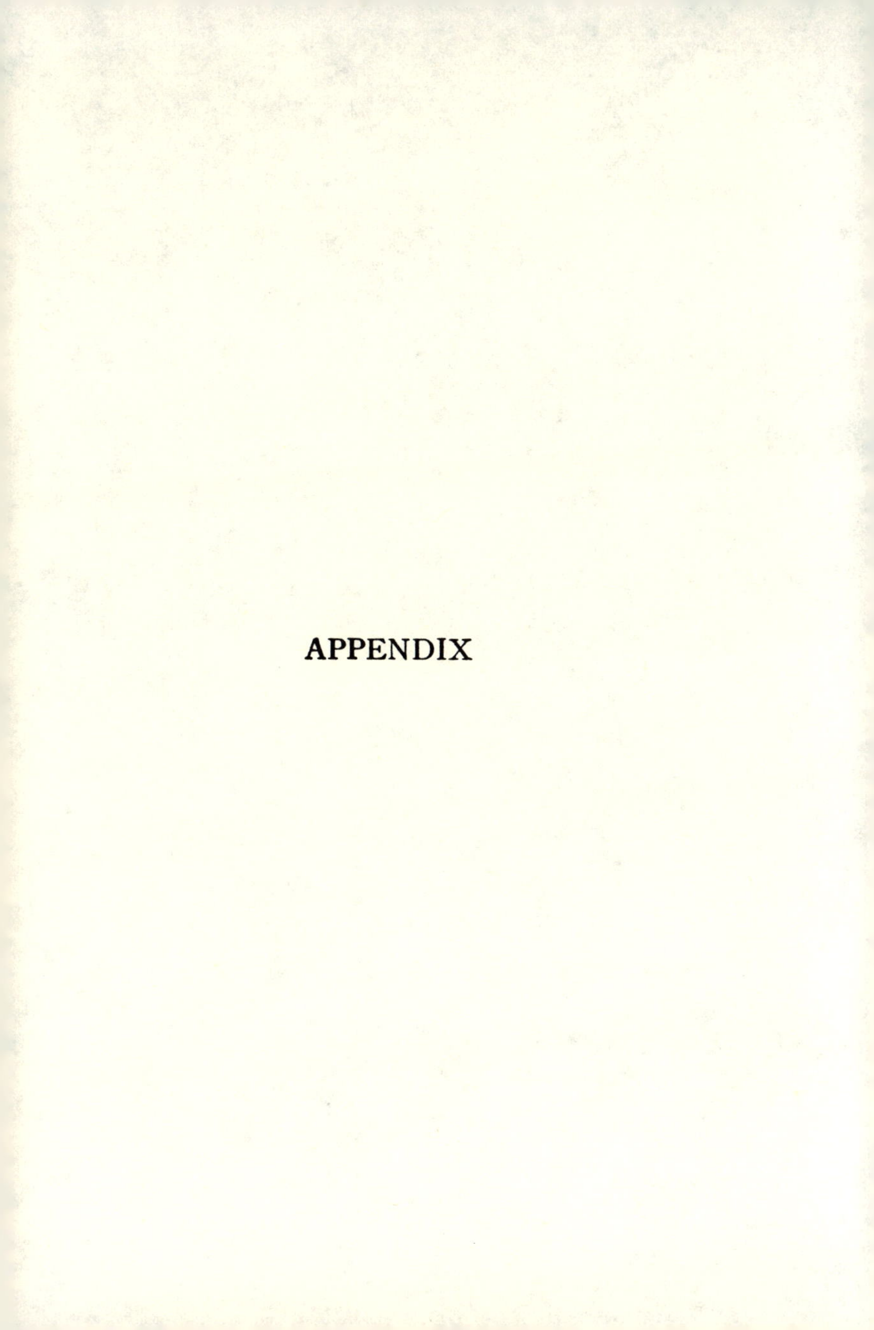

APPENDIX

APPENDIX

TEXT OF QUESTIONNAIRES

In order that readers may know the exact wording used in gathering the data shown in the body of this book, the text of the nineteen questionnaires involved is given here. No attempt is made to indicate arrangement and spacing, although of course these were actually worked out with great care. Forms A, 12, and 14 were printed as return postals. Form 18 was really a letter rather than a questionnaire. Forms 1 through 11, 13, and 15 through 17 were all printed on white sheets 8½x 11, of good quality paper. All the printed matter was on the front of the sheet. The backs were left free for comments and emotions. Return unstamped envelopes were included.

Those who are interested in statistical technique will note that on each of the standard type questionnaires there is a key question, usually towards the end, which is designed to make the correspondent talk; and on a subject on which his opinion will be of real value. In Form 1, for example, the key question was "Would you like to have the same nurse again on a similar case?" There are usually one or two other questions on each sheet which are designed for the same purpose. It is believed that the thought given to the selection and formulation of these particular questions was justified by the exceptionally thoughtful quality of most of the replies received on the backs of the questionnaires.

The total supply and demand study involved the

distribution of 343,772 questionnaires, of which 67,938 were returned at the time tabulations were completed. (Additional returns are being received daily.) The percentage of returns runs from 4 to 70.

FORM A

Return postal. Sent to 59,000 nurses in ten states. Returns: 24,389, or 41%.

(Face of postal)

NOTICE TO ALL NURSES

This card is the first step in a study of the alleged nursing shortage, which is being made by the COMMITTEE ON THE GRADING OF NURSING SCHOOLS. The Committee is a co-operative body of nurses, doctors, health workers, and hospital administrators, attempting to investigate and to find constructive suggestions for improving the present conditions in nursing. The nurse members of the Committee are: Helen Wood, Susan Francis, Elizabeth C. Burgess, Laura R. Logan, Katharine Tucker, and Gertrude Hodgman. The nurse consultant is Janet M. Geister. The plan for making the study is approved by the presidents of the American Nurses' Association, the National League of Nursing Education, and the National Organization for Public Health Nursing.

The study will not be worth while unless large numbers of nurses take part. Please help, by answering the questions on the other part of this postal card, and mailing it as soon as possible, to

THE COMMITTEE ON THE GRADING OF NURSING SCHOOLS

WILLIAM DARRACH, M.D., *Chairman*
MAY AYRES BURGESS, PH.D., *Director*

(Reverse of postal)

1 Name (Mrs., Miss, Mr.)..........
Address: Street..........City..........State..........
2 Name of your training school (if you did not go to a training school omit items 2 and 3)..........
....
3 Year you left training.......... Were you graduated?..........
4 Year you registered in this state..........
5 In how many different states (including Canada) have you worked since you finished training?..........

6 Please check which of the following types of work you expect to do in 1927:

........a. Private duty
........b. Hourly
........c. Visiting nursing
........d. Other public health
........e. Industrial
........f. Hospital nursing staff
........g. Hospital floor duty
........h. Nursing school staff
........i. Anæsthetist
........j. Sanitarium staff
........k. Resident in school, orphanage, etc.
........l. Stay at home
........m. Doctor's office
........n. Dentist's office
........o. Beauty parlor
........p. Demonstrator of drugs, appliances, etc.
........q. Other

7 Which of the different types of nursing listed above have you done since you finished training? (Use a, b, c, etc., instead of writing the words out in full)—

....

Send this in and watch for our next letter!

FORM 1

8½ x 11 sheet. Sent to 38,000 subscribers to the Journal of the American Medical Association in ten states. Returned 1,459, or 4%.

FORM 1

The Doctor and the Private Duty Nurse

DEAR DOCTOR: These questions are to help the Committee on the Grading of Nursing Schools in its study of the nursing shortage. They can be answered in ten minutes. They will not get any nurse into trouble, because you need not give either your name or her name. Please give here the City..........................State.......................
Date..........................and then answer the following questions about your experience with private duty nurses *during the past week.*

1. How many of your patients *needed* private duty nurses last week? How many got them?
2. Of the patients who needed private duty nurses, *but did not get them*, how many failed because they (a) could not find a nurse? (b) could not afford nurse? (c) did not want nurse? (d) called a visiting nurse instead? (e) a relative or friend gave care?
PLEASE CHOOSE ONE OF YOUR PATIENTS WHO HAD A PRIVATE DUTY NURSE LAST WEEK, AND ANSWER THE FOLLOWING QUESTIONS ABOUT THE CASE:
3. Was case (a) surgical, (b) medical, (c) obstetric, (d) pediatric, (e) contagious, (f) mental or nervous? (check which).
4. Was it (a) a short time, or (b) a long time illness? Was it (c) mild, or (d) severe?
5. Was nurse secured through (a) hospital registry; (b) central professional registry; (c) commercial registry; (d) from your private list; (e) from some other doctor; (f) other? or (g) don't you know? (check which).
6. Was it (a) easy; (b) rather difficult; or (c) very difficult to secure the nurse?
7. Was nurse (a) R.N.; (b) practical; or (c) don't you know?
8. Was she on (a) day; (b) night; or (c) 24 hour duty?
9. What did nurse charge per day?
10. Was patient in (a) home, or (b) hospital, or (c) both?
11. In your opinion, was nurse (a) very good; (b) good; (c) fair; (d) poor; (e) very poor?
12. Would you like to have the same nurse again on a similar case?

13. Please check which of the types of nursing given in the list below were particularly needed for this case.

- *a.* Mother's helper and houseworker
- *b.* Responsible adult to take charge of family
- *c.* Skill in giving general care and making patient comfortable
- *d.* Skill in giving special treatments
- *e.* Care in following medical orders
- *f.* Skill in handling people
- *g.* Skill in observing and reporting symptoms
- *h.* Skill in asepsis
- *i.* Ability to work under heavy strain
- *j.* Experience and background
- *k.* Good breeding and attractive personality
- *l.* Familiarity with particular disease
- *m.* Familiarity with hospital routine
- *n.* Familiarity with your personal methods

14. Are you in general practice? If not, what is your specialty?

15. On the other side of this sheet, please make any comments which you think might throw light on the alleged nursing shortage. We should particularly like your reasons for the answer to question 12. You need not sign your name unless you wish; but we should like to have your frank opinion about the nurses who have personally worked with you *during the past week.*

Please Return this Sheet—in the Accompanying Envelope—by Tomorrow if you can—to the Committee on the Grading of Nursing Schools, 370 Seventh Avenue, New York City

FORM 2

8½ x 11 sheet. Sent to each of 38,000 physicians with letter requesting him to hand it to one of his patients who had recently had a special nurse. Returned 617. If only such physicians as answered Form 1 helped in distributing Form 2, this would be a 42% return.

FORM 2

The Patient and the Private Duty Nurse

DEAR DOCTOR: Please give this blank to one of your patients who has recently had a private duty nurse. The questions are to help the Committee on the Grading of Nursing Schools in its study of the alleged nursing shortage. Please fill in the answers to the questions in the first section, and then ask your patient to answer the others, and to mail the report to us. Patients should understand that no names need be used.

For the Doctor to Answer

City..............................State..............................Today's date.............

1. Patient is (a) man (b) woman (c) adolescent (d) child (check which).
2. Was case (a) surgical, (b) medical, (c) obstetric, (d) pediatric, (e) contagious, (f) mental or nervous? (check which).
3. Was it (a) a short time or (b) a long time illness? Was it (c) mild or (d) severe?
4. If patient was in hospital, please state, if you happen to know, its approximate daily average of patients.
5. Does hospital have a training school? Was nurse probably a graduate of it?

For the Patient to Answer

NOTE TO PATIENT: We want to find out what sort of nursing service patients are actually getting. Nothing you say here can make trouble for your nurse, because you need not tell either her name or your name. We do want to know, however, whether or not you liked her, and why. So please answer the following questions:

6. How many days did you have a nurse? About what date did she come? 7. Did you have any special difficulty in getting a nurse?
8. Did you get her from (a) hospital registry (b) central professional registry (c) commercial registry (d) your doctor's list (e) through some other doctor (f) through a friend (g) other (h) or don't you know? (check which).
9. Was she (a) a practical nurse (b) a registered nurse or (c) don't you know? 10. Was she on (a) day, (b) night, or (c) 24 hour service?

11. How much did she charge each day? Did this all go to her, or did she have to pay part of it to some one else?
12. Did you have her (a) in the hospital, (b) at home, or (c) both? 13. If both, was her service in the home (a) more, or (b) less satisfactory than in the hospital? Or (c) was it about equal?
14. Did the nurse seem to know her business? 15. Was she a pleasant person to have around? 16. Were you yourself an easy or a difficult patient to take care of?
17. Did you give the nurse any gifts or tips? If so, did you really want to? Or did you feel she expected you to?
18. What did you like about her? (answer on the back of the page if you need to).
19. What did you not like about her? (answer on the back of the page if you need to).
20. If the case were to happen over again, would you like to have the same nurse?
21. On the back of this sheet please write any comments which you think might help us in our study of what nurses are really like, and what problems arise in connection with their service. We should particularly like your reasons for your answer to question 20.

Please Return this Sheet—in the Accompanying Envelope—by Tomorrow if you can—to the Committee on the Grading of Nursing Schools, 370 Seventh Avenue, New York City

FORM 3

8½ x 11 sheet. Sent to each of 38,000 physicians with letter requesting him to hand it to one of his patients who had recently been in the hospital, but without a special nurse. If only such physicians as answered Form 1 helped in distributing Form 3, this would be a 39% return.

FORM 3

The Patient and the Hospital Nurse

Dear Doctor: Please give this blank to one of your patients *who has recently been in the hospital but did not have a special nurse*—who was cared for, that is, by the regular staff or student nurses. The questions are to help the Committee on the Grading of Nursing Schools in its studies of the alleged nursing shortage. Please fill in the answers to the questions in the first section, and then ask your patient to answer the others, and to mail the report to us. Patients should understand that no names need be used.

For the Doctor to Answer

City.......................... State.......................... Today's Date....................

1. Patient is (a) man (b) woman (c) adolescent (d) child (check which).
2. Was case (a) surgical, (b) medical, (c) obstetric, (d) pediatric, (e) contagious, (f) mental or nervous? (check which).
3. Was it (a) a short time; or (b) a long time illness? Was it (c) mild; or (d) severe?
4. If you happen to know, please state the hospital's approximate daily average of patients. 5. Has it a training school?

For the Patient to Answer

Note to Patient: We want to find out what sort of nursing service patients in hospitals are actually getting. Nothing you say here can make trouble for your nurses or your hospital, because you need not give any names. We do want to know, however, what your experience with nurses has recently been. So please answer the following questions:

6. How many days were you in the hospital? 7. How many beds were in the same room or section with yours or were you alone? 8. Were you cared for mostly by one or two nurses, or was the work distributed among many?
9. At what time were you wakened in the morning? 10. At what time did you have your supper at night?
11. Were you able to get a nurse reasonably quickly when you needed one? 12. Did the nurses seem to take special pains to make you comfortable? 13. Which did the nurses seem to care more about, making you comfortable, or getting the work done?

14. Were you yourself an easy or a difficult patient to take care of?
15. Did nurses seem to have time enough to do their work or were they always in a hurry?
16. Did the nurses seem happy? 17. Were the nurses friendly to you and to your visitors? 18. Did you give the nurses any gifts or tips? If so, did you really want to, or did you feel that they expected you to?
19. Did you feel that you were getting good care or poor care?
20. What did you like about the care you received? (answer on the back of the page if you need to).
21. What did you dislike about the care you received? (answer on the back of the page if you need to).
22. If the case were to happen again, would you like to go back to the same place?
23. On the back of this sheet, please make any comments which you think might throw light on the problem of nurses in hospitals, and the nursing care patients need. We should particularly like your reasons for your answer to question 22. You need not sign your name unless you want to.

Please Return this Sheet—in the Accompanying Envelope—by Tomorrow if you can—to the Committee on the Grading of Nursing Schools, 370 Seventh Avenue, New York City

FORM 4

8½ x 11 sheet. Sent to 9,666 nurses who had returned Form A and indicated that they were private duty nurses. Received back 3,392, or 35%.

FORM 4

The Private Duty Nurse—Her Job!

TO THE PRIVATE DUTY NURSE: A few weeks ago, when you answered one of our postal questionnaries, we asked you to "watch for our next letter." Here it is. These questions are to help the Committee on the Grading of Nursing Schools in its study of private duty nursing. The results will be published in the American Journal of Nursing. NO ONE WILL KNOW WHAT YOU HAVE SAID BECAUSE YOU NEED NOT SIGN YOUR NAME. The questions will not take more than 10 minutes to answer. Please fill in here your City.............................. State........................ ....Date........................ Then: Please give below your work record *for the week which is just finishing* when you receive this letter. Do not choose some "typical" week, choose *last* week. If you didn't work last week, answer as many questions as you can anyway. Remember, a week has 7 days!

1. How many days last week were you on a case? 2. How many days last week were you not on a case? 3. How many days last week were you too sick to work? 4. How many days last week were you on call?
5. How many days last week were you on day duty? Night? 24 hour? 6. How many days last week were you on case in hospital? At patient's home? 7. How many different cases did you have last week?
8. What do you register against?
9. How many calls did you refuse last week on days when you were not working?
10. If you are still on a case, how many days have you been on it? 11. If you have just finished a case, how many days had you been on it?
12. Did you get your last case through (a) hospital registry (b) central professional registry (c) commercial registry (d) doctor (e) friend or former patient (f) other? (check which).
13. How much money did you earn last week? 14. How much did you pay for laundry last week? 15. How much room rent do you pay each month? (If you share an apartment, state only your share of the rent. Do not include food.) 16. Have you had to borrow money to live on during the past twelve months?
17. How much money did you earn in 1926? (If you don't know, say so.) 18. Have you as much as $200 set aside which you could use in case you became ill? $500? $1,000?
19. In what country was your father born? 20. What is, or was,

his occupation? (State what he did, and where he did it, as, "clerk in shoe store," "puddler in steel mill," etc.)

21. Did you finish grammar school? 1st year high school? 2d year? 3d year? 4th year? (If you had additional schooling, state what.)

22. In what state was your training school located? 23. When you were there, about how many patients did the hospital usually care for at one time? 24. In what year did you finish training? Did you get your diploma?

25. In how many different states, including Canada, have you worked since you finished training?

26. Please check any of the following in which you have had experience since you finished training:

a. Private duty
b. Hourly nursing
c. Visiting nursing
d. Other public health
e. Industrial
f. Hospital nursing staff
g. Hospital floor duty
h. Nursing school teacher
i. Anesthetist
j. Sanitarium staff
k. Resident in school, orphanage, etc.
l. Nursing a relative free of charge
m. Doctor's office
n. Dentist's office
o. Beauty parlor
p. Demonstrator of, drugs, appliances etc.
q. Other

27. Do you intend to keep on, indefinitely, in private duty nursing? (Please write your reasons on the back of this sheet. You need not sign the paper unless you want to. But we are anxious to learn what you really think about private duty nursing as a life work, and as compared with the other forms of nursing you have tried.)

Please Return this Sheet—in the Accompanying Envelope—by Tomorrow if you can—to the Committee on the Grading of Nursing Schools, 370 Seventh Avenue, New York City

FORM 5

8½ x 11 sheet. Sent to 154 nurses whose returns on Form A had indicated that they were doing hourly nursing. Returned 49, or 32%. This proved a shot in the dark. Forms 4, 5, 6, and 7 were, of necessity, planned and printed before Form A had had time to come back. It was expected that there would be many more hourly nurses than proved to be the case.

FORM 5

The Hourly Nurse—Her Job!

TO THE HOURLY NURSE: A few weeks ago, when you answered one of our postal questionnaires, we asked you to "watch for our next letter." Here it is. These questions are to help the Committee on the Grading of Nursing Schools in its study of hourly nursing. The results will be published in the American Journal of Nursing. NO ONE WILL KNOW WHAT YOU HAVE SAID BECAUSE YOU NEED NOT SIGN YOUR NAME. The questions will not take more than 10 minutes to answer. Please fill in here your City......................State................ Date..........................Then: Please give below your work record *for the week which is just finishing* when you receive this paper. Do not choose some typical week, choose *last* week. If you didn't work last week, answer as many questions as you can, anyway. Remember, a week has 7 days!

1. How many days last week were you on duty? 2. How many days last week were you not on duty? 3. How many days last week were you too sick to work? 4. How many days last week were you on call?
5. How many nursing visits did you make last week? 6. To how many *different* patients did you give actual nursing care last week?
7. Of the patients you nursed last week, how many did you get through (a) hospital registry (b) central professional registry (c) commercial registry (d) the patient's doctor (e) some other doctor (f) your friend or former patient (g) other?
8. How many calls did you refuse last week on days when you were not working? Of these, how many did you refuse (a) because you wanted to rest? (b) because they were out of your line?
9. How much money did you earn last week? 10. Are you on a yearly salary from some central organization or are you paid so much per hour?
11. During the past month have you done (a) all hourly nursing or (b) some hourly and some private or (c) nearly all private?
12. How much did you pay for laundry last week? 13. How much room rent do you pay each month? (If you share an apartment, state only your share of the rent. Do not include food.) 14.

Have you had to borrow money to live on during the past twelve months?

15. How much money did you earn in 1926? (If you don't know, say so.) 16. Have you as much as $200 set aside which you could use in case you became ill? $500? $1,000? Were you an hourly nurse in 1926?

17. In what country was your father born? 18. What is, or was, his occupation? (State what he did and where he did it, as, "clerk in shoe store," "puddler in steel mill," etc.)

19. Did you finish grammar school? 1st year high school? 2d year? 3d year? 4th year? (If you had additional schooling, state what.)

20. In what state was your training school located? 21. When you were there, about how many patients did the hospital usually care for at one time? 22. In what year did you finish training? Did you get your diploma?

23. In how many different states, including Canada, have you worked since you finished training?

24. Please check any of the following in which you have had experience since you finished training:

a. Private duty
b. Hourly nursing
c. Visiting nursing
d. Other public health
e. Industrial
f. Hospital nursing staff
g. Hospital floor duty
h. Nursing school teacher
i. Anesthetist
j. Sanitarium staff
k. Resident in school, orphange, etc.
l. Nursing a relative free of charge
m. Doctor's office
n. Dentist's office
o. Beauty parlor
p. Demonstrator of drugs, appliances, etc.
q. Other

25. Do you intend to keep on indefinitely in hourly nursing? (Please write your reasons on the back of this sheet. You need not sign the paper unless you want to. But we are anxious to learn what you really think about hourly nursing as a life work, and as compared with the other forms of nursing you have tried.)

Please Return this Sheet—in the Accompanying Envelope—by Tomorrow if you can—to the Committee on the Grading of Nursing Schools, 370 Seventh Avenue, New York City

FORM 6

8½ x 11 sheet. Sent to 3,422 nurses who on Form A had said that they were doing public health nursing. Returned 1,456, or 43%.

FORM 6

The Public Health Nurse—Her Job!

To the Public Health Nurse: A few weeks ago, when you answered one of our postal questionnaires, we asked you to "watch for our next letter." Here it is. These questions are to help the Committee on the Grading of Nursing Schools in its study of the alleged nursing shortage. The results will be published in the Public Health Nurse. No One Will Know What You Have Said Because You Need not Sign your Name. The questions will not take more than 10 minutes to answer. Please fill in here your City.................... State....................Date.................... Then: Please give below your work record *for the week which is just finishing* when you receive this paper. Do not choose some "typical" week, choose *last* week. Remember, a week has 7 days!

1. How many days last week were you on duty? 2. How many days last week were you not on duty? 3. How many days last week were you supposed to be off? 4. How many days last week were you too sick to work?
5. How many visits did you make last week? Of these, how many were primarily for sick-bed care and how many primarily for educational or welfare work?
6. How many *different* patients did you care for last week? Of these, how many received sick-bed care?
7. Are you (a) staff nurse (b) floating nurse (c) supervisor or assistant supervisor (d) director (e) other?
8. How much did you pay for laundry last week? 9. How much room rent do you pay each month? (If you share an apartment, state only your share of the rent. Do not include food.) 10. Have you had to borrow money to live on during the past twelve months?
11. What is your monthly pay? 12. How much money did you earn in 1926? (If you don't know, say so.) 13. Have you as much as $200 set aside which you could use in case you became ill? $500? $1,000?
14. In what country was your father born? 15. What is, or was, his occupation? (State what he did and where he did it, as, "clerk in shoe store," "puddler in steel mill," etc.)
16. Did you finish grammar school? 1st year high school? 2d year? 3d year? 4th year? (If you had additional schooling, state what.)
17. In what state was your training school located? 18. When you were there, about how many patients did the hospital usually

care for at one time? 19. In what year did you finish training? Did you get your diploma?

20. In how many different states, including Canada, have you worked since you finished training?

21. Please check any of the following in which you have had experience since you finished training:

a. Private duty
b. Hourly nursing
c. Visiting nursing
d. Other public health
e. Industrial
f. Hospital nursing staff
g. Hospital floor duty
h. Nursing school teacher
i. Anesthetist
j. Sanitarium staff
k. Resident in school, orphanage, etc.
l. Nursing a relative free of charge
m. Doctor's office
n. Dentist's office
o. Beauty parlor
p. Demonstrator of drugs, appliances, etc.
q. Other

22. Do you intend to continue indefinitely in public health nursing? (Please write your reasons on the back of this sheet. You need not sign your name unless you want to. But we are anxious to learn what you really think about public health nursing as a life work, and as compared with the other forms of nursing you have tried.)

Please Return this Sheet—in the Accompanying Envelope—by Tomorrow if you can—to the Committee on the Grading of Nursing Schools, 370 Seventh Avenue, New York City

FORM 7

8½ x 11 sheet. Sent to 4,296 nurses who on Form A had said that they were doing institutional nursing. Returned 1,908, or 44%.

FORM 7

The Institutional Nurse—Her Job!

To the Institutional Nurse: A few weeks ago, when you answered one of our postal questionnaires, we asked you to "watch for our next letter." Here it is. These questions are to help the Committee on the Grading of Nursing Schools in its study of the nursing shortage. They will not take more than 10 minutes to answer. The results will be published in the American Journal of Nursing. No One will Know What You Have Said, Because you Need not Sign your Name or give the Name of your Hospital. But do, please, answer the questions. Fill in here your City..........................State..........................Date...............and then: Please give below your work record *for the week which is just finishing* when you receive this paper. Do not choose some "typical" week; choose *last* week. Remember, a week has 7 days!

1. How many days last week were you on duty? 2. How many days last week were you not on duty? 3. How many days were you supposed to be off? 4. How many days last week were you too sick to work?
5. About how many hours did you work last week? Of those: 6. About how many hours do you estimate you spent in giving direct nursing care? 7. About how many hours do you estimate you spent in doing educational or supervisory work? 8. About how many hours do you estimate you spent in doing executive or clerical work?
9. Are you (a) superintendent of the hospital (b) superintendent of nurses (c) assistant superintendent (d) instructor or supervisor (e) staff, general duty, or floor nurse (f) head nurse in a department (as surgical, medical, clinic, etc.) (g) on special service (as dietitian, X-ray worker, laboratory worker, etc.) (h) administrative clerical worker (as recorder, librarian, admission clerk, bookkeeper, etc.) (i) matron of home (j) other?
10. What is your annual pay? Does this include maintenance? If you happen to know how much the hospital figures your annual maintenance is worth, please enter it here. 11. If hospital does not provide maintenance, how much room rent do you pay each month? (If you share an apartment, state only your share of the rent. Do not include food.)
12. Have you had to borrow money to live on during the past twelve months? 13. How much money did you earn in 1926? (If you don't know, say so.) 14. Have you as much as $200 set aside which you could use in case you became ill? $500? $1,000?

15. In what country was your father born? 16. What is, or was, his occupation? (State what he did and where he did it, as, "clerk in shoe store," "puddler in steel mill," etc.)
17. Did you finish grammar school? 1st year high school? 2d year? 3d year? 4th year? (If you had additional schooling, state what.)
18. In what state was your training school located? 19. When you were there, about how many patients did the hospital usually care for at one time? 20. In what year did you finish training? Did you get your diploma?
21. In how many different states, including Canada, have you worked since you finished training?
22. Please check any of the following in which you have had experience since you finished training:

a. Private duty
b. Hourly nursing
c. Visiting nursing
d. Other public health
e. Industrial
f. Hospital nursing staff
g. Hospital floor duty
h. Nursing school teacher
i. Anesthetist
j. Sanitarium staff
k. Resident in school, orphanage, etc.
l. Nursing a relative free of charge
m. Doctor's office
n. Dentist's office
o. Beauty parlor
p. Demonstrator of drugs, appliances, etc.
q. Other

23. Do you intend to continue indefinitely in institutional nursing? (Please write your reasons on the back of this sheet. You need not sign your name unless you want to. But we are anxious to learn what you really think about institutional nursing as a life work, and as compared with other forms of nursing you have tried.)

Please Return this Sheet—in the Accompanying Envelope—by Tomorrow if you can—to the Committee on the Grading of Nursing Schools, 370 Seventh Avenue, New York City

FORM 8

8½ x 11 sheet. Sent to 246 public health nursing organizations in ten states. Returned 108, or 44%.

FORM 8

Public Health and the Nursing Supply

To the Director: These questions are to help the Committee on the Grading of Nursing Schools in its study of the alleged nursing shortage. They can be answered in 10 minutes. We want to know what your experience has been in filling vacancies and in securing additional helpers for rush periods. You need not sign your name unless you want to.

Please give here your City..........................State..............................
Date..........................and then answer the following questions:

1. How many nurses are regularly on your staff?
2. *During the past month*, how many staff vacancies for nurses have you had? How many have you filled?
3. About how many applicants did you have for these vacancies?
4. Of the applicants whom you refused, *about how many* were ineligible because they:
   - *a.* Came from the wrong section of the country.
   - *b.* Did not have academic background needed.
   - *c.* Came from too small nursing schools.
   - *d.* Had not had broad enough general nursing experience.
   - *e.* Seemed to be poor bedside nurses.
   - *f.* Had not had theoretical courses in public health work.
   - *g.* Had not had enough practical public health experience.
   - *h.* Seemed to lack understanding of what public health work stands for.
   - *i.* Seemed to lack professional viewpoint.
   - *j.* Had personality difficulty.
   - *k.* Did not seem physically strong enough to do the work.
   - *l.* Other.
5. During the past month, how many extra people have you hired to help out during the rush period?
6. Of these "extras," how many were experienced public health nurses and how many were picked up from the local registries, or other sources, without special qualifications for public health work?
7. Of these "extras," how many would you like to keep on as regular nurses, if there were openings for them on the staff?
8. When you secure new workers for regular staff duty, are you usually able to rely upon their having satisfactory bedside nursing technique or must you teach them that, as well as the educational and preventive aspects peculiar to the public health field?
9. Do you usually have more applicants for staff positions than you need? or is this true only at certain seasons of the year? (When?) or is it almost never true?
10. Do inexperienced nurses resent supervision? Do the more experienced nurses?

11. Please check any of the following which you consider particularly important as means of keeping good workers contentedly on the staff:

a. A sliding salary scale
b. Regular hours
c. Vacations on pay
d. Staff courses and conferences
e. Frequent shifts in assignments of work
f. Sympathetic supervision
g. Hope of promotion to supervisory jobs
h. Opportunity for bedside nursing without idle time on duty.

12. On the other side of this page, please write any suggestions or comments which you think might help us in our study of the alleged nursing shortage. We should particularly like to know what if any difficulty you have in finding and keeping workers of the type you need.

Please Return this Sheet—in the Accompanying Envelope—by Tomorrow if you can—to the Committee on the Grading of Nursing Schools, 370 Seventh Avenue, New York City

FORM 9

8½ x 11 sheet. Sent to 2,892 superintendents of nurses in hospitals with and without schools in ten states. Returned 653, or 23%.

FORM 9

The Hospital and the Graduate Nurse

TO THE SUPERINTENDENT OF NURSES: These questions are to help the Committee on the Grading of Nursing Schools in its study of the alleged nursing shortage. They will not take more than 10 minutes to answer. NOTHING YOU SAY HERE CAN MAKE TROUBLE FOR ANY NURSE, BECAUSE YOU NEED NOT GIVE ANY NAMES. But we are anxious to secure a frank statement of the experiences, good and bad, which hospitals are having with graduate nurses. Please give here your Hospital .... City .... State .... Date .... and then answer the following questions about your recent experience with graduate nurses.

1. How many beds has your hospital? 2. What is its daily average number of patients? 3. Have you a training school? 4. If so, how many students have you?
5. How many graduate nurses does your hospital regularly employ? 6. Of these, how many are doing (a) administrative work (b) clerical work (c) technical laboratory work, etc. (d) supervisory (e) teaching (f) actual bedside nursing (g) other?
7. *During the past week*, about how many patients on the average did you have in each of the following services: (a) Surgical (b) Medical (c) Obstetric (d) Pediatric (e) Other? 8. Was the past week more or less busy than usual? 9. How many private patients did you have *last week*? How many semi-private or ward patients? Total.
10. How many *extra* nurses for general floor duty did you need last week? 11. How many did you get? 12. Did you get them from (a) your own registry (b) central professional registry (c) commercial registry (d) other (e) or don't you know? (check which). 13. Did you have much choice or did you have to take what you could get?
14. Please check whether most of the general "*floor duty*" graduate nurses who have come into your hospital during the past month are:
    - *a.* Well trained or poorly trained
    - *b.* Experienced with your type of work or inexperienced
    - *c.* Reasonably intelligent or stupid
    - *d.* Reasonably careful or careless
    - *e.* Reasonably cooperative or uncooperative
    - *f.* Reasonably adaptable or unadaptable
15. Please check whether most of the "*special*" graduate nurses for private duty patients who have come into your hospital during the past month are:

a. Well trained or poorly trained
b. Experienced with your type of work or inexperienced
c. Reasonably intelligent or stupid
d. Reasonably careful or careless
e. Reasonably cooperative or uncooperative
f. Reasonably adaptable or unadaptable

16. Do you have or want a dining room for the "specials," separate from that for the regular nurses? Why?
17. Do you have or want sitting rooms available for "specials"? Why?
18. In your hospital, (a) About how many patients does a student nurse take care of when the patients are in separate rooms? (b) About how many could she take care of? (c) About how many patients does a "special" nurse take care of when the patients are in separate rooms? (d) About how many could she take care of? (e) What makes the difference? (Answer on the back of the page if you need to.)
19. If you had your choice, which would you rather have to take care of your patients, student nurses or graduate nurses?
20. On the back of this sheet, please make any comments which you think might throw light on the problem of the alleged nursing shortage, especially as found in the employment of graduate nurses for general floor duty, and "special" duty in hospitals. We should particularly like your reasons for your answers to questions 18 and 19.

Please Return this Sheet—in the Accompanying Envelope—by Tomorrow if you can—to the Committee on the Grading of Nursing Schools, 370 Seventh Avenue, New York City

FORM 10

8½ x 11 sheet. Form A had returned 700 names of nurses who were in active practice but in positions not readily classifiable. This form was really the same as Form 6, but was sent accompanied by a letter asking that the recipient answer such questions as were applicable and ignore the rest. Returned 313, or 45%.

The text is not reproduced, because it was practically that of Form 6.

FORM 11

8½ x 11 sheet. Sent to 9,666 private duty nurses, as taken from Form A. There was a heavy toll of undelivered envelopes due to changed addresses. Returns filled out 2,213, or 23%.

FORM 11

More Private Duty Questions!

DEAR R.N.: Here is another questionnaire. *No matter where you are or what you are doing* please fill it in for us and send it back. We particularly want the records of those who are on vacations. (Are you reading your Journal? Every issue of the American Journal of Nursing has somewhere in it a news note showing what we are finding through these studies.) Help us learn more about private duty by answering these six questions:

A. Date..............................City..............................State........................

1. During the week which is just finished: (a) How many days did you work? (b) How many days were you too sick to work? (c) How many days were you on call? (d) How many days were you resting or taking a vacation?
2. Do you help support any people besides yourself? If so, for how many different people besides yourself do you give partial financial support? complete financial support?
3. Give as careful an estimate as you can of the total number of *free days* of nursing care you have given *in the past six months.* (Include in this estimate whatever free service you have given to relatives or friends.)
4. In what year did you first do private duty? How much did you charge *then* for a 24 hour day? for 12 hour day? How much do you charge *now* for a 24 hour day? for a 12 hour day?
5. How do you get most of your cases? From (a) hospital registry, (b) central professional registry, (c) commercial registry, (d) directly from doctor, (e) from former patients, (f) other?
6. Do you find this registry service satisfactory? On the back of this sheet please write your reasons for your answer and any recommendations you can suggest for improvements. You need not sign your name unless you want to.

Please Return this Sheet—in the Accompanying Envelope—by Tomorrow if you can—to the Committee on the Grading of Nursing Schools, 370 Seventh Avenue, New York City

FORM 12

Return postal. Sent to 95,180 members of the American Medical Association in 48 states. Returned 23,500, or 25%.

(Face of postal)

Dear Doctor: This postal is being sent to every member of the American Medical Association. We are trying, *first,* to discover what proportion of the medical profession is directly affected by the private duty nurse situation. *Second,* we want to secure the names and addresses of a large number of doctors who frequently employ nurses for their patients, and who will be willing to report upon the quality of the nursing service which their patients are receiving.

This study is being made by the COMMITTEE ON THE GRADING OF NURSING SCHOOLS, as one of the first steps towards answering the question: "How well does the modern school of nursing prepare the student for private duty service?" The Grading Committee is a national co-operative body, sponsored and supported by

The American Medical Association
The American College of Surgeons
The American Hospital Association
The American Nurses' Association
The National League of Nursing Education
The National Organization for Public Health Nursing
The American Public Health Association

We shall be glad to send you further information about our plans if you so desire. In the meantime, won't you please do us the courtesy of filling out and mailing the other half of this postal card.

Sincerely yours,
WILLIAM DARRACH, M.D., *Chairman*
MAY AYRES BURGESS, PH.D., *Director*

(Reverse of postal)

1. Name..
   ....
   City Street and Number State
2. Are you in active practice?..................
3. Are you a general practitioner?........... If not, what is your specialty?..
4. Do you often employ private duty nurses for your patients? } In hospitals? In homes?
5. If we send you a one page questionnaire, asking for an account of your experience with private duty nurses, will you answer and return it?..

FORM 13

8½ x 11 sheet. Sent to 3,034 R.N. Superintendents in the hospitals of 48 states. Returned 1431, or 47%.

FORM 13

The R.N. Superintendent?

The Committee on the Grading of Nursing Schools is writing to every R.N. Hospital Superintendent in the United States, in order to find out some facts which the Committee needs to know about her work. You will be doing a real favor to the Committee, and to all nurses who are considering hospital administration as a life work, if you will answer the questions on this sheet and mail it back to us. We have made the questions as simple as we can so that they will not take too much of your time to answer. Because we want you to talk freely, *we do not ask you to sign your name!* Please send the sheet back as soon as you can; and watch the American Journal of Nursing for the story of what we find!

1. Are you superintendent (a) of the hospital or (b) of nurses or (c) both?
2. (a) How long have you held your present position? (b) What was your annual salary when you first held this position? (c) What is it now?
3. In addition to your salary do you receive (a) full maintenance? (b) partial maintenance? or (c) no maintenance?
4. (a) Did you finish grammar school? 1st year high school? 2d year? 3d year? 4th year? (if you had any additional schooling, state what) (b) Have you ever taken any courses in hospital or institutional management or business administration? In educational methods or administration?
5. In what year were you graduated from training school?
6. (a) From the time you entered training school until the present day, how many different hospitals have you worked in? (b) About how many patients was the smallest of these hospitals apt to care for at one time? (c) The largest?
7. (a) How many beds has your hospital? (b) What is its daily average number of patients?
8. (a) Have you a training school? If so, how many students have you? (b) Do you need more students? or have you a waiting list?
9. If you have a school, have you raised the entrance requirements within the past 10 years? If so, did that seem to increase or decrease the number of applicants? Did it raise or lower the quality of applicants.
10. (a) If you have a school, do you give all the types of training necessary for registration? or do your students go to some affiliating school for additional experience? (b) Is the affiliating school in your own city? or in some other city? (c) When your students have gone to a school in some other city for affiliation

are they apt to stay in that city after graduation? or do they come back to your own city to work?

11. (a) How many graduate nurses are employed on annual salaries in your hospital? (b) Of these, how many are teachers? supervisors or head nurses? floor duty nurses? Other? (c) How many of your teachers, supervisors, or head nurses have ever done general floor duty in your hospital?
12. (a) What do you pay general duty R.Ns. per month? Do they receive maintenance in addition? What do you pay practical nurses? Orderlies? Ward helpers? Ward maids? (b) How many practicals do you regularly employ? How many orderlies? Ward helpers? Ward maids?
13. (a) Are you responsible to a Board of Trustees? or to a Nursing Committee? or to an individual? (b) If to an individual, what is his position? (c) How many meetings has the Board of Trustees held in 1927? (d) How many of these meetings did you attend?
14. Do you intend to continue in your present line of work? Please write your reasons on the back of this sheet. You need not sign your name unless you want to. But we are anxious to learn what you really think about hospital or nursing administration as a life work, and as compared with other forms of nursing you have tried.

Please Return this Sheet—in the Accompanying Envelope—by Tomorrow if you can—to the Committee on the Grading of Nursing Schools, 370 Seventh Avenue, New York City

FORM 14

Return postal sent to 1,630 superintendents of nurses in 48 states. Returned 893, or 55%.

(Face of postal)

To the Superintendent of Nurses:

Dear Madam: The Committee on the Grading of Nursing Schools is planning to make a study this winter of nurse registries, and in order to secure a list of such registries is sending this postal to all hospitals conducting training schools. It is also anxious to build up a list of schools which have full records of their graduates, as suggested in questions Nos. 5 and 6. It will be a real favor to us in getting these studies under way if you will answer the questions on the other half of this card, and mail it back to us.

Sincerely yours,

May Ayres Burgess,

Director, Committee on the Grading of Nursing Schools

(Reverse of postal)

1. Name of Hospital..
   Your Name..
   City..State..
2. Does your hospital maintain a registry for graduate nurses?..........
   or does it co-operate with....................or give financial support to a central professional registry?..a commercial registry?..................Other?...
3. So far as you know, are there any hospitals in your city which have *no* training school, and yet do conduct a nurses' registry? ....If so, can you give us their names?..............................
   ....
   ....
4. Have you kept a record of past graduates of your school so that you could *easily* tell for each graduate—
   a. The year she was graduated?................ *b.* Whether she is still alive?............ *c.* Whether she is married or single? ....
   d. Whether she is actively nursing or retired?............
5. How many years back does this record go?............

FORM 15

8½ x 11 sheet. Sent to 19,200 physicians who returned Form 12, indicating that they frequently employed private duty nurses and that they would be willing to answer a questionnaire. Returned 2,882, or 15%.

FORM 15

The Doctor and the Private Duty Nurse

DEAR DOCTOR: A while ago you volunteered to help the Committee on the Grading of Nursing Schools in its study of the nursing problem by answering some questions. Here they are. They will not get any nurse into trouble, because you need not give either your name or her name unless you wish. The questions refer to your experience with private duty nurses. (A private duty or special nurse is one who does not belong to a hospital or public health staff, but is hired to take care of an individual patient, either in the home or in the hospital.)

City............................State............................Date........................

1. Are you in general practice? Have you a specialty? What?
2. How many of the patients now under your care NEED private duty nurses? How many have them? Please answer the Following Questions about YOUR MOST RECENT CASE ON WHICH A PRIVATE DUTY NURSE WAS EMPLOYED:
3. Is the private duty nurse on the case now? If not, how many days, weeks ago did she go off it?
4. Was case (a) surgical, (b) medical, (c) obstetric, (d) pediatric, (e) contagious, (f) mental or nervous, (g) other? (check which).
5. Was patient in (a) home, or (b) hospital, or (c) both?
6. How many nurses have you had on this case? (If you had more than one nurse on this case, please answer the following questions *for the one most recently hired.*)
7. Was nurse secured through (a) hospital registry; (b) central professional registry; (c) commercial registry; (d) from your private list; (e) from some other doctor; (f) other? or (g) don't you know? (check which).
8. Was nurse (a) R.N.; (b) practical; or (c) don't you know? 9. Was she on (a) day; (b) night; or (c) 24-hour duty? 10. What did nurse charge per day?
11. In your opinion, was nurse (a) very good; (b) good; (c) fair; (d) poor; (e) very poor?
12. Please check which of the types of nursing given in the list below were particularly needed for this case:

a. Mother's helper and houseworker
b. Responsible adult to take charge of family
c. Skill in giving general care and making patient comfortable
d. Skill in giving special treatments
e. Care in following medical orders
f. Skill in handling people
g. Skill in observing and reporting symptoms
h. Skill in asepsis
i. Ability to work under heavy strain
j. Experience and background
k. Good breeding and attractive personality
l. Familiarity with particular disease
m. Familiarity with hospital routine
n. Familiarity with your personal methods

13. Would you like to have the same nurse again on a similar case?

14. During the past month about how many times have you called a hospital registry, central professional registry, commercial registry and been told that no nurse was available for your case? How many of these calls were for each of the following conditions:

Call for Sunday or holiday
For night duty
For 24-hour duty
For home case
For out-of-town
Maternity
Pediatric
Contagious
Male or GU
Mental or nervous
Alcoholic
Other

15. For most of your patients, which seems to be the more difficult problem, to pay the regular R.N. fee or to secure a really competent and co-operative nurse? 16. For your own patients, which do you prefer, practical nurses or graduate nurses?

17. (a) Is there a strong demand among your own patients for practical nurses? (b) If so, which do you think they want the practicals for *most*, for bedside nursing? or for taking charge of the housework?

18. If competent domestic servants could easily be hired at reasonable rates during sickness periods, do you think it would probably decrease? or almost eliminate? the demand for practicals, or would there probably be no change?

19. How many patients have you had during the past month who have employed a private duty or special nurse?

20. Of these—(a) how many were sick enough to need special skilled nursing care? (b) How many would not have needed to hire a nurse at all if a relative, friend, or competent servant had been available to take care of them in the home? (c) How many could have managed if a visiting nurse could have come into the home for, say, an hour or two each day? (d) How many could have been adequately cared for if they had been in a hospital on regular nursing service without a special nurse?

21. On the other side of this sheet, please make any comments which you think might throw light on the distribution and quality of private duty nursing. We should particularly like your reasons for the answer to question 13. *You need not sign your name unless you wish;* but we should like to have your

frank opinion about the nurses who have personally worked with you during the past few weeks.

Please Return this Sheet—in the Accompanying Envelope—by Tomorrow if you can—to the Committee on the Grading of Nursing Schools, 370 Seventh Avenue, New York City

FORM 16

8½ x 11 sheet. Sent to each of 19,200 physicians with the request that he give it to one of his patients. Returned 1,275. If only those physicians who answered Form 15 co-operated in this distribution, this would be a 44% return.

FORM 16

The Patient and the Private Duty Nurse

DEAR DOCTOR: Please give this blank to one of your patients who has recently had a private duty nurse. We are anxious to secure the patient's viewpoint, and are asking each doctor to co-operate by selecting an intelligent patient, explaining the importance of the study, and asking the patient to give us the benefit of his experience. (Note: If you wish additional copies for other patients, we shall be glad to supply you with as many as you wish.)

At the top of this sheet are three questions which you are asked to answer because a patient's judgment on these points might not be reliable. After you have filled in these answers, please ask the patient (or in cases of children, ask the parent or guardian) to take it, read it all the way through, and answer the questions as fairly as he can. Give each patient one of the envelopes addressed to us, so that he can easily return the report after it is completed. We want the patients to answer frankly and anonymously, so that they will know that even you have not seen their answers. When the study is finished, reports of the findings will be published in the medical, hospital, and nursing journals, and in special pamphlets issued by the Grading Committee. We hope you will keep in touch with the work. Thank you!

For the Doctor to Answer

City........................State........................Today's date......................

1. Patient is (a) man (b) woman (c) adolescent (d) child (check which).
2. Was case (a) surgical, (b) medical, (c) obstetric, (d) pediatric, (e) contagious, (f) mental or nervous? (g) other? (check which).
3. Was it (a) a short time or (b) a long time illness? Was it (c) mild or (d) severe?

For the Patient to Answer

Note to Patient: We want to find out what sort of nursing service patients are actually getting. Nothing you say here can make trouble for your nurse, because you need not tell either her name or your name. We do want to know, however, whether or not you liked her, and why. So please answer the following questions:

4. How many days did you have a nurse? 5. How much did she charge each day?
6. Did you get her from (a) hospital registry (b) central professional registry (c) commercial registry (d) your doctor's list (e) through some other doctor (f) through a friend (g) other or (h) don't you know? (check which).
7. Was she (a) a practical nurse (b) a registered nurse or (c) don't you know? 8. Was she on (a) day, (b) night, or (c) 24-hour service?
9. Did you have her (a) in the hospital, (b) at home, or (c) both? 10. If both, was her service in the home (a) more, or (b) less satisfactory than in the hospital? Or (c) was it about equal?
11. If you had a nurse in your home, why did you need her? Was it mostly because
    a. No one in the family had time to take care of the patient?
    b. The members of the family were too tired to take care of the patient?
    c. Some one was needed to take charge of the housework? Of the children?
    d. The patient wanted to be relieved of all responsibility?
    e. The patient was so ill that expert nursing service was necessary?
12. If you had a special nurse in the hospital, was it
    a. Because most of your friends have special nurses when in the hospitals?
    b. Because the hospital suggested that private patients usually have special nurses?
    c. Because the patient felt that the regular nursing service furnished by the hospital would not be sufficient? If so, was this because the patient had actually tried the regular nursing service of that hospital first? Or was it because of some previous experience or of what people had said?
    d. Because the members of the family wanted to be sure the patient had the best possible care?
    e. Because your doctor felt that the patient was so ill that special nursing care was necessary?
13. Which seems to you the more difficult problem: to meet the cost of nursing care? or to get the right kind of nurse?
14. a. If you had a special nurse in the hospital, would you be interested in a plan by which three or four patients share the cost and services of the same nurse?
    b. If you had a nurse in the home, would you be interested in a

plan by which you could arrange to have her come in for an hour or two each day; charging only for the time she gave?

15. When you had a nurse at home, would you have welcomed an opportunity to talk over her work with a nurse supervisor, if you could have done so without getting the nurse into trouble? Or do you feel that a visit from a nurse supervisor would not have been of any particular help to the nurse or the patient?
16. If the case were to happen over again, would you like to have the same nurse?
17. On the back of this sheet please write any comments which you think might help us in our study of what nurses are really like, and what problems arise in connection with their service. Tell us what you liked about your nurse and what you didn't like. We should particularly like your reasons for your answer to question 16.

Please Return this Sheet—in the Accompanying Envelope—by Tomorrow if you can—to the Committee on the Grading of Nursing Schools, 370 Seventh Avenue, New York City

FORM 17

8½ x 11 sheet. Sent to 879 heads of nurse registries in 48 states. Returned 414, or 47%.

FORM 17

The Nurse and the Registry

TO THE REGISTRAR: This report blank is being sent to hospital, central, commercial, and private registries all over the country in an effort to discover whether unemployment among trained nurses is general everywhere, or only in some particular localities. *Please note that you need not sign your name or give the name or address of your registry unless you wish.* But please do answer the questions and mail them back to us so that we can compare conditions in different parts of the country, and if more nurses are needed in certain cities, can advise those hunting for work where to go. A report of this study will be published in the American Journal of Nursing within the next few months. Please answer as many of the following questions as you can:—

City........................State........................Date..............................

1. Is the registry under the control of (a) a Hospital (b) an Alumnæ Association (c) a District Nurses' Association (d) a Nurses' Club (e) a Medical Society (f) a Health Center (g) a Women's Club (h) a private individual (i) a business firm (j) Other? (check which).
2. Where is it located? (a) In the hospital (b) In the Nurses' Home (c) In a club house (d) In a business building (e) In the home of the registrar (f) In other (check which).
3. a. How many full time people are employed to run the registry? b. How many part time?
4. Who is in charge? (a) Is it a man or a woman (b) Is it a doctor (c) a registered nurse (d) a graduate nurse but not registered (e) a practical nurse (f) a business man or woman (g) a social worker (h) Other? (check which).
5. For the year 1927 did the registry (a) run on a deficit, (b) break about even? or (c) show a profit? 6. Is the person in charge of the registry paid a regular salary or given a share in the profits? Or does she serve without pay?
7. a. Which of the following groups of workers does the registry enroll:

1. Registered nurses
2. Graduate but not registered nurses
3. Male nurses
4. Practical nurses
5. Hospital maids
6. Hospital orderlies
7. Domestic servants
8. Stenographers, clerks, etc.
9. Teachers
10. Doctors
11. Other

b. If the registry is controlled by a hospital, does it serve only graduates of that hospital or others also? c. If it is controlled by the District Nurses' Association, does it serve only members of the Association or others also?

8. a. During the month of December, 1927, how many nurses did you have enrolled on the registry? b. During December about how many calls did you receive, and how many were you able to fill of each of the following kinds?

1. For special or private duty nurses, in hospitals,	calls	received	filled
2. For special or private duty nurses, in homes	"	"	"
3. For public health	"	"	"
4. For instructors in nursing schools	"	"	"
5. For hospital floor duty nurses	"	"	"
6. For other hospital nurses	"	"	"

9. What sorts of calls are hardest to fill?

10. During the month of December, 1927, about how many trained nurses consulted you as to the advisability of their changing from one branch of nursing to another?
11. a. About how many trained nurses are waiting for cases *at the present time* in your registry? b. In general, do you have more or less calls now than you have nurses to fill them?
12. Do you think that employment conditions among nurses are better than at this time last year or worse or about the same?
13. Would you like to have more nurses encouraged to move to your city Or are there enough there now?
14. For which do you have more demand, for graduate nurses? or for practical nurses? 15. Is the demand for practical nurses growing more from year to year or is it falling off? or is it about the same?
16. How many calls did you receive *last week* (a) from hospitals how many did you fill? (b) from homes how many did you fill? (c) Which calls are easier to fill, those from hospitals or from homes?
17. If you care to, will you please enclose with this report a statement of the number of calls received and filled each month in 1927? We should find it of real help.
18. On the back of this sheet, please write anything which you think might throw light on the problems of nurse registries. We should particularly like your reasons for your answer to question 13. (If you answered yes to question 17, don't forget to send us the material!)

Please Return this Sheet—by Tomorrow if you can—in the Accompanying Envelope—to the Committee on the Grading of Nursing Schools, 370 Seventh Avenue, New York City

FORM 18

Letter sent to 607 superintendents of nurses who had answered "Yes" to all the items of question 4, Form 14. Returned with fully annotated notes from 423, or 70%.

FORM 18

January 10, 1928.

To Several Superintendents of Training Schools

In looking through the postals which are coming back to us from superintendents of training schools, I note that quite a number of schools, of which yours is one, seem to be keeping fairly complete records of their graduates. We are trying to find out how long nurses stay in active professional work, because, until we have this figure, we cannot tell how many nursing schools and students of nursing the country really needs. To find the average length of time graduate nurses stay in the profession, we must gather records from as many schools as we can. We do not want to ask you to go to any great labor in gathering figures for us, and if the request which follows would be difficult to meet, I hope you will frankly say so. I am writing to you on the chance that what I need is already easily available in your files.

What we should most like would be a list of your graduates, such as Miss Sally Johnson compiled in 1923 for the graduates of Massachusetts General Hospital. In that report, the graduates are listed, by classes; and opposite the name of each one is a statement showing her status at the time the study was made—which in that case was in 1923.

Would it be possible for you (without too much work) to give us a similar statement, either for each class, or for a few of the classes which have been graduated from your school? If you have ever made a study of that kind in the past, could you send us a copy? Studies made some years ago will be useable, provided we know in each case in what year the study was made.

If no such earlier studies are available, could you conveniently send us a list of your graduates writing for each one

a. The year she was graduated
b. If she married—write "married"
c. If deceased—write "dead." (If she had been married, please state this also)
d. If at home or not nursing—write "inactive" or "at home"
e. If working but not in the nursing profession—write "outside profession" or else state what she is doing
f. If still active in nursing—write "nursing"
g. If you don't know what has become of her—write "?"

For example, if these notations had been used in the study made by Massachusetts General in 1923, the record for the 1901 class would have read like this:

Class of 1901

Bailey, Elvina K.	At home
Cassels, Mary M.	?
Cousart, Carrie V.	Married, at home
Dewar, Annie J.	" " "
Garvey, S. Agnes	Nursing
Goetz, Carrie E.	Married, at home
Hatlow, Elizabeth	Masseuse
Hewitt, Lydia R.	Married, at home
Huse, Julia S.	Deceased
Leighton, Maude W.	At home
Liley, Mary	Married, at home
Mackenzie, Mary A.	Nursing
MacPeake, Edith B.	Married, at home
Manning, Marion A.	Occupational therapy
McDonald, Flora T.	Nursing
Rose, Isabelle C.	Married, at home
Vickery, Elizabeth T.	" " "
Warner, Margaret	At home
Wiggin, Mary R.	" "
Wilkinson, Ella A.	Married, nursing

If we can get as many as fifty lists of this kind we shall be able to secure a reasonably good picture of what is happening in nursing. Will you see whether you can help us out? If information is not at hand for all your graduates, perhaps you could give it for a few classes. Even rather incomplete reports would be much better than none.

As is usual in all our work, this information is something which we are anxious to get within the *next two or three weeks*. Perhaps you have some alumnæ members who would be glad to do this work as a contribution to the Grading Committee. If not, and if it would save time to hire a clerk or typist to help, please do not hesitate to do so, and to send us the bill. The information is so essential to our whole study, and the need for haste is so great that I feel entirely justified in offering to pay reasonable sums for clerical help.

With deep appreciation for whatever assistance you can give, I am

Sincerely yours,

MAY AYRES BURGESS,
Director

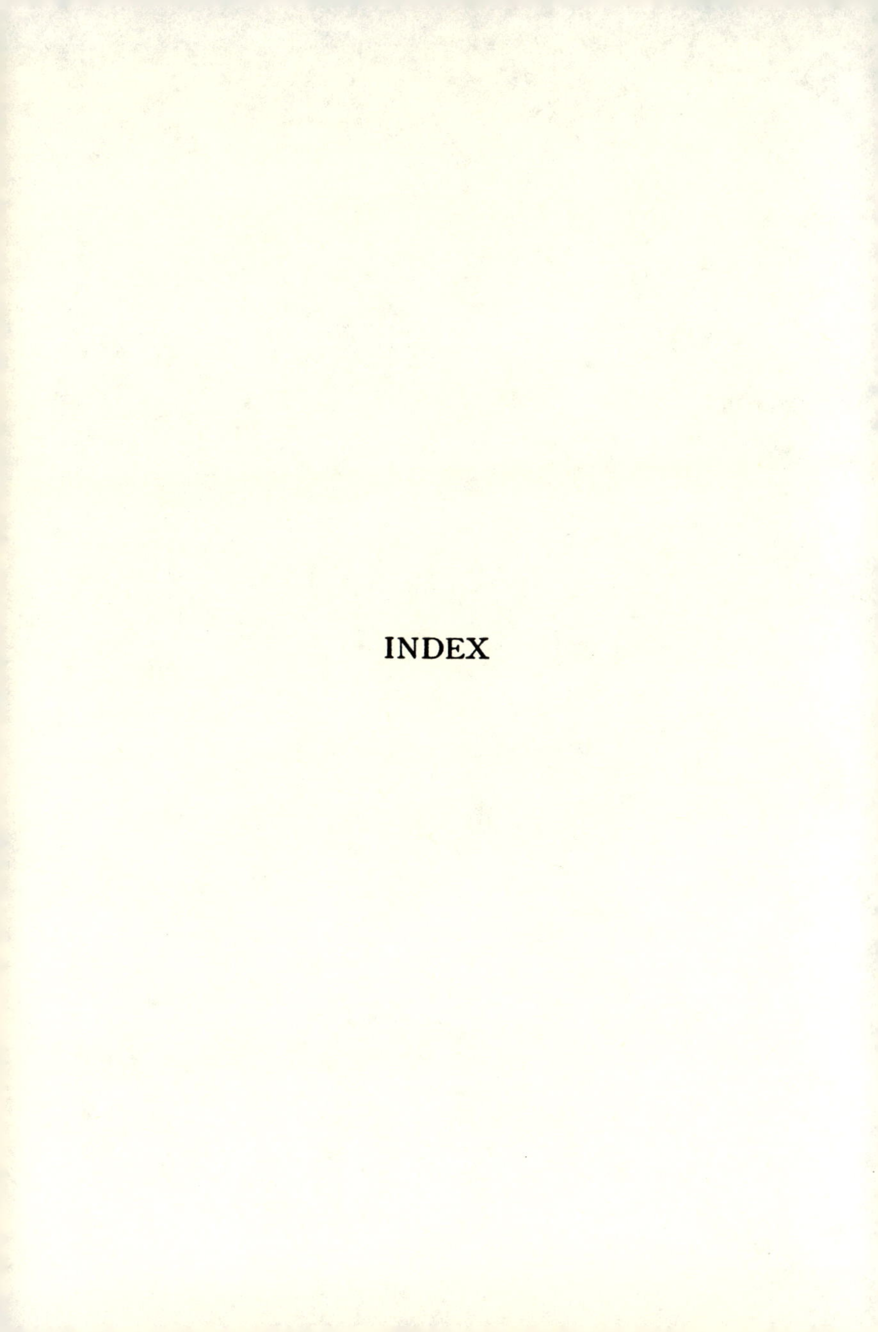

INDEX

INDEX

INDEX

20

Titles in This Series

1 Charlotte Aikens, editor. *Hospital Management*. Philadelphia, 1911.

2 American Society of Superintendents of Training Schools for Nurses. *Annual Conventions*, 1893–1919.

3 John Shaw Billings and Henry M. Hurd, editors. *Hospitals, Dispensaries and Nursing: Papers and Discussion in the International Congress of Charities, Correction and Philanthropy*. Baltimore, 1894.

4 Annie M. Brainard. *The Evolution of Public Health Nursing*. Philadelphia, 1922.

5 Marie Campbell. *Folks Do Get Born*. New York, 1946.

6 *Civil War Nursing:* Louisa May Alcott. *Hospital Sketches*. Boston, 1863. BOUND WITH *Memoir of Emily Elizabeth Parsons*. Boston, 1880.

7 Committee for the Study of Nursing Education. *Nursing and Nursing Education in the United States*. New York, 1923.

8 Committee on the Grading of Nursing Schools. *Nurses, Patients and Pocketbooks*. New York, 1928.

9 Mrs. Darce Craven. *A Guide to District Nurses*. London, 1889.

10 Dorothy Deming. *The Practical Nurse*. New York, 1947.

11 Katharine J. Densford & Millard S. Everett. *Ethics for Modern Nurses*. Philadelphia, 1946.

12 Katharine D. DeWitt. *Private Duty Nursing*. Philadelphia, 1917.

13 Janet James, editor. *A Lavinia Dock Reader*.

14 Annette Fiske. *First Fifty Years of the Waltham Training School for Nurses*. New York, 1984. *BOUND WITH* Alfred Worcester. "The Shortage of Nurses—Reminiscences of Alfred Worcester '83." *Harvard Medical Alumni Bulletin 23*, 1949.

15 Virginia Henderson et al. *Nursing Studies Index, 1900–1959*. Philadelphia, 1963, 1966, 1970, 1972.

16 Darlene Clark Hine, editor. *Black Women in Nursing: An Anthology of Historical Sources*.

17 Ellen N. LaMotte. *The Tuberculosis Nurse*. New York, 1915.

18 Barbara Melosh, editor. *American Nurses in Fiction: An Anthology of Short Stories*.

19 Mary Adelaide Nutting. *A Sound Economic Basis for Schools of Nursing*. New York, 1926.

20 Sara E. Parsons. *Nursing Problems and Obligations*. Boston, 1916.

21 Juanita Redmond. *I Served on Bataan*. Philadelphia, 1943.

22 Susan Reverby, editor. *The East Harlem Health Center Demonstration: An Anthology of Pamphlets*.

23 Isabel Hampton Robb. *Educational Standards for Nurses*. Cleveland, 1907.

24 Sister M. Theophane Shoemaker. *History of Nurse-Midwifery in the United States*. Washington, D.C., 1947.

25 Isabel M. Stewart. *Education of Nurses*. New York, 1943.

26 Virginia S. Thatcher. *History of Anesthesia with Emphasis on the Nurse Specialist*. Philadelphia, 1953.

27 Adah H. Thoms. *Pathfinders—A History of the Progress of Colored Graduate Nurses*. New York, 1929.

28 Clara S. Weeks-Shaw. *A Text-Book of Nursing for the Use of Training Schools, Families, and Private Students*. New York, 1885.

29 Writers Program of the WPA in Kansas, compilers. *Lamps on the Prairie: A History of Nursing in Kansas*. Topeka, 1942.